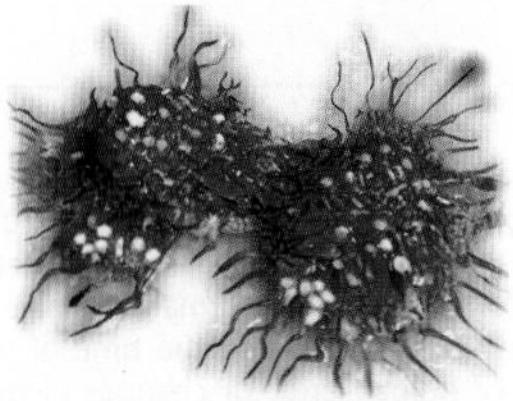

Hematology-Oncology
CLINICAL QUESTIONS

Julie H. Rowe, MD
Putao Cen, MD
Adan Rios, MD
Anneliese O. Gonzalez, MD
Zeyad Kanaan, MD
Hazem El-Osta, MD
Syed H. Jafri, MBBS
Robert J. Amato, DO
Virginia Mohlere

McGovern Medical School
The University of Texas Health Science Center at Houston
Department of Internal Medicine
Division of Oncology

Mc Graw Hill Education

New York Chicago San Francisco Athens London Madrid Mexico City
Milan New Delhi Singapore Sydney Toronto

Hematology-Oncology Clinical Questions

1 2 3 4 5 6 7 8 9 DSS 23 22 21 20 19 18
ISBN 978-1-260-02662-7
MHID 1-260-02662-0

Notice

Medicine is an ever-changing science. As new research and clinical experience broaden our knowledge, changes in treatment and drug therapy are required. The authors and the publisher of this work have checked with sources believed to be reliable in their efforts to provide information that is complete and generally in accord with the standards accepted at the time of publication. However, in view of the possibility of human error or changes in medical sciences, neither the authors nor the publisher nor any other party who has been involved in the preparation or publication of this work warrants that the information contained herein is in every respect accurate or complete, and they disclaim all responsibility for any errors or omissions or for the results obtained from use of the information contained in this work. Readers are encouraged to confirm the information contained herein with other sources. For example and in particular, readers are advised to check the product information sheet included in the package of each drug they plan to administer to be certain that the information contained in this work is accurate and that changes have not been made in the recommended dose or in the contraindications for administration. This recommendation is of particular importance in connection with new or infrequently used drugs.

This book was set in Myriad Pro by Aptara, Inc.
The editors were Karen G. Edmonson and Harriet Lebowitz.
The production supervisor was Richard Ruzycka.
Project management was provided by Dinesh Pokhriyal, Aptara, Inc.
The book designer was Eve Siegel.

Library of Congress Cataloging-in-Publication Data

Names: Rowe, Julie H., author.
Title: Hematology-oncology clinical questions / Julie H. Rowe, Anneliese O. Gonzalez, Sayed H. Jafri, Putao Cen, Zeyad Kanaan, Robert J. Amato, Adan Rios, Hazem El Osta, Virginia Mohlere.
Description: New York : McGraw Hill Education, [2019] | Includes bibliographical references and index.
Identifiers: LCCN 2018024787 | ISBN 9781260026627 (pbk.) | ISBN 1260026620 (pbk.)
Subjects: | MESH: Neoplasms | Hematologic Diseases | Problems and Exercises | Case Reports
Classification: LCC RC266.5 | NLM QZ 18.2 | DDC 616.99/40076–dc23
LC record available at https://lccn.loc.gov/2018024787

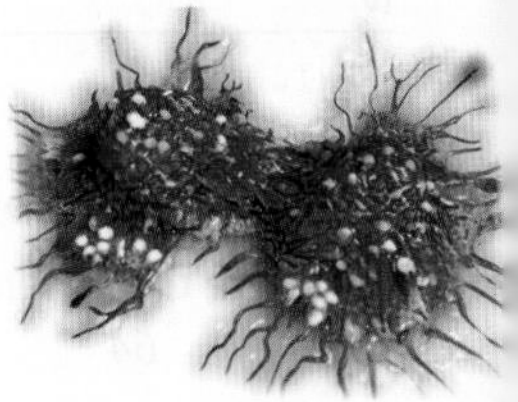

CONTENTS

CONTENTS

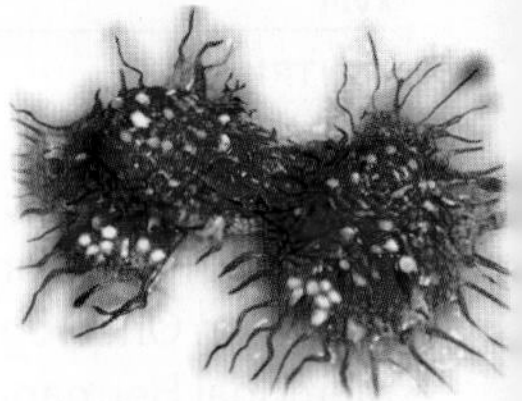

CONTRIBUTORS

Angel Blanco, MD
Medical Director, Radiation Oncology and Gamma Knife Centers
Clinical Associate Professor
McGovern Medical School, The University of Texas Health Science Center at Houston
Basics of Oncology and Pathology
Breast Cancer
Thoracic Cancers

Mehdi Dehghani, MSc, PhD, DABCC
Assistant Professor
Division of Oncology
Department of Internal Medicine
McGovern Medical School, The University of Texas Health Science Center at Houston
Basics of Oncology and Pathology

Brian Dinh, PharmD, BCPS, BCOP
Memorial Hermann Texas Medical Center Cancer Center
Cancer Pharmacology

Jamie M. Everett, MD
Assistant Professor
Department of Pathology and Laboratory Medicine
McGovern Medical School, The University of Texas Health Science Center at Houston
Basics of Oncology and Pathology

Shariq S. Khwaja, MD, PhD
Assistant Professor
Radiation Oncology
Memorial Hermann Cancer Center
McGovern Medical School, The University of Texas Health Science Center at Houston
Genitourinary Cancers

Kathryn Mraz, MS, CGC
Certified Genetic Counselor
Cancer Risk Genetics Program
Division of Oncology
Department of Internal Medicine
McGovern Medical School, The University of Texas Health Science Center at Houston
Genetic and Familial Assessment for Hereditary Cancer Syndromes

Elizabeth Nugent, MD
Assistant Professor of Obstetrics & Gynecology
Division of Gynecologic Oncology
Department of Obstetrics, Gynecology, and Reproductive Sciences
McGovern Medical School, The University of Texas Health Science Center at Houston
Gynecological Malignancies

Tamara E. Saunders, MD, FACS
Assistant Professor of Surgery
Department of Surgery
McGovern Medical School, The University of Texas Health Science Center at Houston
Breast Cancer

Curtis Wray, MD
Associate Professor of Surgery
Department of Surgery
McGovern Medical School, The University of Texas Health
Science Center at Houston
Gastrointestinal Cancers

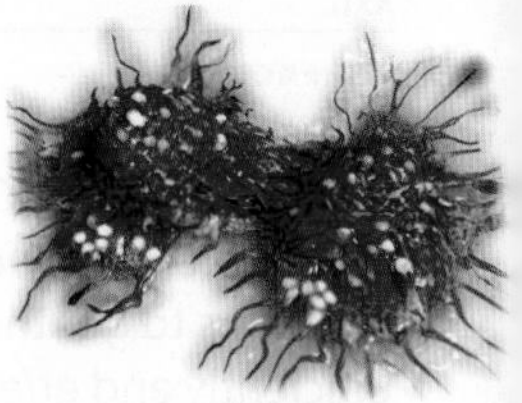

PREFACE

Over the past few decades, there has been an explosion of novel and innovative technology in the diagnostic and therapeutic approaches to cancer. The field of hematology-oncology continues to evolve, and medical oncologists, along with primary care providers and specialists involved in the care of cancer patients, struggle to interpret the latest data and research into concise and practical diagnostic explanations. This book has been developed based on the success of *Cardiology Clinical Questions* by Drs. John P. Higgins, Asif Ali, and David M Filsoff at McGovern Medical School, The University of Texas Health Science Center at Houston, and its popular format, "flow path," as depicted below:

Question → Data → Synthesis → Solution

Through the combined experience of the authors, we have compiled a list of the most commonly asked hematology-oncology questions, which provide the rationale for chapter selection. There are 20 chapters. The initial chapters (Cancer Pharmacology, Basics of Oncology and Pathology, and Most Common Hematology Questions) prepare the learner with the background fundamentals of hematology-oncology. Subsequent chapters are divided by tumor type, beginning with solid tumor types (eg, breast, head and neck, and gastrointestinal cancers) and then hematological malignancies (eg, leukemias and lymphomas).

Aligned with *Cardiology Clinical Questions*, the goal of *Hematology-Oncology Clinical Questions* is to empower clinicians to get their patients to the best solution as efficiently and effectively as possible. Each chapter provides a **Key Concept** section, which describes the basics of the question. The **Clinical Scenario** provides a clinical vignette in which these questions can be applied. The **Action Items** highlight important "must know" facts, and the **Discussion** provides further details. The **Pearls** are the takeaway points of the key concept and often consider a common question asked by faculty of their students at the bedside.

The authors hope that this volume will be a powerful tool to help learners from all points of the clinical spectrum to understand basic concepts of caring for a cancer patient.

CHAPTER 1

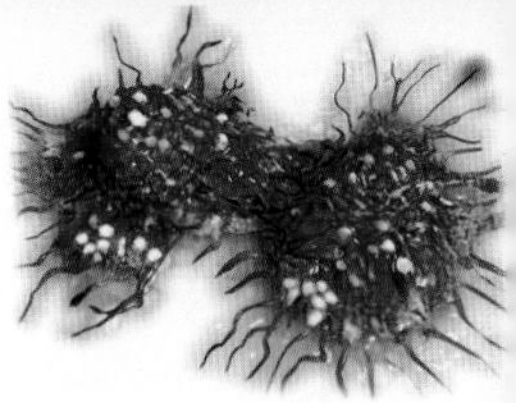

Cancer Pharmacology

Which chemotherapeutic agents cause hypersensitivity reaction, and how do we treat it?

Key concept	Hypersensitivity reactions (HRs) can occur with chemotherapeutic agents such as • taxanes (paclitaxel, docetaxel) • platinums (oxaliplatin, carboplatin, and cisplatin) • epipodophyllotoxins (teniposide and etoposide) • asparaginase • anthracyclines (doxorubicin, daunorubicin, idarubicin, and epirubicin) • alkylating agents (procarbazine, dacarbazine, chlorambucil, melphalan, cyclophosphamide, and ifosfamide)[1] Severe HRs associated with chemotherapeutic agents are rare and occur in <5% of patients.[2] The most common mechanism of HRs to chemotherapeutic agents is usually type I, which is IgE-mediated and results in release of histamines, leukotrienes, and prostaglandins. Common clinical manifestations include urticarial rash, angioedema, shortness of breath, bronchospasm, and hypotension.[2] Monoclonal antibodies (mAb, eg, cetuximab, rituximab, trastuzumab, gemtuzumab, and alemtuzumab) have higher incidence rates of HRs, varying from 5% with fully humanized panitumumab to 77% with rituximab. However, the highest incidences of reactions occur during the first infusion.[2] The mechanism of hypersensitivity reactions to mAbs is due to cytokine release and antibody production against the mAb.[2]

Clinical scenario	A 58-year-old postmenopausal woman is currently receiving paclitaxel for adjuvant therapy for her breast cancer. This is her 6th week. Thirty minutes into administration of paclitaxel, she develops severe shortness of breath, urticaria, and wheezing. What drugs should be administered to treat this hypersensitivity reaction?

Action items	Management of acute HRs[1,2]:
	• Discontinue infusion
	• Administer:
	  • High-flow oxygen
	  • Fluid resuscitation
	  • H1 and H2 antihistamines (diphenhydramine or famotidine)
	  • Corticosteroids (hydrocortisone or methylprednisolone)
	  • If severe, epinephrine or vasopressors
	  • Glucagon if persistent hypotension (if patient is taking a beta-blocker)

Pearls	• Paclitaxel is associated with anaphylactoid-like hypersensitivity reaction due to its solvent, polyethoxylated castor oil, which induces histamine release and hypotension[2] • Desensitization protocols can be used to continue treatment in patients who are benefiting from therapy[1]
References	1. Syrigou E, Makrilia N, Koti I, et al. Hypersensitivity reactions to antineoplastic agents: an overview. Anti-Cancer Drugs 2009; 20(1):1-6. 2. Heinz-Josef L. Management and preparedness for infusion and hypersensitivity reactions. Oncologist 2007;12:601-9.

How do we prevent and treat chemotherapy-induced peripheral neuropathy (CIPN)?

Key concept	The incidence of CIPN is ~40% in patients who have been treated with multiple agents.[1] The chemotherapeutic agents most commonly associated with CIPN include platinum agents (ie, oxaliplatin), vinca alkaloids, bortezomib, and taxanes (ie, paclitaxel).[1] Clinical trials have provided limited data on the effective prevention and management of CIPN.[1]
Clinical scenario	A 63-year-old man with stage 3 colon cancer is undergoing adjuvant chemotherapy with FOLFOX (5-fluororacil, leucovorin, and oxaliplatin). He is currently on cycle #6 and reports having some numbness of his fingertips and toes. He is still able to do his daily activities but has noted that he had been dropping things more frequently. What treatment would you recommend?
Discussion	• CIPN usually presents in symmetric, distal, sensory symptoms described either as "numbness or tingling" or "glove and stocking" and is usually dose-dependent. Nerve conduction studies have demonstrated decreased amplitude of sensory nerve action potentials[1] • Oxaliplatin and paclitaxel are associated with acute neuropathy syndromes (along with CIPN), which usually occur within hours to days after administration[1] • Oxaliplatin induces a cold sensitivity when touching cold items or swallowing cold liquids and throat discomfort; paclitaxel produces an acute myalgia and arthralgia syndrome • Numerous clinical trials have been conducted to evaluate agents that can used to prevent CIPN, including acetylcysteine, amitriptyline, calcium and magnesium, carbamazepine, glutamate, nimodipine, venlafaxine, and vitamin E; however, none of the studies showed sufficient evidence of benefit[1] • A phase 3 trial of duloxetine (30 mg by mouth daily vs. placebo) for treatment of CIPN found that 59% of those receiving duloxetine vs. 38% of the placebo arm had decreased pain[2]

Pearls	• There are no good preventive agents for CIPN[1] • Duloxetine can be used for treatment of CIPN[2]
References	1. Hershman DL, Lacchetti C, Dworkin RH, et al. Prevention and management of chemotherapy-induced peripheral neuropathy in survivors of adult cancers: American Society of Clinical Oncology clinical practice guideline. J Clin Oncol 2014;32(18):1941-67. 2. Smith EM, Pang H, Cirrincione C, et al. Effect of duloxetine on pain, function, and quality of life among patients with chemotherapy-induced painful peripheral neuropathy: a randomized clinical trial. JAMA 2013;309(13):1359-67.

What are the acute and severe toxicities of methotrexate (MTX)?

Key concept	MTX is an antimetabolite that inhibits dihydrofolate reductase, therefore inhibiting folate metabolism and preventing purine nucleoside and thymidylate biosynthesis. Acute toxicities include nausea, stomatitis, abnormal liver function tests, fatigue, and myelosuppression. Severe toxicities include nephrotoxicity, pulmonary toxicity, and hepatotoxicity. Leucovorin and glucarpidase can be used to treat acute MTX toxicities and delayed renal clearance.
Clinical scenario	A 47-year-old Hispanic man is diagnosed with primary central nervous system (CNS) lymphoma and is planned for treatment with high-dose MTX. He is receiving bicarbonate-containing fluids, and his urine is monitored to achieve urine pH >7. He receives high-dose MTX, and the next morning, he is found to have creatinine of 2.5. What are the next steps to manage his nephrotoxicity?
Action items	• High-dose MTX (HD-MTX) is defined as doses of ≥500 mg/m^2 (usually given in hematologic malignancies and sarcomas) • Prevention of MTX toxicity includes increased hydration (rates of 150–200 mL of bicarbonate-containing fluids), alkaline pH of urine, and avoidance of medications (ie, nonsteroidal anti-inflammatory drugs, penicillin, trimethoprim-sulfamethoxazole, proton-pump inhibitors, and levetiracetam) that could potentially interfere with MTX excretion • Monitoring serum MTX concentrations should be monitored after administration of HD-MTX with concurrent hydration, leucovorin rescue, and continued alkalinization of urine until MTX level is 0.05–0.1 μM • **Treatment of MTX toxicity includes leucovorin and/or glucarpidase and if severe, hemodialysis.**

Discussion	• Acute renal toxicity occurs in around 2%–12% of patients receiving HD-MTX, and the injury is mediated through crystal nephropathy as a result of precipitation of metabolites • Hepatotoxicity includes elevations in liver enzymes (60% transient hepatitis and 25% hyperbilirubinemia) • Neurotoxicity (~11%) includes confusion, seizures, somnolence, and headaches • Pulmonary toxicity is rare and associated with chemical-induced pneumonitis • Leucovorin is readily converted to tetrahydrofolate, "rescuing" host cells • Glucarpidase, a recombinant bacterial enzyme, rapidly metabolizes extracellular MTX into two nontoxic metabolites (DAMPA and glutamate), providing an alternative non-renal pathway for MTX elimination
Pearls	• Administration of leucovorin rescues host cells from intracellular MTX; therefore, it should be continued concomitantly with hemodialysis and/or glucarpidase • Evaluate whether there are any third-space fluids (ascites/effusions) that could prolong MTX elimination, increasing toxicity
References	1. Howard SC, McCormick J, Pui CH, et al. Preventing and managing toxicities of high-dose methotrexate. Oncologist 2016;21(12):1471-82.

What is the anthracycline lifetime cumulative dose limit for a given patient?

Key concept	Anthracycline therapy (doxorubicin, daunorubicin, idarubicin, epirubicin, and the anthraquinone mitoxantrone) is associated with an increase in the risk for developing heart failure, with significant associated morbidity and mortality.
Clinical scenario	A 50-year-old woman is diagnosed with a stage III follicular lymphoma. You review the NCCN guidelines for therapeutic options and elect to treat the patient with an anthracycline-containing regimen (R-CHOP). The clinical history reveals that this patient has history of congestive heart failure with a cardiac ejection fraction of 40%. Based on this finding and review of the guidelines, a non–anthracycline-containing regimen is chosen.
Action items	When treating a patient with an anthracycline-containing regimen, the following factors are of paramount importance: • Accurate cardiac history and status • Current evaluation of cardiac function as inferred from the cardiac ejection fraction evaluated by any validated method (echocardiography is the most widely used of the cardiac imaging techniques currently available) • Optimal management of cardiovascular risk factors prior to anthracycline exposure, including management of arterial hypertension and of metabolic disorders • Smoking cessation, weight loss, and physical activity should always be encouraged, whenever feasible

Discussion

Although it is known that anthracyclines can be associated with the development of heart failure, they are key components of many chemotherapy regimens. Thus, their use must be accompanied by great care in selecting the patients in whom these agents are used. In general, the optimal clinical situation is a patient with no history of cardiac failure, normal cardiac function at the time of initiating treatment as evaluated by an accepted method, and with optimization of the cardiac function (good control of blood pressure and metabolic disorders).

Of all the approaches used to prevent anthracycline toxicity, infusion vs. rapid bolus administration of the anthracycline and the use of chemical protection with dexrazoxane are known to have a favorable impact on cardiac function after anthracycline therapy. Due to its potential negative effect on outcome, the FDA has restricted the use of dexrazoxane to patients with metastatic breast cancer who have received at least 300 mg/m^2 of doxorubicin and who have an ongoing indication to receive doxorubicin-based chemotherapy. The infusional protection against cardiotoxicity is a more general and practical method of preventing cardiac anthracycline toxicity. From a pharmacokinetics point of view, the peak concentration level that accompanies short infusions (15–30 minutes) is probably responsible, together with the total lifetime cumulative dose, for the deleterious cardiac effect of anthracyclines. Therefore, a longer time of anthracycline infusion is better for avoiding cardiac toxicity. In certain protocols, such as DA-EPOCH (dose-adjusted etoposide, doxorubicin, and cyclophosphamide with vincristine and prednisone), the drug is administered through an indwelling central catheter over prolonged infusion times. From a practical point of view, any range of infusion time that diminishes the peak concentration effect is favorable; thus, even infusions of 2 hours' duration are potentially protective of the cardiac function.

(continued on following page)

	(continued from previous page) The lifetime cumulative doses of the different anthracyclines can be summarized as follows: • Doxorubicin (adriamycin): 450 mg/m^2 • Idarubicin: >90 mg/m^2 • Epirubicin: >900 mg/m^2 • Mitoxantrone: >120 mg/m^2 • Liposomal anthracyclines: >900 mg/m^2 (not commonly used due to the development of hand-foot syndrome)
Pearls	A decrease in left ventricle ejection fraction (LVEF) is defined as follows: • Decrease in absolute value of at least 20% in LVEF from baseline or • Decrease in absolute value of at least 10% in LVEF from baseline and to below the institution's lower limit of normal or • Post-baseline decline in absolute value of at least 5% in LVEF below the institution's lower limit of normal or • Heart failure

References

1. Von Hoff DD, Layard MW, Basa P, et al. Risk factors for doxorubicin-induced congestive heart failure. Ann Intern Med 1979;91: 710-8.
2. Cardinale D, Colombo A, Bacchiani G, et al. Early detection of anthracycline cardiotoxicity and improvement with heart failure therapy. Circulation 2015;131:1981-8.
3. Lang RM, Badano LP, Mor-Avi V, et al. Recommendations for cardiac chamber quantification by echocardiography in adults: an update from the American Society of Echocardiography and the European Association of Cardiovascular Imaging. J Am Soc Echocardiogr 2015;28:1-39.
4. Zamorano JL, Lancellotti P, Rodriguez Muñoz D, et al. 2016 ESC Position Paper on cancer treatments and cardiovascular toxicity developed under the auspices of the ESC Committee for Practice Guidelines: The Task Force for cancer treatments and cardio-vascular toxicity of the European Society of Cardiology (ESC). Eur Heart J 2016;37:2768-801.
5. Legha SS, Benjamin RS, Mackay B, et al. Adriamycin therapy by continuous intravenous infusion in patients with metastatic breast cancer. Cancer 1982;49:1762-6.

What are monoclonal antibodies, and how are they used in treating cancer?

Key concept	Monoclonal antibodies (mAbs or moAbs) are antibodies made by identical immune cells (plasma cells), all of which are clones of a unique parent cell. mAbs bind to the same epitope (the part of an antigen that is recognized by the antibody). This is known as monovalent affinity. In contrast, polyclonal antibodies bind to multiple epitopes and are made by plasma cells of different lineages. mAbs can be engineered, increasing the therapeutic targets of one single monoclonal antibody to two epitopes (bispecific monoclonal antibodies).
Clinical scenario	A 72-year-old woman with a history of rheumatoid arthritis is evaluated by her primary care physician for persistent cough and shortness of breath. CT of the chest with contrast is ordered shows right lower lobe pneumonia. However, incidentally, there are enlarged retroperitoneal lymph nodes noted, with the largest measuring 3 cm. She denies any symptoms of weight loss or night sweats but does endorse fatigue. She undergoes biopsy of the enlarged lymph node under the guidance of interventional radiology. Pathology demonstrates follicular lymphoma, grade 1. What are the possible treatment options for this patient?
Discussion	mAbs are used as effective strategies in cancer immunotherapy. An antibody is composed of two distinct functional units: the fragment of antigen binding (Fab) and the constant fragment (Fc). The Fc unit is linked to immune effector function. The mechanisms of action of monoclonal antibodies include: antibody-dependent cellular cytotoxicity (ADCC), complement-dependent cytotoxicity, and induction of adaptive T cell immunity (Figure 1-1)[1]: • ADCC results from the binding of an antibody-coated tumor (eg, IgG) to an Fc receptor (FcγR), which initiates immune effector cells such as natural killer cells, dendritic cells, and neutrophils; effector cells secrete perforin and granzymes that promote cell death • Phagocytosis can occur through binding of an antibody-coated tumor to an Fc receptor of macrophages, which leads to lysosomal degradation • After tumor lysis, there is cross-presentation of tumor peptides to MHC class II antigen-presenting cells (APCs), leading to CD4+ T cell activation. Subsequently, the tumor peptides are presented to MHC class I APCs, which then activates CD8+ cytotoxic T cells

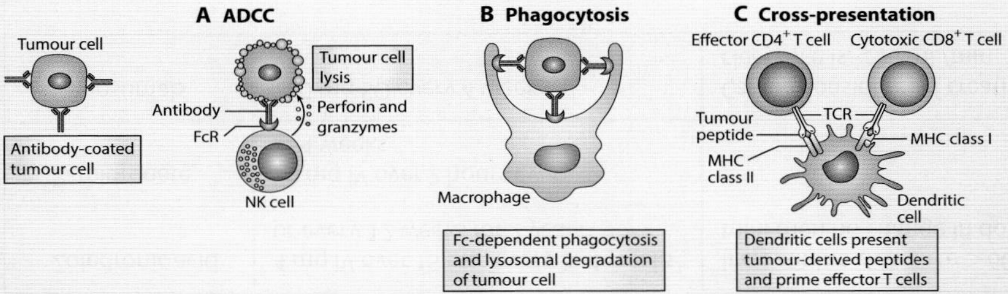

Figure 1-1. Mechanisms of monoclonal antibodies in cancer immunotherapy. (Reproduced with permission from Springer Nature: Weiner LM, Surana R, Wang S. Monoclonal antibodies: versatile platforms for cancer immunotherapy. Nat Rev Immunol 2010;10(5):317-327. Copyright © 2010.)

Pearls

The nomenclature of monoclonal antibodies is based on the source from which the antibodies were derived[1,2]:

SOURCE	INFIX	EXAMPLE AND TARGET
Mouse	-o-	Y^{90}-Ibritumomab, CD20
Chimeric	-xi-	Rituximab, CD20
Humanized	-zu-	Bevacizumab, VEGFA
Human	-u-	Panitumumab, EGFR

References

1. Weiner LM, Surana R, Wang S. Monoclonal antibodies: versatile platforms for cancer immunotherapy. Nat Rev Immunol 2010;10(5):317-27.
2. Lawrence TS, Rosenberg SA, eds. *DeVita, Hellman, and Rosenberg's Cancer: Principles & Practice of Oncology*. Philadelphia: Lippincott Williams & Wilkins; 2015.

What are the different bone-modifying agents for malignancies?

Key concept	Bony metastases are often the sequelae of multiple solid tumors including breast, multiple myeloma, prostate, and others.[1] Skeletal-related events (SREs) encompass fractures—including pathologic, vertebral, and/or non-vertebral—radiation therapy or surgery to bone, and spinal cord compression.[1] Bone-modifying agents (BMAs) are denosumab and bisphosphonates, including zoledronic acid, pamidronate, and others.[1] The mechanism of action of bisphosphonates is inhibition of osteoclast-mediated bone resorption.[1] Denosumab is a fully human monoclonal antibody to receptor activator of the nuclear factor κB ligand.[1]
Clinical scenario	A 72-year-old man with metastatic prostate cancer with multiple osteoblastic lesions is presenting with a T12 compression fracture with creatinine clearance 29 mL/min. What bone-modifying agent is recommended? What are the side effects associated with BMAs?
Action items	

TYPE OF BMA	DOSAGE	PEARLS
Intravenous		
Zoledronic acid	4 mg IV over 15 min every 3–4 weeks[1] or every 12 weeks for 2 years[2]	If creatinine clearance >60 mL/min, then no change in dosage
Pamidronate	90 mg IV over 2 hours every 3–4 weeks	
Denosumab	120 mg SQ every 4 weeks	Can be considered if creatinine clearance is <30 mL/min

	Oral[3]		
	Alendronate Etidronate Ibandronate Risedronate	Variable dosages; refer to https://online.lexi.com	• Medications should be taken with water and >30 min before ingestion of food or medications • Should not lie down within 30 min of taking dose due to potential side effects of GI irritation
Pearl	• If plan for use of BMA, all patients should undergo a dental examination prior to initiation of treatment • Side effects of bisphosphonates include nephrotoxicity and hypocalcemia; side effects of denosumab include fatigue, nausea, hypophosphatemia, and hypocalcemia • A more rare side effect for both bisphosphonates and denosumab is osteonecrosis of the jaw, characterized by necrosis of the maxillofacial or mandibular region resulting in exposed bone that does not heal within 8 weeks		
References	1. Van Poznak CH, Temin S, Yee GC, et al. American Society of Clinical Oncology executive summary of the clinical practice guideline update on the role of bone-modifying agents in metastatic breast cancer. J Clin Oncol 2011;29(9):1221-7. 2. Himelstein AL, Foster JC, Khatcheressian JL, et al. Effect of longer-interval vs. standard dosing of zoledronic acid on skeletal events in patients with bone metastases. a randomized clinical trial. JAMA 2017;317(1):48-58. 3. Drake MT, Clarke BL, Khosla S. Bisphosphonates: mechanism of action and role in clinical practice. Mayo Clinic Proc 2008;83(9):1032-45.		

DRUG FACTS TABLES

DRUG FACTS: Traditional cytotoxic agents

CATEGORY	CLASS	DRUGS	MECHANISMS OF ACTION	ACTION IN CELL CYCLE PHASE	MAJOR SIDE EFFECTS
ANTIMETABOLITES	Cytidine analogs	Cytarabine, gemcitabine	• Pyrimidine analogs, phosphorylated to active forms within cancer cells • Interfere with DNA synthesis, repair, and function by incorporating into DNA and inhibiting DNA polymerase and ribonucleotide reductase	S phase	Myelosuppression, nausea & vomiting (n/v), diarrhea, mucositis, tumor lysis syndrome (TLS), flu-like syndrome, rash, cerebellar toxicity, conjunctivitis, elevated liver transaminases
	DNA hypomethylating agents	Azacitidine, decitabine	• Incorporate into DNA and inhibit DNA methyltransferase, blocking DNA synthesis and hypomethylation (which promotes cell differentiation, reactivates epigenetically silenced tumor suppressor genes, stimulates immune mechanisms, and suppresses tumor growth)	G2–M phase	Myelosuppression & infection, fatigue, n/v, diarrhea, musculoskeletal symptoms (arthralgias), cough, dyspnea

	Folate antagonists	Methotrexate, pemetrexed, pralatrexate	• Inhibit dihydrofolate reductase, resulting in depletion of intracellular reduced folates (tetrahydrofolates) essential for thymidylate and purine synthesis, interfering with DNA synthesis, repair, and cellular replication	S phase	Myelosuppression, mucositis, renal failure, central nervous system (CNS) toxicity, hepatotoxicity, mucositis, rash **PEARL:** Pemetrexed includes additional antifolate targets resulting in inhibition of BOTH purine and thymidine nucleotide and protein synthesis
	Purine analogs	Cladribine, fludarabine, pentostatin	• Cladribine and fludarabine are purine analogs activated via phosphorylation and incorporated into DNA, resulting in DNA breakage and shutdown of DNA synthesis and repair • Inhibit DNA synthesis by depleting nicotinamide adenine dinucleotide and adenosine triphosphate and inhibition of DNA polymerase and ribonucleotide reductase • Pentostatin is a purine antimetabolite that inhibits adenosine deaminase, causing accumulation of deoxyadenosine and deoxyadenosine 5′-triphosphate, resulting in reduced purine metabolism and inhibiting DNA synthesis	Cell-cycle nonspecific	Myelosuppression, fever, immunosuppression, severe opportunistic infections, diarrhea, CNS toxicity, pulmonary toxicity, TLS

(continued on following page)

DRUG FACTS: Traditional cytotoxic agents

(continued from previous page)	Pyrimidine analogs	Capecitabine, 5-fluorouracil	• Fluorinated uracil analogs act as false pyrimidines and undergo sequential phosphorylation • Phosphorylated active metabolites interfere with cell growth by incorporating into RNA replacing uracil, and inhibiting thymidylate synthetase, depleting thymidine synthetase, depleting thymidine triphosphate, a necessary component of DNA synthesis	S phase	Mucositis, diarrhea, hand-foot syndrome (HFS), myelosuppression, n/v, hyperpigmentation, photosensitivity, ocular toxicity, myocardial ischemic symptoms
	Thiopurines	Mercaptopurine, thioguanine	• Guanine analog metabolized by thiopurine methyltransferase and hypoxanthine phosphoribosyl transferase into substrates that inhibit purine biosynthesis and incorporate into DNA and RNA, inhibiting synthesis and function	S phase	Myelosuppression, dry skin, rash, photosensitivity, hepatotoxicity, n/v, mucositis, diarrhea
ALKYLATING AGENTS	Alky sulfonates	Busulfan	• Methanesulfonate-type bifunctional agent that, once hydrolyzed, releases methanesulfonate groups, creating DNA cross-linking that results in inhibition of DNA synthesis and function	Cell-cycle nonspecific	Myelosuppression, skin hyperpigmentation, pulmonary fibrosis, gynecomastia, adrenal insufficiency, seizures, hepatic veno-occlusive disease, severe n/v

	Nitrogen mustards	Bendamustine, chlorambucil, cyclophosphamide, ifosfamide, melphalan	• Forms cross-links with DNA, resulting in single- and double-strand breaks and inhibition of DNA synthesis and function • Bendamustine may have some antimetabolite activity from benzimidazole ring	Cell-cycle nonspecific	Myelosuppression, infection, dermatologic reactions, TLS, infusion reactions, n/v, mucositis, diarrhea, alopecia, risk of secondary malignancies, infertility & sterility **PEARL:** Cyclophosphamide and ifosfamide ONLY: hemorrhagic cystitis, syndrome of inappropriate antidiuretic hormone (SIADH, typically with high doses of cyclophosphamide), CNS toxicity (ifosfamide)
	Nitrosoureas	Carmustine, lomustine	• Forms cross-links with DNA, resulting in single- and double-strand breaks and inhibition of DNA synthesis and function • Inhibits several key enzymatic processes by carbamylation of amino acids in proteins	Cell-cycle nonspecific	Myelosuppression, severe n/v, cumulative nephrotoxicity, pulmonary fibrosis, facial flushing during infusion **PEARL:** Lipid-soluble, can cross the blood-brain barrier

(continued on following page)

DRUG FACTS: Traditional cytotoxic agents

(continued from previous page)					
	Platinum compounds	Carboplatin, cisplatin, oxaliplatin	• Forms intrastrand and interstrand cross-links with DNA, resulting in single- and double-strand breaks and inhibition of DNA synthesis and function	Cell-cycle nonspecific	Myelosuppression, nephrotoxicity, potassium & magnesium wasting, severe n/v (acute or delayed onset), peripheral neuropathy, ototoxicity, risk of hypersensitivity reactions at higher cumulative doses, pharyngolaryngeal dysesthesias
	Triazines/ methylating agents	Dacarbazine, procarbazine, temozolomide	• Demethylation to monomethyl triazeno-imidazole-carboxamide, which interrupts DNA replication by causing methylation of guanine • Temozolomide is the oral equivalent that spontaneously converts to the active drug	Cell-cycle nonspecific	Myelosuppression, severe n/v, diarrhea, neurotoxicity, increased liver enzymes, flu-like syndrome, facial flushing, photosensitivity, secondary malignancies, infertility & sterility
ANTI-MICROTUBULAR AGENTS	Halichondrin B analog	Eribulin	• Inhibits tubulin polymerization by inhibiting microtubule growth without affecting shortening phase and sequesters tubulin into nonproductive aggregates • Disrupts mitotic spindles, causing apoptotic cell death after prolonged mitotic blockage	G2–M phase	Myelosuppression, peripheral neuropathy, asthenia, alopecia, nausea, constipation

	Taxanes	Cabazitaxel, docetaxel, paclitaxel, albumin-bound paclitaxel	• Induce tubulin polymerization, promoting microtubule assembly and interfering with microtubule disassembly, resulting in formation of inappropriately stable, nonfunctional microtubules	M phase	Myelosuppression, hypersensitivity reactions, n/v, diarrhea, fatigue, peripheral neuropathy, myalgias & arthralgias, mucositis, cardiac arrhythmias, fluid retention & edema, rash, alopecia, renal failure
	Vinca alkaloids	Vinblastine, vincristine, vinorelbine	• Binds to tubulin, inhibiting its polymerization and interfering with formation of the mitotic spindle, causing cells to accumulate in mitosis, leading to apoptosis	M phase	Myelosuppression, mucositis, neurotoxicity (peripheral neuropathy, paresthesias, ileus, urinary retention, facial palsies), myalgias, SIADH, vesicant
TOPOISOMERASE INHIBITORS	Topoisomerase-I inhibitors	Irinotecan, topotecan	• Stabilize the topoisomerase I–DNA complex and prevent re-ligation of DNA after it has been cleaved by topoisomerase I • Collision between this stable cleavable complex and the advancing replication fork results in double-strand DNA breaks and cellular death	Cell-cycle nonspecific	Myelosuppression, n/v, alopecia, fatigue, increased liver enzymes, mucositis **PEARL:** The acute diarrhea from irinotecan is related to cholinergic effects *(continued on following page)*

DRUG FACTS: Traditional cytotoxic agents

(continued from previous page)	Topoisomerase-II inhibitors	Etoposide, teniposide	• Inhibit topoisomerase II by stabilizing the topoisomerase II–DNA complex and preventing unwinding of DNA, causing single-strand breaks	S and G2 phases	Myelosuppression, n/v, alopecia, mucositis, hypotension (infusion rate–related), hypersensitivity reactions, risk of secondary malignancies
	Anthracyclines	Daunorubicin, doxorubicin, liposomal doxorubicin, epirubicin, idarubicin	• Induce formation of covalent topoisomerase II–DNA complexes, inhibiting re-ligation of DNA during DNA replication causing DNA strand breaks • Form oxygen free radicals and cross-links between base pairs in DNA, leading to DNA breaks	Cell-cycle nonspecific	Myelosuppression, mucositis, n/v, alopecia, vesicant **PEARL:** Acute cardiac toxicities: arrhythmias, pericarditis Chronic cardiac injury to myocardium associated with cumulative doses: • Daunorubicin >550 mg/m^2 • Doxorubicin and liposomal doxorubicin >450–550 mg/m^2 • Epirubicin >900 mg/m^2 • Idarubicin >90 mg/m^2
	Miscellaneous/ other	Mitoxantrone	• Induces formation of covalent topoisomerase II–DNA complexes inhibiting re-ligation of DNA during DNA replication, causing DNA strand breaks • Forms cross-links between base pairs in DNA, leading to DNA breaks • Does not form oxygen free radicals	Cell-cycle nonspecific	Myelosuppression, n/v, mucositis, alopecia, less cardiotoxic than anthracyclines

ANTI-TUMOR ANTIBIOTICS	*Streptomyces* species	Bleomycin, dactinomycin, mitomycin C	• Form oxygen free radicals and cross-links to guanine-cytidine base pairs, resulting in cross-link, leading to inhibition of DNA, RNA, and protein synthesis	• Bleomycin: G2 phase • Dactinomycin and mitomycin C: cell-cycle nonspecific	Myelosuppression, mucositis, n/v, diarrhea, alopecia Bleomycin: Anaphylaxis & hypersensitivity reactions, fever & flu-like symptoms, pulmonary fibrosis Dactinomycin: dermatologic reactions, photosensitivity, vesicant Mitomycin C: delayed & prolonged myelosuppression, pulmonary fibrosis, hemolytic anemia & uremic syndrome, vesicant

References
Chabner BA, Longo DL, eds. *Cancer Chemotherapy and Biotherapy.* 5th ed. Philadelphia: Lippincott Williams & Wilkins; 2011.
DeVita VT Jr, Lawrence TS, Rosenberg SA, ed. *Cancer: Principles and Practices of Oncology.* 9th ed. Philadelphia: Lippincott Williams & Wilkins; 2011.
Fischer DS, ed. *Cancer Chemotherapy Handbook*. Norwalk: Appleton & Lange; 1994.
Lexi-Comp, Inc. Lexi-Comp Clinical Reference Library. Available at: www.lexi.com.
Shord SS, Cordes LM. Cancer treatment and chemotherapy. In: DiPiro JT, et al., eds. *Pharmacotherapy: A Pathophysiologic Approach.* 10th ed. New York, NY: McGraw-Hill; 2016. Available at: http://accesspharmacy.mhmedical.com/content.aspx?bookid=1861&sectionid=146074145.

DRUG FACTS: Adverse effects of traditional cytotoxic agents

<table>
<tr><th>ADVERSE EFFECT (AE)</th><th>AGENT</th><th>PREVENTATIVE MEASURES TO PREVENT OR REDUCE AE</th></tr>
<tr>
<td>CARDIOTOXICITY
<table>
<tr><th>ONSET</th><th>SYMPTOMS</th></tr>
<tr><td>Acute</td><td>Electrocardioarrhythmias such as sinus tachycardia, QT prolongation, supraventricular beats, or acute myocardial infarction (rarely)</td></tr>
<tr><td>Subacute</td><td>Pericarditis or myocarditis</td></tr>
<tr><td>Chronic</td><td>Congestive heart failure</td></tr>
</table>
</td>
<td>ANTHRACYCLINES[1]
<table>
<tr><th>ANTHRACYCLINE</th><th>CONVERSION FACTOR</th><th>%CARDIOTOXICITY AT CUMULATIVE DOSE</th></tr>
<tr><td>Doxorubicin</td><td>1</td><td>5% risk at 450 mg/m²</td></tr>
<tr><td>Daunorubicin</td><td>0.5</td><td>5% risk at 900 mg/m²</td></tr>
<tr><td>Epirubicin</td><td>0.5</td><td>5% risk at 935 mg/m²</td></tr>
<tr><td>Idarubicin</td><td>2</td><td>5% risk at 160 mg/m²</td></tr>
<tr><td>Mitoxantrone</td><td>2.2</td><td>5% risk at 200 mg/m²</td></tr>
</table>
</td>
<td>DEXRAZOXANE[2,3]
• Proposed mechanism of toxicity from anthracyclines is release of reactive oxygen species (ROS) associated with free cellular iron, which induces cardiomyocyte death
• Dexrazoxane acts as an iron-chelating agent that prevents free ROS
• 10:1 ratio of dexrazoxane:doxorubicin
• Administer within 30 min prior to anthracycline administration</td>
</tr>
<tr>
<td>CENTRAL NERVOUS SYSTEM (CNS) TOXICITY[4]
• CNS complications include headaches, seizures, encephalopathy, cerebrovascular disease, and cerebellar dysfunction/ataxia
• Peripheral nervous system complications include plexopathy, peripheral neuropathy, and inflammatory demyelinating polyneuropathy</td>
<td>
<table>
<tr><th colspan="2">COMMON CNS COMPLICATIONS</th></tr>
<tr><th>AGENTS</th><th>SYMPTOMS</th></tr>
<tr><td>Nucleotide analogs (fludarabine), methotrexate, retinoic acid, tamoxifen, temozolomide, etoposide, intrathecal (IT) chemotherapy</td><td>Headache</td></tr>
</table>
</td>
<td>Recognize CNS toxicity and consider drug discontinuation or dose adjustment
PEARL: Methylene blue can be used for ifosfamide-induced encephalopathy[5]</td>
</tr>
</table>

	Busulfan, cisplatin, cytarabine, dacarbazine, etoposide, 5-fluorouracil (5-FU), fludarabine, gemcitabine, ifosfamide, paclitaxel, vincristine, IT chemotherapy	Seizure	
	5-Azacytidine, cisplatin, cytarabine, etoposide, fludarabine, gemcitabine, methotrexate, mitomycin C, nitrosoureas, anti–vascular endothelial growth factor agents (bevacizumab, sorafenib, sunitinib), immunomodulatory agents (sirolimus, tacrolimus), biologic agents (CAR T cell infusion, rituximab, ipilimumab, interferon-α)	Encephalopathy	
	L-Asparaginase, cyclosporine, doxorubicin, estramustine, methotrexate, and platinum-based treatments	Cerebrovascular disease (eg, stroke and thrombosis)	
	High-dose cytarabine (cumulative doses >36 g/m^2), capecitabine, 5-FU, vincristine, hexamethylmelamine, nelarabine, oxaliplatin	Cerebellar dysfunction, ataxia	
	Platinum-based agents (carboplatin, cisplatin, and oxaliplatin), vinca alkaloids (vinblastine, vincristine, vindesine, vinorelbine), taxanes (cabazitaxel, docetaxel, nab-paclitaxel), alkylators (ifosfamide, procarbazine), anti-metabolites (cytarabine, gemcitabine, nelarabine)	Peripheral neuropathy	*(continued on following page)*

<table>
<tr><td>(continued from previous page)
HEMORROHAGIC CYSTITIS[6,7]</td><td>Ifosfamide, cyclophosphamide (most common agents), busulfan, thiotepa, temozolomide, and radiation</td><td>• Continuous bladder irrigation (decreases the duration of exposure to toxins, reducing toxicity)
• Hydration
• Parenteral or oral mesna, which is excreted by the urinary tract, where the sulfhydryl group of mesna complexes with the terminal methyl group of acrolein forming a nontoxic thioether</td></tr>
<tr><td>PULMONARY TOXICITY[8,9]<table><tr><th>ONSET</th><th>ENTITY</th><th>SYMPTOMS</th></tr><tr><td>Acute</td><td>Inflammatory interstitial pneumonitis</td><td>Nonproductive cough, progressive dyspnea, and, in some patients, low-grade fevers (generally <101°F or 38.3°C)</td></tr></table></td><td>Bleomycin (cumulative doses of 400–500 mg/m^2), mitomycin, cyclophosphamide (cumulative doses or 150–250 mg), busulfan, methotrexate, cytosine arabinoside, carmustine, procarbazine, vinca alkaloids</td><td>• Baseline evaluation of lung function, if there are risk factors for pulmonary toxicity
• Oral steroids</td></tr>
</table>

<table>
<tr><td>
<table>
<tr><td>Late</td><td>Pulmonary fibrosis</td><td>Insidious onset of dyspnea associated with a nonproductive cough and characterized by pulmonary function tests, demonstrating a restrictive pattern, with decreases in lung volumes and diffusing lung capacity for carbon</td></tr>
<tr><td></td><td colspan="2">Pulmonary veno-occlusive disorder, pulmonary nodules bronchiolitis obliterans with organizing pneumonia, pleural effusion</td></tr>
</table>
</td><td></td><td></td></tr>
<tr><td>
RENAL TOXICITY[10]
<table>
<tr><th>ENTITY</th><th>MANIFESTATIONS</th></tr>
<tr><td>Tubulopathies</td><td>Salt or magnesium wasting, syndrome of inappropriate antidiuretic hormone</td></tr>
<tr><td>Acute kidney injury</td><td>Acute tubular necrosis, crystal nephropathy, and thrombotic microangiopathy</td></tr>
<tr><td>Nephritic and nephrotic syndrome</td><td>Thrombotic microangiopathy, minimal change disease</td></tr>
<tr><td>Chronic kidney disease</td><td>Chronic interstitial nephritis, glomerulosclerosis</td></tr>
</table>
</td><td>Platinum agents (eg, cisplatin), ifosfamide, cetuximab, panitumumab, vincristine, methotrexate (MTX), nitrosoureas, anti-angiogenesis agents, gemcitabine, mitomycin C</td><td>• Correct dosage based on renal function, which includes creatinine clearance (24-h collection and Cockcroft-Gault calculation)
• Correction of hypovolemia:
  • Urinary alkalinization with isotonic sodium bicarbonate for MTX (reduces intratubular crystal formation)
  • Intravenous isotonic or hypertonic saline for cisplatin

(continued on following page)</td></tr>
</table>

DRUG FACTS: Adverse effects of traditional cytotoxic agents

<table>
<tr><td>(continued from previous page)</td><td></td><td>• Specific antidotes
<table><tr><th>Antidote</th><th>Agent</th></tr><tr><td>Sodium thiosulfate, amifostine</td><td>Cisplatin</td></tr><tr><td>Leucovorin, glucarpidase</td><td>5-FU, MTX</td></tr></table></td></tr>
<tr><td>DERMATOLOGIC MANIFESTATION[11,12]
• Infusion reactions
• Diffuse or localized cutaneous pigmentary changes
• Radiation dermatitis
• Hand-foot syndrome
• Nail changes (changes in pigmentation, onycholysis, paronychia)
• Mucosal changes
• Stomatitis,
• Alopecia
• Photosensitivity
• Cutaneous erythematosus lupus
• Drug rashes
• Acneiform or papulo-pustular eruption
• Telangiectasias
• Exfoliative dermatitis
• Erythema multiforme</td><td>Signal transduction inhibitors (epidermal growth factor receptor antagonists—gefitinib, cetuximab, erlotinib, panitumumab), multikinase inhibitors (imatinib, dasatinib, nilotinib, sorafenib, sunitinib), proteasome inhibitors (bortezomib), taxanes, vinca alkaloids, antimetabolites, alkylating agents, anthracyclines</td><td>• Topical emollients (non-alcoholic emollients, urea creams), hydrocortisone, and antibiotics
• Oral antibiotics
• Oral antihistamines
• Depending on severity, oral corticosteroids</td></tr>
</table>

References

1. Wojtacki J, Lewicka-Nowak E, Leśniewski-Kmak K. Anthracycline-induced cardiotoxicity: clinical course, risk factors, pathogenesis, detection and prevention - review of the literature. Med Sci Monit 2000;6(2):RA411-20.
2. Zinecard® (dexrazoxan for injection). Available at: https://www.accessdata.fda.gov/drugsatfda_docs/label/2012/020212s013lbl.pdf.
3. Popelová O, Štěrba M, Hašková P, et al. Dexrazoxane-afforded protection against chronic anthracycline cardiotoxicity in vivo: effective rescue of cardiomyocytes from apoptotic cell death. Br J Cancer 2009;101(5):792-802.
4. Stone JB, DeAngelis LM. Cancer-treatment-induced neurotoxicity focus on newer treatments. Nat Rev Clin Oncol 2016;13(2):92-105.
5. Patel PN. Methylene blue for management of ifosfamide-induced encephalopathy. Ann Pharmacother 2006;40(2):299-303.
6. Manikandan R, Kumar S, Dorairajan LN. Hemorrhagic cystitis: a challenge to the urologist. Indian J Urol 2010;26(2):159-66.
7. Hensley ML, Hagerty KL, Kewalramani T, et al. American Society of Clinical Oncology 2008 clinical practice guideline update: use of chemotherapy and radiation therapy protectants. J Clin Oncol 2009;27(1):127-45.
8. Abid SH, Malhotra V, Perry MC. Radiation-induced and chemotherapy-induced pulmonary injury. Curr Opin Oncol 2001;13(4):242-8.
9. Lehne G, Lote K. Pulmonary toxicity of cytotoxic and immunosuppressive agents: a review. Acta Oncol 1990;29(2):113-24.
10. Perazella MA, Moeckel GW. Nephrotoxicity from chemotherapeutic agents: clinical manifestations, pathobiology, and prevention/therapy. Semin Nephrol 2010;30(6):570-81.
11. Heidary N, Naik H, Burgin S. Chemotherapeutic agents and the skin: an update. J Am Acad Dermatol 2008;58(4):545-70.
12. Fabbrocini G, Panariello L, Caro G, et al. Acneiform rash induced by EGFR inhibitors: review of the literature and new insights. Skin Appendage Disord 2015;1(1):31-7.

DRUG FACTS: Targeted cytotoxic agents

CLASS	DRUG	INDICATION	MECHANISM OF ACTION	MAJOR SIDE EFFECTS
BCL-2 inhibitor	Venetoclax (Venclexta®)	Chronic lymphocytic leukemia (CLL)	Selectively inhibits the anti-apoptotic protein BCL-2, which is overexpressed in CLL cells and results in displacement of pro-apoptotic proteins and restoring the apoptotic process	Myelosuppression, tumor lysis syndrome (TLS), diarrhea, nausea, upper respiratory tract infection **PEARL:** BCL-2 mediates tumor cell survival and has been associated with chemotherapy resistance
Cyclin-dependent kinase (CDK) inhibitor	Palbociclib (Ibrance®)	Breast	Reversible small-molecule CDK inhibitor, selective for CDK 4 and 6, that reduces proliferation of tumor cell lines by preventing progression from the G1 to the S phase	Thromboembolic events, infection, bone marrow suppression, gastrointestinal toxicity
Hedgehog inhibitors	Sonidegib (Odomzo®)	Basal cell cancer	Selective Hedgehog pathway inhibitor that binds to and inhibits Smoothened homolog (SMO), the transmembrane protein involved in Hedgehog signal transduction	Fatigue, alopecia, amenorrhea, musculoskeletal toxicity, teratogenic effects
	Vismodegib (Erivedge®)	Basal cell cancer	Selective Hedgehog pathway inhibitor that binds to and inhibits SMO, the transmembrane protein involved in Hedgehog signal transduction	Muscle spasms, alopecia, dysgeusia, fatigue, nausea, vomiting, diarrhea, decreased appetite, constipation, arthralgias, teratogenic effects
Histone deacetylase (HDAC) inhibitors	Belinostat (Beleodaq®)	Peripheral T cell lymphoma	Catalyzes acetyl group removal from protein lysine residues (of histone and some non-histone proteins); HDAC inhibition results in accumulation of acetyl groups, leading to cell cycle arrest and apoptosis	Pyrexia, nausea, fatigue, anemia, hepatotoxicity, infection, TLS

	Panobinostat (Farydak®)	Multiple myeloma	Inhibits enzymatic activity of HDAC, resulting in increased acetylation of histone proteins; accumulation of acetylated histones and other proteins induces cell-cycle arrest and/or apoptosis of some transformed cells	Cardiotoxicity, nausea, vomiting, diarrhea, hemorrhage, infection, hepatotoxicity
	Romidepsin (Istodax®)	Cutaneous T cell lymphoma, peripheral T cell lymphoma	Catalyzes acetyl group removal from protein lysine residues (including histone and transcription factors); HDAC inhibition results in accumulation of acetyl groups, leading to alterations in chromatin structure and transcription factor activation causing termination of cell growth (induces arrest in cell cycle at G1 and G2/M phases), leading to cell death	Neutropenia, lymphopenia, thrombocytopenia, infection, nausea, fatigue, vomiting, anorexia, anemia, ECG T-wave changes
	Vorinostat (Zolinza®)	Cutaneous T cell lymphoma	Inhibits HDAC enzymes (HDAC1, HDAC2, HDAC3, and HDAC6), which catalyze acetyl group removal from protein lysine residues (including histones and transcription factors); HDAC inhibition results in accumulation of acetyl groups, which alters chromatin structure and transcription factor activation; cell growth is terminated and apoptosis occurs	Diarrhea, fatigue, nausea, thrombocytopenia, anorexia, dysgeusia, thromboembolic events, hyperglycemia

(continued on following page)

DRUG FACTS: Targeted cytotoxic agents

(continued from previous page) Mammalian target of rapamycin (mTOR) kinase inhibitors	Everolimus (Afinitor®)	Breast, neuroendocrine tumors, renal cell carcinoma (RCC)	Macrolide immunosuppressant that has antiproliferative and antiangiogenic properties; reduces angiogenesis by inhibiting vascular endothelial growth factor (VEGF) and hypoxia-inducible factor (HIF-1) expression	Angioedema, myelosuppression, edema, hepatic artery thrombosis, infection, secondary malignancies, hyperglycemia, hyperlipidemia, hypertriglyceridemia, mucositis, nephrotoxicity, interstitial lung disease (ILD), pneumonitis, delayed wound healing
	Temsirolimus (Torisel®)	RCC	mTOR inhibition exhibits anti-angiogenesis activity by reducing levels of HIF-1 and HIF-2α and VEGF	Angioedema, edema, infection, hyperglycemia, hyperlipidemia, hypertriglyceridemia, nephrotoxicity, ILD, pneumonitis, delayed wound healing
Poly (ADP-ribose) polymerase (PARP) inhibitors	Niraparib (Zejula®)	Ovarian, fallopian tube, primary peritoneal cancer	Highly selective for PARP-1 and PARP-2, which are involved in detecting DNA damage and promote repair; inhibiting PARP enzymatic activity results in DNA damage, apoptosis, and cell death	Myelosuppression, hypertension, nausea, vomiting, constipation, mucositis, secondary malignancy, rash, fatigue
	Olaparib (Lynparza®)	Ovarian cancer		Myelosuppression, edema, nausea, vomiting, constipation, mucositis, secondary malignancy, rash, musculoskeletal pain, fatigue
	Rucaparib (Rubraca®)	Ovarian cancer		Myelosuppression, nausea, vomiting, constipation, mucositis, secondary malignancy, musculoskeletal pain, fatigue, renal toxicity, hepatotoxicity, hyperlipidemia

Phosphatidylinositol 3-kinase (PI3K) inhibitor	Idelalisib (Zydelig®)	CLL, follicular lymphoma, small lymphocytic lymphoma	Inhibits the delta isoform of PI3K, resulting in apoptosis of malignant tumor cells, and several other signaling pathways, including B cell receptor, CXCR4, and CXCR5	GI disorders, pneumonitis, neutropenia, fever, rash, elevated liver enzymes, dermatologic toxicity
Retinoids	Bexarotene (Targretin®)	Cutaneous T cell lymphoma	Selectively binds to and activates retinoid X receptors (RXRs), which then function as transcription factors to regulate the expression of genes that control cellular differentiation and proliferation	Peripheral edema, insomnia, headache, fever, increased triglycerides & cholesterol, hypothyroidism, leukopenia & anemia, dry skin, increased liver enzymes, pancreatitis, photosensitivity
	Tretinoin (ATRA)	Acute promyelocytic leukemia (APL)	Binds $\geq$1 nuclear receptors, decreasing proliferation and inducing differentiation of APL cells; initially produces maturation of primitive promyelocytes and repopulates marrow and peripheral blood with normal hematopoietic cells to achieve complete remission	Headache, dry skin & mucous membranes, mucositis, increased liver enzymes & bilirubin **PEARL:** Patients treated with ATRA may develop differentiation syndrome ("ATRA syndrome"), which is characterized by pulmonary symptoms, fever, hypotension, & pleural effusions and can be life threatening if not recognized early
Small molecule inhibitors/immunomodulators	Lenalidomide (Revlimid®)	Mantle cell lymphoma, multiple myeloma, myelodysplastic syndrome with deletion 5q	Immunomodulatory, antiangiogenic, and antineoplastic characteristics via multiple mechanisms; selectively inhibits secretion of proinflammatory cytokines (potent inhibitor of tumor necrosis factor [TNF]–α secretion); enhances cell-mediated immunity by stimulating proliferation of anti-CD3 stimulated T cells (resulting in increased interleukin [IL]–2 and interferon [IFN]–γ secretion); inhibits trophic signals to angiogenic factors in cells	Fetal toxicity, fatigue, peripheral neuropathy, neutropenia & thrombocytopenia, thromboembolic events

(continued on following page)

(continued from previous page)				
	Pomalidomide (Pomalyst®)	Multiple myeloma	Induces cell-cycle arrest and apoptosis directly in multiple myeloma cells; enhances T cell– and natural killer (NK) cell–mediated cytotoxicity, inhibits production of proinflammatory cytokines TNF-α, IL-1, IL-6, and IL-12, and inhibits angiogenesis	Myelosuppression, dizziness, confusion, hepatotoxicity, hypersensitivity, ILD, neuropathy, secondary malignancy, thromboembolic events, fetal toxicity, TLS
	Thalidomide (Thalidomid®)	Multiple myeloma	Exhibits immunomodulatory and anti-angiogenic characteristics; associated with an increase in NK cells and increased levels of IL-2 and IFN-γ; other proposed mechanisms of action include suppression of angiogenesis, prevention of free radical–mediated DNA damage, increased cell-mediated cytotoxic effects, and altered expression of cellular adhesion molecules	Fetal toxicity, somnolence, constipation, dizziness or orthostatic hypotension, rash, peripheral neuropathies, thromboembolic events
VEGF inhibitor	Ziv-aflibercept (Zaltrap®)	Colorectal cancer	Recombinant fusion protein which is composed of portions of binding domains for VEGF receptors 1 and 2, attached to the Fc portion of human IgG1; acts as a decoy receptor for VEGF-A, VEGF-B, and placental growth factor, which prevents VEGF receptor binding/activation to receptors (an action critical to angiogenesis), leading to anti-angiogenesis and tumor regression	Neutropenia, diarrhea, proteinuria, hepatotoxicity, stomatitis, fatigue, thrombocytopenia, hypertension, decreased weight, decreased appetite, epistaxis, abdominal pain, dysphonia, increased serum creatinine, headache, hemorrhage, GI perforation, compromised wound healing, arterial thromboembolic events, fistula formation

References

Chabner BA, Longo, DL, ed. *Cancer Chemotherapy and Biotherapy.* 5th ed. Philadelphia: Lippincott Williams & Wilkins; 2011.
DeVita VT Jr, Lawrence TS, Rosenberg SA, ed. *Cancer: Principles and Practices of Oncology.* 9th ed. Philadelphia: Lippincott Williams & Wilkins; 2011.
Fischer DS, Durivage HJ, Knobf MT et al., eds. *Cancer Chemotherapy Handbook.* Norwalk: Appleton & Lange; 1994.
Lexi-Comp, Inc. Lexi-Comp Clinical Reference Library. www.lexi.com
Shord SS, Cordes LM. Cancer treatment and chemotherapy. In: DiPiro JT, et al., eds. *Pharmacotherapy: A Pathophysiologic Approach.* 10th ed. New York: McGraw-Hill; 2016.

DRUG FACTS: Monoclonal antibodies for cancer treatment

CLASS	DRUG	INDICATION	MECHANISM OF ACTION	MAJOR SIDE EFFECTS
Human epidermal growth factor receptor 2 (HER2) inhibitor	Ado-trastuzumab emtansine (Kadcyla®)	Breast	HER2 antibody–drug conjugate that incorporates the HER2-targeted actions of trastuzumab with the microtubule inhibitor DM1, which allows for selective delivery into HER2 overexpressing cells, resulting in cell-cycle arrest and apoptosis	Cardiovascular toxicity, thrombocytopenia, hemorrhage, hepatotoxicity, infusion reactions, extravasation reactions, peripheral neuropathy, interstitial lung disease, fatigue, musculoskeletal pain, gastrointestinal distress
	Pertuzumab (Perjeta®)		Recombinant humanized monoclonal antibody that targets the extracellular HER2 dimerization domain, inhibiting HER2 dimerization and blocking HER downstream signaling, halting cell growth and initiating apoptosis	Diarrhea, nausea, alopecia, rash, neutropenia, fatigue, peripheral neuropathy, embryo & fetal toxicity, left ventricular dysfunction, infusion-related reactions **PEARL:** Cardiovascular toxicity (especially if combined with trastuzumab)
	Trastuzumab (Herceptin®)		Binds to the extracellular domain of the HER2; mediates antibody-dependent cellular cytotoxicity by inhibiting proliferation of cells that overexpress HER2 protein	Cardiovascular toxicity: congestive cardiomyopathy, usually reversible with medical management; infusion-related reaction
Vascular endothelial growth factor (VEGF) inhibitor	Bevacizumab (Avastin®)	Cervical, colorectal (CRC), glioblastoma multiforme, non–small cell lung cancer (NSCLC), ovarian, renal cell carcinoma (RCC), gastric	Humanized monoclonal antibody that binds to and neutralizes VEGF, preventing its association with tumor receptors and inhibiting angiogenesis	Decreased bone mineral density, hypercholesterolemia, gastrointestinal distress, hot flashes, thromboembolic events, edema, gastrointestinal hemorrhage or perforation (rare)

	Ramucirumab (Cyramza ®)	CRC, gastric, NCSLC	Recombinant monoclonal antibody that inhibits VEGFR2; binds to and blocks VEGFR ligands, which inhibit activation of VEGFR2, resulting in decreased tumor proliferation and migration	Gastrointestinal hemorrhage or perforation (rare), impaired wound healing, hypertension, proteinuria, thyroid dysfunction, thromboembolic events, hemorrhage
Epidermal growth factor receptor (EGFR) inhibitor	Cetuximab (Erbitux®)	CRC, head and neck	Recombinant chimeric monoclonal antibody that binds to EGFR, competitively inhibiting the binding of epidermal growth factor (EGF) and other ligands. Binding to EGFR blocks phosphorylation and down-stream signal activation of receptor-associated kinases, resulting in inhibition of cell growth and induction of apoptosis; EGFR signal transduction results in RAS wild-type activation—cells with RAS mutations appear to be unaffected by EGFR inhibition	Acneiform rash, paronychial cracking in fingers or toes, fatigue, weakness, abdominal pain, nausea, constipation, diarrhea, infusion-related reactions, electrolyte wasting, cardiopulmonary arrest
	Necitumumab (Portrazza®)	NSCLC	Recombinant human IgG1 EGFR monoclonal antibody that binds with high affinity to the ligand binding site of EGFR to prevent receptor activation and downstream signaling	Acneiform rash, paronychial cracking in fingers or toes, asthenia, abdominal pain, nausea, constipation, diarrhea, infusion & hypersensitivity reactions, electrolyte wasting, cardiopulmonary arrest

(continued on following page)

DRUG FACTS: Monoclonal antibodies for cancer treatment

(continued from previous page)				
	Panitumumab (Vectibix®)	CRC	Recombinant chimeric monoclonal antibody that binds to EGFR, competitively inhibiting the binding of EGF and other ligands; binding to EGFR blocks phosphorylation and downstream signal activation of receptor-associated kinases, resulting in inhibition of cell growth and induction of apoptosis; EGFR signal transduction results in RAS wild-type activation—cells with RAS mutations appear to be unaffected by EGFR inhibition	Acneiform rash, paronychial cracking in fingers or toes, asthenia, abdominal pain, nausea, constipation, diarrhea, infusion and hypersensitivity reactions, electrolyte wasting, cardiopulmonary arrest
Platelet-derived growth factor receptor (PDGFR) inhibitor	Olaratumab (Lartruvo®)	Soft tissue sarcoma	Human IgG1 antibody that expressly binds to PDGFR-α to prevent binding of PDGF ligands, blocking receptor activation and disrupting PDGF receptor signaling; inhibition of the PDGF-α receptor exerts activity on tumor cells in cell differentiation, growth, and angiogenesis	Fatigue, musculoskeletal pain, dermatitis, nausea/vomiting, upper respiratory infections, anemia, pneumonitis, secondary malignancies (myelodysplastic syndrome/acute myeloid leukemia [MDS/AML])
Programmed death-1 (PD-1) inhibitor	Atezolizumab (Tecentriq®)	NSCLC, urothelial	Humanized monoclonal antibody immune checkpoint inhibitor that binds to PD-L1 to selectively prevent interaction between the PD-1 and B7.1 receptors, restoring antitumor T cell function	Adrenal insufficiency, cardiovascular toxicity, diabetes mellitus, immune-mediated toxicities (pneumonitis, colitis, hepatitis, nephritis, thyroid dysfunction), pancreatitis, urinary tract infection, pneumonia, infusion-related reactions, interstitial lung disease, hypoalbuminemia, hyponatremia, fatigue

Avelumab (Bavencio®)	Merkel cell, urothelial	Fully human monoclonal antibody immune checkpoint inhibitor that binds to PD-L1 to selectively prevent interaction between the PD-1 and B7.1 receptors, restoring antitumor T cell function	Adrenal insufficiency, diabetes mellitus, immune-mediated toxicities (pneumonitis, colitis, hepatitis, nephritis, thyroid dysfunction), nephrotoxicity, urinary tract infection, infusion-related reactions, fatigue, rash, peripheral edema, musculoskeletal pain
Durvalumab (Imfinzi®)	NSCLC, urothelial	Human immunoglobulin G (IgG)–1 kappa monoclonal antibody immune checkpoint inhibitor that binds to PD-L1 to selectively prevent interaction between the PD-1 and B7.1 receptors, restoring antitumor T cell function	Adrenal insufficiency, immune-mediated toxicities (pneumonitis, colitis, hepatitis, nephritis, thyroid dysfunction), infection, nephrotoxicity, urinary tract infection, infusion-related reactions, fatigue, peripheral edema, musculoskeletal pain
Nivolumab (Opdivo®)	CRC (if microsatellite instability-high or mismatch repair deficit), head and neck, hepatocellular cancer (HCC), melanoma, Hodgkin lymphoma, NSCLC, RCC, urothelial	Fully human IgG4 monoclonal antibody that selectively inhibits programmed cell death-1 (PD-1) activity by binding to the PD-1 receptor to block the ligands PD-L1 and PD-L2 from binding; this releases PD-1 pathway-mediated inhibition of the immune response, including the antitumor immune response	Fatigue, immune-mediated toxicities (pneumonitis, colitis, hepatitis, nephritis, thyroid dysfunction)

(continued on following page)

DRUG FACTS: Monoclonal antibodies for cancer treatment

(continued from previous page)	Pembrolizumab (Keytruda®)	Gastric, head and neck, Hodgkin lymphoma, melanoma, NSCLC, microsatellite instability-high cancer, urothelial	Fully human IgG4 monoclonal antibody that selectively inhibits PD-1 activity by binding to the PD-1 receptor to block the ligands PD-L1 and PD-L2 from binding. This releases PD-1 pathway-mediated inhibition of the immune response, including the antitumor immune response	Fatigue; immune-mediated toxicities (pneumonitis, colitis, hepatitis, nephritis, thyroid dysfunction)
Anti-cytotoxic T lymphocyte–associated antigen 4 (CTLA-4) inhibitor	Ipilimumab (Yervoy®)	Melanoma	Recombinant human IgG1 monoclonal antibody that binds to CTLA-4; blocking CTLA-4 allows for enhanced T cell mediate immune responses against tumors	Fatigue, diarrhea, pruritus, rash, immune-mediated reactions (enterocolitis, dermatitis, neuropathy, endocrinopathy, hepatitis)
Anti-CD19	Blinatumomab (Blincyto)	Acute lymphoblastic leukemia	Bispecific T cell engager that binds to CD19 (expressed on B cells) and CD3 (expressed on T cells) and activates endogenous T cells by connecting CD3 in the T cell receptor complex with CD19 on B cells, forming a cytolytic synapse between a cytotoxic T cell and the cancer target B cell; this complex mediates the production of cytolytic proteins, release of inflammatory cytokines, and proliferation of T cells, resulting in lysis of CD19-positive cells	Infusion reactions, cytokine release syndrome, neurologic toxicities, infections, fever, headache, peripheral edema, rash, tumor lysis syndrome (TLS), hepatotoxicity, bone marrow suppression, pancreatitis

Anti-CD20	Ibritumomab (Zevalin®)	Non-Hodgkin lymphoma	Anti-CD20 antibody conjugated to chelator tiuxetan, which acts as a specific chelation site for yttrium-90 and acts as a delivery system to direct the radioactive isotope to the targeted cells; beta-emission induces cellular damage through the formation of free radicals	Delayed hematologic toxicity, infusion-related reactions, fatigue, nausea, cutaneous & mucocutaneous reactions, extravasation & radiation necrosis, secondary malignancies **PEARL:** Delayed, prolonged, and severe cytopenias can result after treatment; do not administer to patients with ≥25% lymphoma marrow involvement or with impaired bone marrow reserve
	Obinutuzumab (Gazyva®)	Chronic lymphocytic leukemia (CLL), follicular lymphoma	Anti-CD20 monoclonal antibody that activates complement-dependent cytotoxicity, antibody-dependent cellular cytotoxicity (ADCC) and antibody-dependent cellular phagocytosis, resulting in cell death	Infusion reactions, myelosuppression, nausea, diarrhea, progressive multifocal leukoencephalopathy, hepatitis B virus reactivation
	Ofatumumab (Arzerra®)	CLL	Monoclonal antibody that binds the CD20 molecule, resulting in potent complement-dependent cell lysis and ADCC	Neutropenia, pneumonia, pyrexia, cough, diarrhea, anemia, fatigue, dyspnea, rash, nausea, bronchitis, upper respiratory infection

(continued on following page)

DRUG FACTS: Monoclonal antibodies for cancer treatment

(continued from previous page)				
	Rituximab (Rituxan®)	CLL, follicular lymphoma, diffuse large B cell lymphoma (DLBCL)	Monoclonal antibody directed against the CD20 antigen on the surface of B lymphocytes and binds to the antigen on the cell surface, activating complement-dependent B cell cytotoxicity, and to human Fc receptors, mediating cell killing through ADCC	Hypersensitivity reactions & infusion-related reactions, TLS, myelosuppression & infection, rare reports of progressive multifocal leukoencephalopathy, severe skin reactions, myalgias, tachycardia **PEARL:** Screen all patients for hepatitis B virus (HBV) infection PRIOR to start of treatment due to possible HBV reactivation and possible severe complications such as fulminant hepatitis, liver failure, and death
	Rituximab and hyaluronidase	CLL, follicular lymphoma, DLBCL	Monoclonal antibody directed against the CD20 antigen on the surface of B lymphocytes, activating complement-dependent B cell cytotoxicity, and to human Fc receptors, mediating cell killing through ADCC; hyaluronidase increases the absorption rate of rituximab-containing products by increasing permeability of subcutaneous tissue through temporary depolymerization of hyaluronan	Bowel obstruction/perforation, hypersensitivity reactions & infusion-related reactions, TLS, myelosuppression & infection, rare reports of progressive multifocal leukoencephalopathy, severe skin reactions, myalgias, tachycardia, HBV reactivation

Anti-CD22	Inotuzumab ozogamicin (Besponsa®)	Acute lymphoblastic leukemia	Humanized CD22-directed monoclonal antibody-drug conjugate composed of the antibody inotuzumab, a calicheamicin component; after the antibody-drug conjugate binds to CD22, the CD22-conjugate complex is internalized and releases calicheamicin, which binds to the minor groove of DNA to induce double strand cleavage and subsequent cell-cycle arrest and apoptosis	Hematologic toxicity, hemorrhage, hepatotoxicity, hypersensitivity, infection, infusion-related reactions, QT prolongation, increased serum amylase & lipase, fatigue
Anti-CD30	Brentuximab vedotin (Adcetris®)	Hodgkin lymphoma, anaplastic large cell lymphoma (ALCL), mycosis fungoides	Antibody drug conjugate linking a CD30-specific chimeric IgG1 antibody and a microtubule-disrupting agent, monomethylauristatin E (MMAE) that binds CD30-expressing tumor cells and forms a complex that is internalized within the cell and releases MMAE, which binds to the tubules and disrupts the cellular microtubule network, inducing cell cycle arrest and apoptosis	Neutropenia, peripheral neuropathy, fatigue, nausea or vomiting, anemia, diarrhea, rash, thrombocytopenia, infusion-related reactions, TLS, progressive multifocal leukoencephalopathy, dermatologic toxicity, pancreatitis, hepatotoxicity, infection

(continued on following page)

DRUG FACTS: Monoclonal antibodies for cancer treatment

(continued from previous page)

Anti-CD33	Gemtuzumab ozogamicin (Mylotarg®)	Acute myeloid leukemia	Humanized CD-33 directed monoclonal antibody-drug conjugate composed of the IgG4 kappa antibody gemtuzumab linked to a cytotoxic calicheamicin derivative which binds the CD33 antigen, resulting in internalization of the antibody-antigen complex; after internalization, the calicheamicin derivative is released inside the myeloid cell and the calicheamicin derivative binds to DNA, resulting in double strand breaks, inducing cell-cycle arrest and apoptosis	Myelosuppression, prolonged thrombocytopenia, hemorrhage, hepatotoxicity, hypersensitivity/ infusion-related reaction, QT interval prolongation, TLS, infection, nausea, constipation, mucositis
Anti-CD52	Alemtuzumab (Campath®)	CLL	Humanized monoclonal antibody that binds to the CD52+ cells, resulting in an antibody-dependent lysis of tumor cells	Prolonged myelosuppression & immunosuppression, autoimmune conditions, infection, infusion-related reactions, nausea, vomiting, rash, headache, fatigue, secondary malignancies
Anti-signaling lymphocytic activation molecule family member 7 (SLAMF7)	Elotuzumab (Empliciti)	Multiple myeloma	Humanized IgG1 immunostimulatory monoclonal antibody directed against SLAMF7 which directly activates natural killer cells through both the SLAMF7 pathway and Fc receptors, resulting in antibody-dependent cellular cytotoxicity	Fatigue, pyrexia, diarrhea or constipation, respiratory infections, peripheral neuropathy, hepatotoxicity, infusion-related reactions, second primary malignancies

References
Chabner BA, Longo, DL, ed. *Cancer Chemotherapy and Biotherapy.* 5th ed. Philadelphia: Lippincott Williams & Wilkins; 2011.
DeVita VT Jr, Lawrence TS, Rosenberg SA, ed. *Cancer: Principles and Practices of Oncology.* 9th ed. Philadelphia: Lippincott Williams & Wilkins; 2011.
Fischer DS, Durivage HJ, Knobf MT et al., eds. *Cancer Chemotherapy Handbook*. Norwalk, CT: Appleton & Lange; 1994.
Lexi-Comp, Inc. Lexi-Comp Clinical Reference Library. www.lexi.com
Shord SS, Cordes LM. Cancer treatment and chemotherapy. In: DiPiro JT, et al., eds. *Pharmacotherapy: A Pathophysiologic Approach.* 10th ed. New York: McGraw-Hill; 2016.
Tecentriq® (atezolizumab) injection prescribing information. South San Francisco, CA: Genentech, Inc.
Bavencio® (avelumab) injection prescribing information. Rockland, MA: EMD Serono, Inc.
Blincyto® (blinatumomab) injection prescribing information. Thousand Oaks, CA: Amgen Inc.

DRUG FACTS: Tyrosine kinase inhibitors (TKIs)

CLASS	DRUG	INDICATION	MECHANISM OF ACTION	MAJOR SIDE EFFECTS
Anaplastic lymphoma kinase (ALK) inhibitors	Alectinib (Alecensaro)	Non–small cell lung cancer (NSCLC)	Inhibits ALK phosphorylation and ALK-mediated activation of downstream signaling and expression, resulting in decreased cellular proliferation and survival in tumors	Bradycardia, edema, rash, hyperglycemia, electrolyte abnormalities, hepatotoxicity, myalgia, interstitial lung disease (ILD), photosensitivity, renal toxicity
	Ceritinib (Zykadia)		Inhibits ALK phosphorylation and ALK-mediated activation of downstream signaling and expression, resulting in decreased cellular proliferation and survival in tumors; also inhibits insulin-like growth factor 1 receptor (IGF-1R), insulin receptor, and ROS1	Gastrointestinal toxicity, increases in liver enzymes, fatigue, visual disturbances, QT prolongation, bradycardia, hyperglycemia
	Crizotinib (Xalkori®)		Inhibits ALK phosphorylation and ALK-mediated activation of downstream signaling and expression, resulting in decreased cellular proliferation and survival in tumors	Nausea & vomiting (n/v), diarrhea, constipation, fatigue, increases in liver enzymes, visual disorders, edema, ILD, QT prolongation, bradycardia
BCR-ABL inhibitors	Bosutinib (Bosulif®)	Philadelphia chromosome-positive (Ph+) chronic myelogenous leukemia (CML)	Binds site on the BCR-ABL tyrosine kinase ATP-binding domain; inhibits SRC kinases	n/v, edema, pleural effusions & ascites, myelosuppression, congestive heart failure (CHF), arthralgias, rash, diarrhea, increased liver enzymes, hypophosphatemia

	Dasatinib (Sprycel®)	Ph+ CML, Ph+ acute lymphocytic leukemia (ALL)	Binds site on the BCR-ABL tyrosine kinase ATP-binding domain; inhibits SRC kinases	Edema, n/v, pleural effusions & ascites, myelosuppression, CHF, arthralgias, fatigue, rash, diarrhea, increased liver enzymes, QT prolongation, hypophosphatemia & hypocalcemia
	Imatinib mesylate (Gleevec®)	Ph+ CML	Binds site on the BCR-ABL tyrosine kinase ATP-binding domain	Edema, n/v, pleural effusions & ascites, myelosuppression, CHF, arthralgias, rash, diarrhea, increased liver enzymes, hypophosphatemia
	Nilotinib (Tasigna®)	Ph+ CML	Binds site on the BCR-ABL tyrosine kinase ATP-binding domain	Edema, n/v, myelosuppression, increased lipase, hyperglycemia, arthralgias, rash, diarrhea, increased liver enzymes, QT prolongation
	Ponatinib (Iclusig®)	Ph+ CML, Ph+ ALL	Binds site on the BCR-ABL tyrosine kinase ATP-binding domain; inhibits mutated (T315I) BCR-ABL; also inhibits vascular endothelial growth factor (VEGF) and platelet-derived growth factor (PDGF), the SRC families of kinases, and c-KIT and FMS-like tyrosine kinase 3 (FLT3)	Myelosuppression, hypertension, rash, abdominal pain, fatigue, headache, dry skin, constipation, arthralgia, nausea, pyrexia, thromboembolic events, hepatotoxicity, CHF, pancreatitis, hemorrhage (secondary to thrombocytopenia), fluid retention
BRAF inhibitors	Dabrafenib (Tafinlar®)	BRAF-V600E-mutated melanoma, NSCLC	Selectively inhibits some mutated forms of the protein kinase B-raf (BRAF); through BRAF inhibition, inhibits tumor cell growth	Papilloma, arthralgia, alopecia, fatigue, headache, palmar-plantar erythrodysesthesia (also called hand-foot syndrome [HFS]), pyrexia

(continued on following page)

DRUG FACTS: Tyrosine kinase inhibitors (TKIs)

(continued from previous page)	Vemurafenib (Zelboraf)	BRAF-V600E-mutated melanoma	Inhibits tumor growth by inhibiting kinase activity of mutated forms of BRAF, including BRAF with V600E mutation, blocking cellular prolifera-tion of tumor cells with the mutation	Papilloma, arthralgia, alopecia, fatigue, headache, photosensitivity reaction, hypersensitivity reactions, QT prolongation
Bruton's tyrosine kinase (BTK) inhibitors	Acalabrutinib (Calquence)	Mantle cell lymphoma (MCL)	Covalently and irreversibly cysteine residue in the active BTK site to inhibit BTK enzyme activity, resulting in decreased malignant B cell prolifera-tion and survival	Diarrhea, neutropenia, myalgias, headache, fatigue, hemorrhage, sec-ondary malignancies, atrial fibrillation & flutter
	Ibrutinib (Imbruvica®)	MCL, CLL	Irreversible inhibitor of BTK	Diarrhea, fatigue, musculoskeletal pain, nausea, rash, atrial fibrillation, hemorrhage, tumor lysis syndrome, bone marrow suppression
Epidermal growth factor receptor (EGFR) inhibitors	Afatinib (Giotrif)	EGFR mutation+ NSCLC	Covalently and irreversibly binds to the intracellular tyrosine kinase domain, resulting in tumor growth inhibition and tumor regression	Acneiform eruption, skin rash, diar-rhea, stomatitis, hepatotoxicity, renal failure, ILD
	Erlotinib (Tarceva®)	EGFR mutation+ NSCLC, pancreatic	Inhibits intracellular phosphorylation of several tyrosine kinases associated with transmembrane cell surface receptors, including those associated with the EGFR; this may decrease the growth, invasion, metastasis, angio-genesis, and resistance to apoptosis of tumor cells	Rash, diarrhea, ILD, hepatic & renal failure

	Gefitinib (Iressa®)	EGFR mutation+ NSCLC	Inhibits intracellular phosphorylation of several tyrosine kinases associated with transmembrane cell surface receptors, including those associated with the EGFR; this may decrease the growth, invasion, metastasis, angiogenesis, and resistance to apoptosis of tumor cells	Rash, diarrhea, ILD, hepatic & renal failure
	Osimertinib (Tagrisso)	EGFR mutation+ NSCLC	Irreversible EGFR TKI that binds to select mutant forms of EGFR, including T790M, L858R, and exon 19 deletion at lower concentrations than wild-type	Gastrointestinal toxicity, dermatologic toxicity, ILD/pneumonitis, pneumonia, pulmonary embolism, cardiomyopathy, QT prolongation
FLT3 inhibitors	Midostaurin (Rydapt)	Acute myeloid leukemia, mast cell leukemia	Inhibits FLT3 receptor signaling and cell proliferation and induces apoptosis in internal tandem duplication (ITD)– and tyrosine-kinase domain (TKD)–mutant expressing leukemic cells, as well as in cells overexpressing wild-type FLT3 and PDGF receptor (PDGFR); also inhibits other receptors, such as wild-type FLT3, FLT3 mutant kinases ITD and TKD, and KIT, and may inhibit KIT signaling, cell proliferation, histamine release and induce apoptosis in mast cells	Myelosuppression, nausea, vomiting, diarrhea, abdominal pain, hypersensitivity reaction, ILD, pneumonitis

(continued on following page)

DRUG FACTS: Tyrosine kinase inhibitors (TKIs)

(continued from previous page)				
Human epidermal growth factor receptor (HER)–2 inhibitor	Lapatinib (Tykerb®)	Breast	Inhibits EGFR (ErbB1) and HER2 (ErbB2) by reversibly binding to tyrosine kinase, blocking phosphorylation and activation of downstream second messengers (Erk1/2 and AKT), regulating cellular proliferation and survival in ErbB- and ErbB2-expressing tumors	Diarrhea, rash, nausea, vomiting, fatigue, decreases in left ventricular ejection fraction, hepatotoxicity, QT prolongation, ILD
Mitogen-activated extracellular kinase (MEK) inhibitor	Trametinib (Mekinist®)	Melanoma, NSCLC	Reversibly and selectively inhibits MEK1 and -2 activation and kinase activity; MEK is a downstream effector of the protein kinase BRAF	Neutropenia, cardiac toxicity, dermatologic toxicity, fever, colitis, GI perforation, hemorrhage, hepatotoxicity, hyperglycemia, primary cutaneous malignancies, ocular toxicity, ILD/pneumonitis **PEARL:** Obtain baseline TTE for evaluation of potential cardiac toxicity at baseline, 1 month after initiation of treatment, and every 2–3 months thereafter
Multi-kinase inhibitors	Brigatinib (Alunbrig)	NSCLC	Broad-spectrum multi-kinase inhibitor with activity against ALK, ROS1, insulin-like growth factor-1 receptor (IGF-1R), and FLT3, as well as EGF receptor deletion and point mutations	Hypertension, creatine phosphokinase elevation, pancreatic enzyme elevations, GI toxicity, hyperglycemia, visual disturbances, ILD, pneumonitis

Cabozantinib (Cometriq®)	Renal cell carcinoma (RCC), thyroid	Small-molecule inhibitor of numerous receptor kinases, most importantly the rearranged during transfection receptor (RET), VEGF receptor (VEGFR)–2, and MET membrane receptor	Diarrhea, stomatitis, HFS, decreased weight, decreased appetite, nausea, fatigue, oral pain, hair color changes, dysgeusia, hypertension, abdominal pain, constipation, increased liver enzymes, proteinuria, lymphopenia, neutropenia, thrombocytopenia, hypocalcemia, hypophosphatemia, GI perforations & fistulas
Lenvatinib (Lenvima)	RCC, thyroid	Multitargeted TKI of VEGF receptors VEGFR1 (FLT1), VEGFR2 (KDR), and VEGFR3 (FLT4); fibroblast growth factor (FGF) receptors FGFR1, 2, 3, & 4; PDGFRα; KIT; and RET—inhibition of these receptor tyrosine kinases leads to decreased tumor growth and slowing of cancer progression	Cardiac toxicity, hypertension, hypothyroidism, GI perforation & fistula, nausea, vomiting, diarrhea, hemorrhage, hepatotoxicity, hypocalcemia, HFS, proteinuria, thromboembolic events
Neratinib (Nerlynx)	Breast	Irreversible inhibitor of HER1, HER2, HER4, and EGF receptor, which reduces autophosphorylation and downstream MAPK and AKT signaling pathways	Severe diarrhea, hepatotoxicity, fatigue, rash, nausea, vomiting, abdominal pain
Pazopanib (Votrient®)	RCC, sarcoma	Inhibitor of multiple receptor tyrosine kinases, including PDGFR, VEGFR, C-KIT, interleukin-2 receptor inducible T cell kinase, leukocyte-specific protein tyrosine kinase, and transmembrane glycoprotein receptor tyrosine kinase	Diarrhea, hypertension, hair/skin hypopigmentation, nausea, anorexia, vomiting, decreased weight, fatigue, musculoskeletal pain, dysgeusia, dyspnea, hypothyroidism, proteinuria, fatal hepatotoxicity, thromboembolic events

(continued on following page)

DRUG FACTS: Tyrosine kinase inhibitors (TKIs)

(continued from previous page)	Regorafenib (Stivarga®)	CRC, gastrointestinal stromal tumor (GIST), hepatocellular carcinoma (HCC)	Inhibitor of multiple receptor tyrosine kinases, including those involved in the regulation of tumor angiogenesis (VEGFR-1, 2, and 3), oncogenes and downstream targets (c-KIT, RET, RAF1, and BRAF), as well as PDGFR and FGFR	Asthenia, fatigue, decreased appetite, HFS, diarrhea, mucositis, weight loss, infection, hypertension, dysphonia, hepatotoxicity, hemorrhage
	Sorafenib (Nexavar®)	HCC, RCC, thyroid	Inhibitor of multiple receptor tyrosine kinases, including PDGFR, VEGFR, stem cell factor receptor, and kinases in the RAF/MEK pathway	Diarrhea, rash, HFS, fatigue, hypertension, prolonged QT interval, cardiac events (including myocardial infarction), drug-induced hepatitis
	Sunitinib malate (Sutent®)	GIST, pancreatic neuroendocrine tumor, RCC	Inhibitor of multiple receptor tyrosine kinases, including PDGFR, VEGFR, stem cell factor, and others involved in tumor growth and metastasis	Diarrhea, rash, bleeding, CHF & cardiac effects, QT prolongation, fatigue, hypertension, hepatotoxicity, thyroid dysfunction
	Vandetanib (Caprelsa®)	Thyroid	Inhibitor of VEGFR, EGFR, and RET tyrosine kinases; through inhibition of MEK 1 and 2 kinase activity causes decreased cellular proliferation, cell cycle arrest, and increased apoptosis	Diarrhea, rash, acne, nausea, hypertension, headache, fatigue, upper respiratory tract infections, decreased appetite, abdominal pain, prolonged QT interval, torsades de pointes & sudden death, ILD, hemorrhage, increased liver enzymes

VEGF inhibitor	Axitinib (Inlyta®)	RCC	Selectively inhibits VEGFR-1, -2, and -3, blocking angiogenesis and tumor growth	Diarrhea, rash, HFRS, bleeding, thrombotic events, hypertension, hepatotoxicity, hypothyroidism, proteinuria, GI perforation, fatigue, rare reports of progressive multifocal leukoencephalopathy
MISCELLANEOUS TARGETED AGENTS				
Proteasome inhibitors	Bortezomib (Velcade®)	Multiple myeloma, MCL	Inhibits proteasome enzyme complexes, which regulate protein homeostasis within the cell; reversibly inhibits chymotrypsin-like activity at the 26S proteasome, leading to activation of signaling cascades, cell-cycle arrest, and apoptosis	Fatigue or malaise, nausea, diarrhea, anorexia, constipation, vomiting, myelosuppression (especially thrombocytopenia), hyponatremia, hypokalemia, cumulative & dose-related peripheral neuropathy, fever
	Carfilzomib (Kyprolis®)	Multiple myeloma	Inhibits proteasomes, which are responsible for intracellular protein homeostasis; a potent, selective, and irreversible inhibitor of chymotrypsin-like activity of the 20S proteasome, leading to cell-cycle arrest and apoptosis	Fatigue, anemia, thrombocytopenia, nausea, diarrhea, dyspnea, pyrexia, infusion-related reactions, rare reports of cardiac arrest, CHF, & myocardial infarction

References

Chabner BA, Longo DL, eds. *Cancer Chemotherapy and Biotherapy.* 5th ed. Philadelphia: Lippincott Williams & Wilkins; 2011.

DeVita VT Jr, Lawrence TS, Rosenberg SA, eds. *Cancer: Principles and Practices of Oncology.* 9th ed. Philadelphia: Lippincott Williams & Wilkins; 2011.

Fischer DS, Durivage HJ, Knobf MT et al., eds. *Cancer Chemotherapy Handbook.* Norwalk, CT: Appleton & Lange; 1994.

Lexi-Comp, Inc. Lexi-Comp Clinical Reference Library. Available at: http://www.lexi.com

Shord SS, Cordes LM. Cancer treatment and chemotherapy. In: DiPiro JT, et al., eds. *Pharmacotherapy: A Pathophysiologic Approach.* 10th ed. New York: McGraw-Hill; 2016.

Gilotrif® (afatinib) tablets prescribing information. Ridgefield, CT: Boehringer Ingelheim Pharmaceuticals, Inc.

DRUG FACTS: Hormonal agents for cancer treatment

CLASS	DRUG	INDICATION	MECHANISM OF ACTION	MAJOR SIDE EFFECTS
Antiestrogens	Tamoxifen citrate (Soltamox®)	Breast, endometrial	Inhibit nuclear binding of the estrogen receptor, blocking estrogen stimulation of cancer cells and inhibiting DNA synthesis	Hot flashes, nausea & vomiting (n/v), vaginal bleeding, decreased bone mineral density, weakness, arthralgia, menstrual irregularities, hepatotoxicity, mood changes, depression, increased risk of uterine or endometrial cancer, thromboembolic events
Aromatase inhibitors	Anastrozole (Arimidex®)	Breast, endometrial, uterine, ovarian	Selective nonsteroidal aromatase inhibitor that prevents the conversion of androstenedione to estrone, and testosterone to estradiol; this decreases mass and growth in tumors responsive to hormones	Decreased bone mineral density, hypercholesterolemia, gastrointestinal distress, hot flashes, thromboembolic events, edema
	Exemestane (Aromasin®)	Breast	Steroidal aromatase inhibitor that irreversibly blocks the active site of the aromatase enzyme, preventing conversion of androgens to estrogens	Decreased bone mineral density, gastrointestinal distress, hot flashes, thromboembolic events, edema, fatigue, hyperhidrosis, lymphedema, arthralgia, myalgia
	Letrozole (Femara®)	Breast	Nonsteroidal competitive inhibitor of the aromatase enzyme, leading to significant reduction in plasma estrogen without changing corticosteroid synthesis	Decreased bone mineral density, hypercholesterolemia, headache, nausea, hot flashes, diaphoresis, thromboembolic events, edema, fatigue, weakness, arthralgia, myalgia

Antiandrogens	Bicalutamide (Casodex®)	Prostate	Nonsteroidal androgen receptor inhibitor that competes with dihydrotestosterone and testosterone binding, preventing testosterone stimulation of tumor cell growth	Gynecomastia, hot flashes, hepatotoxicity, n/v, diarrhea, pain, anemia, tumor flare
	Flutamide (Eulexin®)	Prostate	Nonsteroidal antiandrogens that competitively inhibit the binding of androgens to the peripheral receptors	Gynecomastia, hot flashes, galactorrhea, decreased libido, impotence, hepatotoxicity, vomiting, diarrhea, tumor flare
	Nilutamide (Nilandron®)	Prostate	Nonsteroidal antiandrogens that competitively inhibit the binding of androgens to the receptor	Gynecomastia, hot flashes, hepatotoxicity, interstitial pneumonitis, n/v, diarrhea, anemia, tumor flare, vision disturbances
LH-RH analogs and antagonists	Degarelix (Firmagon®)	Prostate	Gonadotropin-releasing hormone (GnRH) antagonist reversibly blocks GnRH receptors located on the anterior pituitary gland decreasing secretion of luteinizing hormone (LH) and follicle stimulation hormone (FSH), decreasing testosterone production; *tumor flare is not experienced*	Hot flashes, erectile dysfunction, gastrointestinal disturbances, injection site reactions, gynecomastia, anemia, decreased bone marrow density, increased serum transaminases
	Goserelin (Zoladex®)	Prostate	GnRH analog that competes for binding to the hypothalamus causing an initial surge in release of LH and FSH followed by down-regulation of the receptor through a negative feedback loop	Decreased bone mineral density, hot flashes, hypercalcemia, hyperglycemia, peripheral edema, headache, emotional lability, depression, acne vulgaris, injection site reactions, vaginitis, peripheral edema, tumor flare, gynecomastia

(continued on following page)

DRUG FACTS: Hormonal agents for cancer treatment

(continued from previous page)				
	Leuprolide (Lupron®)	Prostate	GnRH analog that competes for binding to the hypothalamus causing an initial surge in release of LH and FSH followed by down-regulation of the receptor through a negative feedback loop	Cardiovascular toxicity, decreased bone mineral density, hyperglycemia, emotional lability, injection site reactions, tumor flare
Other hormonal agents	Abiraterone acetate (Zytiga®)	Prostate	Selectively and irreversibly inhibits CYP17 blocking the enzymatic formation of androgens in testicular, adrenal, and prostatic tumor tissues, thereby lowering testosterone concentrations to castrate levels	Adrenocortical insufficiency, diarrhea, dyspepsia, edema, hepatotoxicity, hypertriglyceridemia, hyperglycemia, hypokalemia, hot flashes, hypertension, joint swelling, mineralocorticoid excess, myalgias, upper respiratory tract infection, urinary tract infection
	Enzalutamide (Xtandi®)	Prostate	Androgen receptor signaling inhibitor that inhibits nuclear translocation of the androgen receptor, DNA binding, and co-activator recruitment	Arthralgia and muscle pain, weakness, hot flashes, peripheral edema, hypertension, upper respiratory tract infection, headache, dizziness, spinal cord compression, hematuria, hypertension, gastrointestinal disturbances

	Estramustine (Emcyt®)	Prostate	Estradiol and nornitrogen mustard carbamate-linked combination exhibits antiandrogen effects (due to estradiol) and antimicrotubule effects (due to nornitrogen mustard), which results in a decrease in plasma testosterone and an increase in estrogen levels	Edema, n/v, cardiovascular toxicity, thromboembolic events, gynecomastia, impotence, hepatotoxicity, impaired glucose tolerance
Reference: UpToDate. Available at: https://www.uptodate.com.				

DRUG FACTS: FDA-approved checkpoint inhibitors

DRUG (US COMMERCIAL NAME)	TARGET	INDICATIONS AND DOSE
Ipilimumab (Yervoy®)	CTLA-4	• Metastatic melanoma: 3 mg/kg every 3 weeks for 4 doses alone or in combination with nivolumab • Adjuvant therapy in stage III melanoma: 10 mg/kg every 3 weeks for 4 doses, then every 12 weeks for up to 3 years
Nivolumab (Opdivo®)	PD-1	• Metastatic progressive non–small cell lung cancer: 240 mg every 2 weeks • Recurrent or metastatic head and neck squamous cell carcinoma: 3 mg/kg every 2 weeks • Metastatic or unresectable melanoma: 240 mg every 2 weeks when used alone • 1 mg/kg every 3 weeks for 4 doses in combination with ipilimumab, then 240 mg every 2 weeks alone • Relapsed or progressive classic Hodgkin lymphoma: 3 mg/kg every 2 weeks • Advanced recurring or progressive renal cell carcinoma: 240 mg every 2 weeks • Advanced recurring or progressive urothelial carcinoma: 240 mg every 2 weeks • Metastatic recurring or progressive colorectal cancer with microsatellite instability (MSI) or mismatch repair deficiency: 240 mg every 2 weeks • Progressive hepatocellular carcinoma: 240 mg every 2 weeks
Pembrolizumab (Keytruda®)	PD-1	• Metastatic progressive non–small cell lung cancer (PD-L1 ≥1%): 200 mg every 3 weeks • Metastatic non–small cell lung cancer first-line therapy (PD-L1≥50%): 200 mg every 3 weeks • Metastatic non-squamous non–small cell lung cancer first-line therapy: 200 mg every 3 weeks in combination with carboplatin/pemetrexed for 4 cycles, then pemetrexed/pembrolizumab maintenance • Recurrent or metastatic head and neck squamous cell carcinoma: 200 mg every 3 weeks • Recurring or progressive classical Hodgkin lymphoma: 200 mg every 3 weeks • Unresectable or metastatic melanoma: 200 mg every 3 weeks • Metastatic recurring or progressive colorectal cancer with microsatellite instability (MSI) or mismatch repair deficient: 200 mg every 3 weeks • Advanced recurring or cisplatin-ineligible urothelial carcinoma: 200 mg every 3 weeks • Advanced recurring gastric or gastroesophageal (GE) junction carcinoma with PD-L1 ≥1%: 200 mg every 3 weeks

Atezolizumab (Tecentriq®)	PD-L1	• Metastatic progressive non–small cell lung cancer: 1200 mg every 3 weeks • Advanced recurring or cisplatin-ineligible urothelial carcinoma: 1200 mg every 3 weeks
Avelumab (Bavencio®)	PD-L1	• Advanced recurring urothelial carcinoma: 10 mg/kg every 2 weeks • Metastatic Merkel cell carcinoma: 10 mg/kg every 2 weeks
Durvalumab (Imfinzi®)	PD-L1	• Advanced recurring urothelial carcinoma: 10 mg/kg every 2 weeks

DRUG FACTS: Immune-related adverse events (irAEs) associated with the use of checkpoint inhibitors

TYPE OF TOXICITY	MANIFESTATIONS	MANAGEMENT	COMMENTS
Mucocutaneous	Rash, pruritus, dry mouth, vitiligo, Stevens-Johnson syndrome (severe but very rare)	• Topical steroids, oral antihistamine • Severe cases may require systemic steroids, immunosuppression, and treatment discontinuation	Most common irAE

Colonic	Diarrhea, colitis (abdominal pain, distension, nausea, vomiting)	• Grade 1: symptomatic management, close monitoring for worsening
		• Grade 2: withhold treatment until toxicity is grade ≤1, oral corticosteroid if no improvement
		• Grade 3 or 4:
		  • Hospitalization
		  • Discontinue treatment
		  • Initiate high-dose corticosteroids
		  • Antibiotics coverage
		  • Consult GI
		  • Taper off steroid once toxicity is downgraded to grade ≤1
		  • If corticosteroid refractory, give immunosuppressive agents (eg, infliximab or mycophenolate)
			Rule out infectious etiology

Hepatic	Elevated AST and ALT, rarely elevated bilirubin, jaundice, fever	• Same as above • Avoid infliximab due to its hepatotoxicity	Rule out other etiologies (eg, viral, alcohol, other medications)
Pulmonary	Cough, dyspnea, radiological infiltrates	Same as above	Rare but can be serious; rule out other etiologies (eg, lymphangitic, carcinomatosis, infectious)

Endocrinologic	Hypothyroidism (nonspecific), hyperthyroidism, hypophysitis (fatigue, headache, inflammation changes on MRI), adrenal insufficiency (dehydration, hypotension, electro-lytes abnormalities), type 1 diabetes	• Hormone replacement if necessary • Endocrine consultation • High-dose corticosteroid • Treatment discontinuation in severe cases	The most common primary endocrinopathy is hypothy-roidism; TSH is usually elevated, unlike hypothyroidism secondary to hypophysitis, when TSH is low
Others	Neurologic, pancreatic, cardiac, ocular, renal, rheumatologic	Per protocol	

References
UpToDate. Available at: https://www.uptodate.com/home.
Risk evaluation and mitigation strategy (REMS). Available at: https://www.fda.gov/downloads/Drugs/DrugSafety/PostMarketDrugsafetyInformationforPatientsand-Providers/UCM249435.pdf.

This table is not comprehensive, but describes the pertinent immune-related toxicities associated with checkpoint inhibitors. The management of immune-related adverse events is detailed in general guidelines.
ALT, alanine transaminase; AST, aspartate transaminase; TSH, thyroid-stimulating hormone.

CHAPTER 2

Basics of Oncology and Pathology

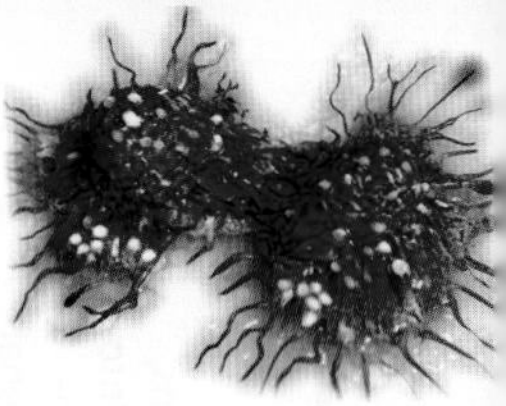

What are the different treatment modalities in radiation therapy?

Key concept	Radiation therapy techniques have evolved for more than a century. At present, the majority of patients are treated with teletherapy (ie, external radiation). Teletherapy treatment modalities include electromagnetic radiation (ie, X-rays and gamma rays) and particulate radiation (electrons, protons, neutrons, and heavy ions). Brachytherapy involves implantation of radioactive sources into the tumor tissues, on either a temporary or a permanent basis. Dose escalation and hypofractionation can benefit patients with radiation-resistant tumor types, including sarcoma, melanoma, renal cell carcinoma, and colorectal metastases.[1]
Clinical scenario	A 54-year-old woman is diagnosed with inoperable FIGO stage IIIB squamous cell carcinoma of the uterine cervix on the basis of pelvic wall involvement. As per NCCN[2] guidelines, she is dispositioned for cisplatin-based chemoradiation with curative intent.
Action items	• Radiation treatment planning and delivery: Optimal radiation therapy for cervical carcinoma involves both teletherapy and brachytherapy components, with the brachytherapy component being essential for optimal cure rates, as this modality allows for dose escalation to the tumor while minimizing the dose to adjacent healthy structures[1] • A customized treatment plan is developed that includes intensity-modulated radiation therapy (IMRT) to the pelvis followed by multisession intracavitary brachytherapy to the cervical tumor[1]
Discussion	Owing to advances in computational delivery, and in parallel to the development of sophisticated 3-dimensional volumetric imaging (including CT, PET, and MRI), radiation therapy has quickly evolved from 2-dimensional treatment planning to 3- and 4-dimensional delivery over the past 2 decades.[1]

	At present, dose delivery is tailored to the 3-dimensional volume of the tumor. The most sophisticated techniques use inverse planning methods, whereby dose delivery is optimized through computer-generated fluence maps.[1] IMRT remains the most common treatment modality for advanced teletherapy delivery. Particulate delivery with protons and heavy ions is also being evaluated, with physical advantages noted for certain specific applications (including pediatric brain tumors and chordomas at the base of the skull), owing to specific energy deposition differences in those modalities. The use of proton therapy for other tumor sites is under investigation.[1]
Pearls	A number of sophisticated radiation treatment modalities allow for increasing treatment options for treatment of multiple disease sites.
References	1. National Comprehensive Cancer Network (NCCN) guidelines. Version 2.2017. Available at: www.nccn.org. 2. Halperin EC, Brady LW, Perez CA, et al. *Perez and Brady's Principles and Practice of Radiation Oncology*. 6th ed. Philadelphia: Lippincott Williams & Wilkins; 2013.

What is the clinical scope and management for brain metastases?

Key concept	Brain metastases are common sequelae of solid tumors (lung, breast, melanoma, renal, and colorectal). Lung cancer has the highest number of brain metastases; however, melanoma has the highest propensity to metastasize to brain. Although their exact incidence is unknown, about 8%–10% of patients with cancer will manifest brain metastasis, with an expected growing incidence as a function of increased life expectancy.[1,2] Management is primarily local, owing to limited penetration of most systemic agents through the blood-brain barrier. The historical standard of care (whole-brain radiation therapy [WBRT]) is being rapidly replaced by focal techniques such as stereotactic radiosurgery (SRS) and surgical resection, alone or in combination.[1,3]
Clinical scenario	A 48-year-old woman with a history of stage 2 triple-negative (ER– PR– Her-2-Neu–) breast cancer treated 3 years prior presents with headache and seizure. Imaging demonstrates a solitary 2-cm lesion in the left motor cortex.

Action items	• Assess prognosis; although the historical expected survival duration for patients with brain metastases is <1 year, at present multiple factors are used to assess prognosis, including
	  • the extent of intracranial disease (number and volume of metastases)
	  • the extent of extracranial disease (primary site control and/or presence of extracranial metastases)
	  • histology and radiosensitivity
	  • performance status[1,3]
	• A customized treatment plan should be tailored for each patient based on the above factors and should be discussed in a multidisciplinary team including medical oncology, radiation oncology, and neurosurgery[1,3]

Discussion	SRS offers a convenient method for the treatment of brain metastases that differs from traditional fractionated WBRT in both scope and adverse-effect profile. Published studies describe local control rates ranging from 70% to 90% for brain tumors smaller than 2 cm, dependent on histology. The control rates are lower for larger lesions, and sometimes a decision is made to combine surgery with SRS for such tumors.[1,3] SRS is preferred to WBRT due to comparable long-term overall survival,[3] as well to decreased neurocognitive decline. Studies, including the most recent North Central Cancer Treatment Group N0574 trial, have demonstrated a decline in cognitive function in patients who received WBRT and SRS versus SRS alone.[4] A recently published meta-analysis denoted decreased overall survival for patients receiving WBRT versus SRS alone, presumably due to neurocognitive dysfunction.[5] Trials are being performed to determine the maximum number of lesions that can safely be treated with SRS. At present, the number is typically 4, but recent series have described a favorable safety profile in treating up to 10 brain metastases.[6]
Pearls	• SRS is an emerging option for the treatment of brain metastases • Palliative WBRT remains the standard of care for widely disseminated central nervous system disease, leptomeningeal disease, or poor performance status[1,3]
References	1. National Comprehensive Cancer Network (NCCN) guidelines for central nervous system cancers. Version 1.2017. Available at: https://www.nccn.org. 2. Barnholtz-Sloan JS, Sloan AE, Davis FG, et al. Incidence proportions of brain metastases in patients diagnosed (1973 to 2001) in the Metropolitan Detroit Cancer Surveillance System. J Clin Oncol 2004;22(14):2865-72. 3. Lin X, DeAnglis LM. Treatment of brain metastases. J Clin Oncol 2015;33(30):3475-84. 4. Badiyan SN, Regine WF, Mehta M. Stereotactic radiosurgery for treatment of brain metastases. J Oncol Pract 2016;12(8):703-12. 5. Sahgal R, Aoyama H, Kocher M, et al. Phase 3 trials of stereotactic radiosurgery with or without whole-brain radiation therapy for 1 to 4 brain metastases: individual patient data meta-analysis. Int J Radiat Oncol Biol Phys 2015;91(4):710-7. 6. Li J, Brown PD. The diminishing role of whole-brain radiation therapy in the treatment of brain metastases. JAMA Oncol 2017;3(8):1023-4.

What malignancies are associated with infectious etiology? Are there any preventative measures for these malignancies?

Key concept	There are multiple cancers that are linked to infectious etiology, including viruses and bacteria.[1] There are 3 FDA-approved human papillomavirus (HPV) vaccinations—Gardasil, Gardasil 9, and Cervarix—that prevent infections with high-risk HPV types 16 and 18, which causes about 70% of cervical cancers and other HPV-related malignancies.[2,3] Extranodal marginal zone lymphoma of mucosa-associated lymphoid tissue (MALT lymphoma), if localized, can be treated with primary antibiotic therapy directed at *Helicobacter pylori* infection.[4]
Clinical scenario	A 27-year-old woman is visiting her obstetrician-gynecologist for her well-woman examination, and she asks for more information about HPV and cervical cancer. She asks whether she is a candidate for vaccination.

TYPE OF CANCER	INFECTIOUS ETIOLOGY	PATHOGENESIS
Gastric adenocarcinoma	*Helicobacter pylori*	• Pathways involving cellular inflammatory response to *H. pylori* and the role of cytotoxin-associated gene A protein in carcinogenesis • Chronic gastritis occurs from chronic *H. pylori* infection leading to lymphocytic response in the stomach[4]

• Anal cancer • Cervical cancer • Oropharyngeal cancer • Less common: penile, vulvar, and vaginal	Human papillomavirus (HPV) • Most commonly HPV type 16 and 18	Expression of viral oncogenes E6 and E7 interact with p53 and retinoblastoma, which immortalizes epithelial cells[5]

Extranodal MALT lymphoma	*H. pylori*	• Similar pathogenesis as above in gastric adenocarcinoma:
		  • Chronic gastritis occurs from chronic *H. pylori* infection leading to lymphocytic response in the stomach
		  • This subsequently leads to continued antigenic stimulation and ultimately neoplastic transformation[4]

(continued on following page)

(continued from previous page)

• Nasopharyngeal carcinoma • Hodgkin lymphoma • Non-Hodgkin lymphoma (eg, Burkitt lymphoma, diffuse-large B cell lymphoma)	Epstein–Barr virus (EBV)	EBV infection leads to chromosomal abnormalities and gene alterations[6]
Hepatocellular carcinoma	• Hepatitis B virus (HBV) • Hepatitis C virus (HCV)	Due to HBV or HCV infection, oncoproteins lead to carcinogenesis and subsequent hepatocyte transformation
Kaposi sarcoma	Kaposi sarcoma herpes virus (KSHV or HHV8)	Due to HHV8 infection, oncoproteins lead to carcinogenesis with broad tropism to variety of cell types, including B cells, endothelial cells, macrophages, and epithelial cells
Peripheral T cell lymphoma	• Human T cell lymphotropic virus, type-1 (HTLV-1) • EBV	

Pearls	Based on randomized controlled trials, HPV vaccinations[#] are effective in reduction of HPV-related disease incidence and can be considered in patients aged 9–26[2,3] *H. pylori* eradication therapy is the standard treatment for MALT
References	1. Chen C-J, Hsu W-L, Yang H-I, et al. Epidemiology of virus infection and human cancer. In: Chang M, Jeang KT, eds. *Viruses and Human Cancer. Recent Results in Cancer Research,* vol. 193. Berlin: Springer; 2014:11-32. 2. National Cancer Institute. Human papillomavirus (HPV) vaccines. Available at: https://www.cancer.gov/about-cancer/causes-prevention/risk/infectious-agents/hpv-vaccine-fact-sheet. 3. Saslow D, Andrews KS, Manassaram-Baptiste D, et al. Human papillomavirus vaccination guideline update: American Cancer Society guideline endorsement. CA Cancer J Clin 2016;66(5):375-85. 4. Thieblemont C, Zucca E. Clinical aspects and therapy of gastrointestinal MALT lymphoma. Best Pract Res Clin Haematol 2017;30(1-2):109-17. 5. Hausen HZ. Papillomaviruses causing cancer: evasion from host-cell control in early events in carcinogenesis. J Natl Cancer Inst 2000;92(9):690-8. 6. Lo KW, Chung GTY, To KF. Deciphering the molecular genetic basis of NPC through molecular, cytogenetic, and epigenetic approaches. Semin Cancer Biol 2012;22(2):79-86.

[#]Vaccination recommendations vary due to new vaccine formulations: Gardasil (HPV types 6, 11, 16, 18) is recommended in children and adults 9–26 years old. Gardasil 9 (HPV types 6, 11, 16, 18, 31, 33, 45, 52, and 58) is recommended in girls and women 9–26 years old and boys 9–15 years old. Cervarix (HPV types 16 and 18) is recommended in girls and women 9–25 years old.

What are the features of a normal peripheral blood smear?

Key concept	A peripheral blood smear can be a valuable tool in reaching a diagnosis or excluding potential diagnoses prior to the availability of results from advanced testing. In fact, a review of the peripheral blood smear can guide further testing and potentially eliminate the need for costly testing.
Clinical scenario	A 54-year-old woman presents to her primary care physician for a routine evaluation and reports fatigue. A complete blood count is performed and a peripheral blood smear obtained.
Action items	• Blood samples are collected from a peripheral vein into an EDTA-containing tube • A drop of blood is placed on the slide and smeared across the slide with an inclined spreader, optimally within 2 hours of collection • The smear is then air dried, fixed with alcohol, and stained • Each smear contains a head, a tail (or feathered edge), and a body • Initial examination should begin at the body of the smear and progress systematically • Findings can be readily reported; however, the interpretation of these findings should take into account the clinical context[1]

Discussion

Figure 2-1 shows an example of a normal blood smear.

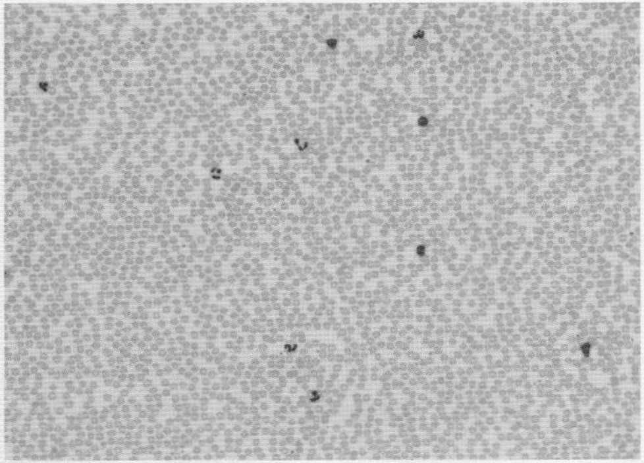

Figure 2-1. Normal peripheral blood smear. (Reproduced with permission from Lei Chen, MD and Hanadi El Achi, MD.)

Normal blood smear elements have the following features:

Red blood cells (RBCs)
- Pink in color due to eosin staining of hemoglobin[2]
- Size equal to size of the nucleus of a mature lymphocyte
- Central pallor approximately one-third of RBC diameter
- No cytoplasmic inclusions
- No wide variations in RBC sizes

(continued on following page)

What are the features of a normal peripheral blood smear?

(continued from previous page)

White blood cells (WBCs)[3]
- 2–5 leukocytes per high-power field
- Predominantly polymorphonuclear cells (PMNs)

Neutrophils
- Segmented with 3–5 connected lobes
- Pink or colorless cytoplasm
- Moderate azurophilic granules

Lymphocytes
- Small round cells
- High nuclear-to-cytoplasmic ratio
- Scant dark blue cytoplasm

Eosinophils
- Larger than PMNs
- Bi-lobed nuclei
- Red cytoplasmic granules

Basophils
- Smaller than PMNs
- Deep blue (basophilic) cytoplasmic granules that may obscure the nucleus

	Monocytes • Large cells • Bluish cytoplasm • Large nucleus, variable shapes **Platelets** • Small cells with coarse cytoplasmic granules • 7–15 cells per 100× field
Pearls	• The feathered edge can be viewed to evaluate platelet clumping or large cells such as monocytes and blasts • A nucleated RBC can be interpreted as a WBC by automated counters • A left shift describes neutrophilia along with neutrophil precursors, mainly bands; a right shift describes neutrophil hypersegmentation such as in megaloblastic anemias • Activated lymphocytes are large, with an irregular nucleus, and contain abundant cytoplasm • A method to estimate a platelet count is to count the number of platelets in 10 oil-immersion fields, divide the total by 10 (average per field), and multiply by 20,000[4] • Spurious thrombocytopenia can occur due to EDTA-induced platelet aggregation
References	1. Bain B. Diagnosis from the blood smear. N Engl J Med 2005;353:498-507. 2. Tkachuk DC, Hirschmann JV, eds. Approach to the microscopic evaluation of blood and bone marrow. In: *Wintrobe Atlas of Clinical Haematology.* Philadelphia: Lippincott Williams & Wilkins; 2007:275-327. 3. Bain BJ. Blood cell morphology in health and disease. In: Bain BJ, Bates I, Laffan MA, et al., eds. *Dacie and Lewis Practical Hematology.* 12th ed. London: Churchill Livingstone; 2017: 61-92. 4. Malok M, Titchener EH, Bridgers C, et al. Comparison of two platelet count estimation methodologies for peripheral blood smears. Clin Lab Sci 2007;20(3):154-60.

Does this peripheral blood smear explain the patient's anemia?

Key concept	A careful review of the morphology of blood elements on a peripheral blood smear can yield clues to diagnosing patients with anemia (Figure 2-2). A systematic approach should be followed and multiple fields inspected. Findings should attempt to explain the patient's clinical presentation. Automation of peripheral blood cell counting has largely replaced manual efforts; however, morphologic evaluation remains a required skill to confirm automated interpretations and eliminate false-positive and false-negative findings. 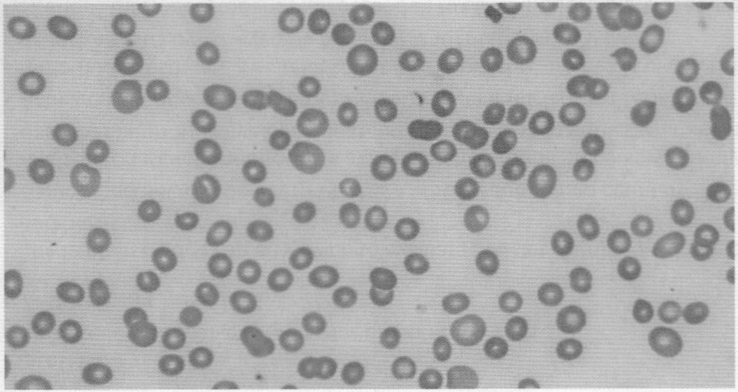 **Figure 2-2.** Anemia smear. (Reproduced with permission from Amer Wahed, MD and Aakash, MD.)
Clinical scenario	A 77-year-old man is found to have a hemoglobin level of 10.1 g/dL and a mean corpuscular volume of 109 fL.

Action items

RED BLOOD CELL (RBC) MORPHOLOGY	EXAMPLES[1]
Target cells	Liver disease, asplenia, hemoglobinopathies (sickle cell disease, hemoglobin C disease), iron-deficiency anemia
Bite cells	Glucose-6-phosphate dehydrogenase (G6PD) deficiency
Blister cells	G6PD deficiency
Pencil cells	Iron-deficiency anemia
Spherocytes	Hemolytic anemia, including hereditary spherocytosis
Elliptocytes	Hereditary elliptocytosis
Fragmented cells (schistocytes, helmet cells)	Disseminated intravascular coagulation (DIC), thrombotic thrombocytopenic purpura (TTP), hemolytic uremic syndrome (HUS), mechanical heart valves
Sickle cells	Sickle cell anemia
Stomatocytes	Liver disease, alcoholism, artifactual
Burr cells (echinocytes)	Uremia, malnutrition, artifactual

(continued on following page)

Does this peripheral blood smear explain the patient's anemia?

(continued from previous page)

Spur cells (acanthocytes)	Renal failure, liver disease, abetalipoproteinemia, spur cell anemia, pyruvate kinase deficiency
Tear drop cells (dacrocytes)	Myelophthisic conditions, myelofibrosis, myelodysplastic syndromes, severe iron-deficiency anemia, thalassemia, megaloblastic anemia
Rouleaux	Elevated plasma protein conditions such as paraproteinemia and elevated fibrinogen
Nucleated RBC	Severe bone marrow stress due to anemia, hypoxia, sepsis, leukemia, etc.
RBC inclusions	*Howell-Jolly bodies (DNA remnants):* asplenia, severe hemolytic anemia *Heinz bodies (denatured hemoglobin):* G6PD deficiency *Pappenheimer bodies (iron):* thalassemia, sideroblastic anemia, post-splenectomy, hemolytic anemia *Basophilic stippling (ribosomes):* lead poisoning, sickle cell anemia, thalassemia *Organisms: Plasmodium* spp., *Babesia* spp.

Discussion	Figure 2-2 shows an example of a megaloblastic anemia secondary to folate deficiency. The diagnosis was made by noting hypersegmented neutrophils on this peripheral blood smear. Neutrophils with >5 lobes are considered hypersegmented. This results from impaired nucleic acid metabolism secondary to deficiencies in vitamin B12, folate, or copper or secondary to drugs that affect nucleic acid metabolism.
Pearls	• The presence of nucleated RBCs and neutrophil precursors on a peripheral blood smear is termed leukoerythroblastosis, seen in bone marrow disorders, severe sepsis, and severe anemia • Schistocytes can be seen in healthy individuals; however, the presence of >1% schistocytes on a peripheral blood smear should raise a suspicion for thrombotic microangiopathies[2]
References	1. Ryan DH. Examination of the blood. In: Beutler E, Lichtman MA, Coller BS, et al., eds. *Williams Hematology*. 6th ed. New York: McGraw-Hill Professional; 2001:12-4. 2. Zini G, d'Onofrio G, Briggs C, et al. ICSH recommendations for identification, diagnostic value, and quantitation of schistocytes. Int J Lab Hematol 2012;34(2):107-16.

Can acute leukemias be diagnosed by peripheral blood smear review under light microscopy?

Key concept	Reviewing leukocyte morphology and numbers on a peripheral blood smear under light microscopy can provide a rapid diagnosis of acute leukemia (Figure 2-3); however, morphologic features alone may not reliably determine the lineage and type of acute leukemia, necessitating advanced diagnostics. 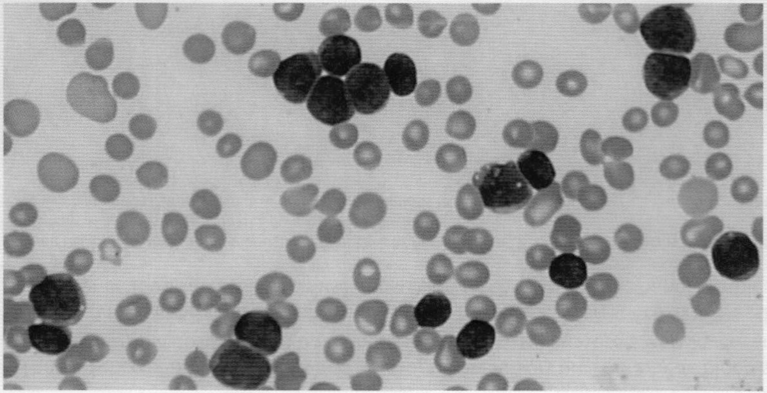 **Figure 2-3.** Leukemic blood smear. (Reproduced with permission from Nghia Nguyen, MD.)

Clinical scenario	A 34-year-old man presents to the emergency room with gingival bleeding, epistaxis, and melena of 48 hours duration. A complete blood count reveals a white blood cell count of 287×10^9/L, a platelet count of 9000/µL, and a hemoglobin level of 2.8 g/dL. A peripheral blood smear is obtained.
Action items	• In addition to evaluating the abnormal leukocytes in patients with acute leukemia, attention should also be given to red blood cell (RBC) and platelet morphology and numbers • Conditions such as disseminated intravascular coagulopathy can be seen in patients with acute myeloid leukemia (AML), especially in cases of acute promyelocytic leukemia (APL), and should be suspected in peripheral smears with thrombocytopenia, anemia, and fragmented RBCs
Discussion	Figure 2-3 depicts AML with minimal differentiation. The myeloblasts are less distinguishable from lymphoblasts than in other AML subtypes. The diagnosis was confirmed by immunophenotyping using flow cytometry prior to initiation of induction chemotherapy. *(continued on following page)*

(continued from previous page)

Relative differences between myeloid and lymphoid precursors (blasts)[1]

Myeloid blast
- Nucleus with fine chromatin
- 2–5 nucleoli
- Basophilic cytoplasm, less basophilic than lymphoblasts
- Agranular cytoplasm (majority)
- Auer rods may be present

Lymphoid blast
- Coarser chromatin and clumping near the nuclear membrane
- Fewer nucleoli
- Basophilic cytoplasm
- Scant cytoplasm

Promyelocyte
- Slightly larger than myeloblasts
- Abundant granules, Auer rods can be seen
- Condensed chromatin and nucleoli
- Abnormal folding of nucleus, can appear binucleate

Pearls	• It may be particularly difficult to differentiate myeloblasts from L2 lymphoblasts morphologically • Auer rods are seen more commonly in AML of neutrophilic precursors and are rare in AML of monocytic, erythroid, or megakaryocytic precursors; abundant Auer rods can be seen in APL[2]
References	1. Adewoyin AS, Nwogoh B. Peripheral blood film—a review. Ann Ib Postgrad Med 2014;12(2):71-9. 2. Stass S, Lanham G. Auer rods in mature granulocytes: a unique morphologic feature of acute myelogenous leukemia with maturation. Am J Clin Pathol 1984;81:662-5.

What is the significance of this red blood cell (RBC) formation on a peripheral blood smear?

Key concept	Variable patterns of RBC aggregation can be seen in blood films and should be distinguished from one another. This requires careful selection of the area of the film to be examined.[1]
Clinical scenario	A 72-year-old man presents to the emergency room with progressive shortness of breath. He is found to have bilateral pulmonary emboli. He has a serum total protein level of 12 g/dL and a globulin level of 10.3 g/dL (normal, 2.7–4.2 g/dL). Further characterization reveals an IgM protein level of 8300 mg/dL (normal, 60–263 mg/dL) and a serum viscosity >5 relative to saline (normal, 1.6–1.9).
Action items	• Negatively charged carboxyl groups of sialic acids in the RBC membranes cause the RBCs to repel each other, preventing aggregation • Positively charged plasma proteins (eg, globulins or fibrinogen) reduce the negative charge of RBC membranes, leading to their aggregation[2]
Discussion	Rouleaux formation, as seen in Figure 2-4, is typically seen in varying degrees in wet preparations of whole blood and must be distinguished from autoagglutination. 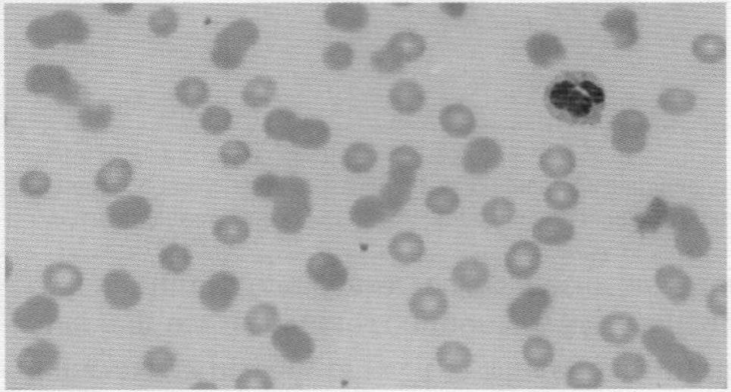 **Figure 2-4.** Rouleaux formation of red blood cells. (Reproduced with permission from Nghia Nguyen, MD.)

	Rouleaux[1] • RBCs are arranged side by side, giving them the classic "stacked coins" morphology • Rouleaux occur in the presence of acute phase proteins, mainly globulins and fibrinogen • Extensive rouleaux may appear similar to RBC agglutination • Disease states associated with rouleaux include inflammatory states (eg, infections or connective tissue disorders) and paraproteinemia (eg, multiple myeloma or Waldenstrom macroglobulinemia) ***Agglutination***[1] • Clumping of RBCs, in which individual RBCs cannot be distinguished • Occurs in the presence of cold agglutinins • Disease states associated with RBC agglutination include cold agglutinin disease and paroxysmal cold hemoglobinuria
Pearls	• The erythrocyte sedimentation rate test is based on the concept of increased rouleaux formation in the presence of acute-phase reaction proteins in which RBCs "stack" sediment more readily due to their increased density[1]
References	1. Bain B. Preparation and staining methods for blood and bone marrow films. In: Bain BJ, Bates I, Laffan MA, et al., eds. *Dacie and Lewis Practical Hematology.* 12th ed. London: Churchill Livingstone; 2017:50-60. 2. Fernandes H, Cesar C, Barjas-Castro M. Electrical properties of the red blood cell membrane and immunohematological investigation. Rev Bras Hematol Hemother 2011;33(4):297-301.

What are the key elements in evaluating a bone marrow aspirate and biopsy?

Key concept	Evaluation of the bone marrow is key in diagnosing hematologic disorders and is often provoked by abnormal peripheral blood findings. It allows for the evaluation of precursors of blood elements and their maturation and morphology. Review of bone marrow samples often includes additional special testing beyond morphology, such as cytogenetics, flow cytometry, and immunohistochemical staining, which aid in confirming the suspected diagnosis.
Clinical scenario	A 72-year-old man with macrocytic anemia and normal serum vitamin B12 and folic acid is seen by a hematologist. Examination of blood smear shows macrocytic hypochromic anemia with marked aniso-poikilocytosis, slight polychromasia, normal number and morphology of platelets, and neutrophilia without the presence of hypersegmented polymorphonuclear cells. Blasts are not seen. He undergoes a bone marrow aspiration and biopsy procedure. The samples are reviewed with the hemato-pathologist. The bone marrow aspirate is adequate with the presence of spicules. Trilineage representation of hematopoiesis and adequate hematopoietic maturation are seen. No increase in blasts is seen. Erythropoiesis is increased, representing 50% of nucleated bone marrow cells with a few dysplastic forms seen. The decalcified bone marrow biopsy is 0.2 cm in length. A bone marrow cellularity of 30% is estimated from the biopsy. No evidence of granuloma or abnormal cellular infiltrates is seen in the clot section. Iron stores from the clot section are increased with no ring-sideroblasts. Myelodysplasia (refractory anemia) cannot be ruled out with current morphological findings. Correlation with cytogenetics is suggested to rule out myelodysplasia.
Action items	• A bone marrow aspiration and biopsy is a low-risk sterile procedure that entails the insertion of a hollow needle into the cortex of a bone • The most common sites are the superior posterior iliac spine and the sternum (aspirate only) • Marrow aspirate is collected using a syringe into labeled tubes, and a cylindrical bone marrow core is obtained • The presence of spicules (particles) suggests an adequate bone marrow aspirate sample, and an aspicular aspirate suggests hemodilution from sinusoidal blood rather than bone marrow

Discussion	An adequate bone marrow sample includes a bone marrow aspirate smear, a bone marrow clot, and a bone marrow biopsy. Each component is evaluated for separate features.[1] ***Bone marrow biopsy*** • Useful for the quantitative evaluation of the marrow: cellularity, myeloid-to-erythroid ratio, and number of megakaryocytes • Useful for the evaluation of tumor infiltration and granulomas • Useful for the evaluation of fibrosis and necrosis ***Bone marrow clot*** • Useful for the quantitative evaluation of the marrow, especially if the biopsy is suboptimal • May be more useful than the biopsy for the evaluation of erythropoiesis • Useful for the evaluation of immunohistochemical staining patterns ***Bone marrow aspirate smear*** • Useful for the qualitative evaluation of the marrow: cell identification, dysplasia, maturation, and cytologic abnormalities
Pearls	• A dry tap results from failure to obtain bone marrow on aspiration; a bone marrow touch preparation technique may be used to obtain results that would have otherwise been obtained from the aspirate • The normal range for bone marrow cellularity is 30%–70%, often estimated by using a simple equation: 100 – age = cellularity %[2]
References	1. Hyun BH, Stevenson AJ, Hanau CA. Fundamentals of bone marrow examination. Hematol Oncol Clin North Am 1994;8(4):651-63. 2. Burkhardt R, Kettner G, Bohm W, et al. Changes in trabecular bone, hematopoiesis and bone marrow vessels in aplastic anemia, primary osteoporosis, and old age: a comparative histomorphometric study. Bone 1987;8:157-64.

What are some of the applications of flow cytometry in the evaluation of hematologic conditions?

Key concept	Flow cytometry is a technique in which cell characteristics are measured as they pass ("flow") single file through a beam of light in a fluid stream. The light scatter determines the size and granularity of the cell. Additionally, the same technique can be used to identify cell surface or cytoplasmic proteins, which are used to characterize a group of cells, a function termed "immunophenotyping."
Clinical scenario	A 61-year-old man who presented with pancytopenia undergoes bone marrow aspiration and biopsy. Flow cytometric cell surface marker analysis of the bone marrow aspirate specimen discloses a CD45-intermediate population situated in the "blast" region of the histogram comprising 85% of total analyzed events. Cells in this population express CD19, CD20 (partial), CD22 (cytoplasmic), CD10 (partial), CD38, HLA-DR, CD34, and TdT. Myeloperoxidase is not significantly expressed. The flow cytometric immunophenotypic profile is consistent with B-lymphoblastic leukemia/lymphoma.
Action items	• The light scatter patterns generated from flow cytometry can identify cells as either neutrophils, lymphocytes, or monocytes • Immunophenotyping of a selected population of cells (eg, lymphocytes) can then be used to determine the presence or absence of specific cellular proteins • The majority of the cell surface proteins are designated cluster of differentiation (CD) markers

Discussion

The various hematological disorders each have a relatively specific immunophenotypic pattern that is used as a signature in diagnosing these conditions with flow cytometry techniques. Below is a list of hematological malignancies and select markers associated with them.

ACUTE MYELOID LEUKEMIA (AML)[1]	
Precursor AML	CD34, CD38, CD117, CD133, HLA-DR
Granulocytic AML	CD13, CD15, CD16, CD33, CD65, cytoplasmic myeloperoxidase
Monocytic AML	Nonspecific esterase, CD11c, CD14, CD64, lysozyme, CD4, CD11b, CD36, neuron-glial antigen 2 homolog
Megakaryocytic AML	CD41, CD61, CD42
Erythroid AML	CD235a
B-ACUTE LYMPHOBLASTIC LEUKEMIA (ALL)[2]	
Pro-B ALL	Positive: terminal deoxynucleotidyl transferase (TdT), CD19 Negative: CD10, CD20, cytoplasmic IgM, surface immunoglobulin (Ig)
Pre-pre-B ALL	Positive: TdT, CD19, CD10 Negative: CD20, cytoplasmic IgM, surface Ig

(continued on following page)

(continued from previous page)

Pre-B ALL	Positive: TdT, CD19, CD10, cytoplasmic IgM, ±CD20 Negative: surface Ig
Early B-ALL (Burkitt leukemia)	Positive: CD19, CD10, CD20, surface Ig Negative: TdT, cytoplasmic IgM
T-ALL[2]	
Prothymocyte ALL	Positive: TdT, CD7, CD2, cytoplasmic CD3 Negative: CD5, CD1, surface CD3, CD4, CD8
Immature thymocyte ALL	Positive: TdT, CD7, CD2, CD5, cytoplasmic CD3 Negative: CD1, surface CD3, CD4, CD8
Common thymocyte ALL	Positive: TdT, CD7, CD2, CD5, CD1, surface CD3, cytoplasmic CD3, CD4, CD8
Mature thymocyte ALL	Positive: CD7, CD2, CD5, surface CD3, cytoplasmic CD3, CD4 or CD8 Negative: TdT, CD1
Mature T cell ALL	Positive: CD7, CD2, CD5, surface CD3, cytoplasmic CD3, CD4 or CD8 Negative: TdT, CD1

B CELL NEOPLASMS[2]	
Chronic lymphocytic leukemia	Positive: CD20, CD5, CD23, CD43, surface Ig, CD79b Negative: CD10, cyclin D1, FMC7
Follicular lymphoma	Positive: CD20, surface Ig, CD79, CD10, B cell lymphoma-2 (bcl-2) Negative: CD5, CD23, CD43, cyclin D1
Mantle cell lymphoma	Positive: CD20, CD79, FMC7, surface Ig, cyclin D1 (bcl-1), CD5, CD43, FMC7 Negative: CD10, CD23
Large B cell lymphoma	Positive: ±surface Ig, ±cytoplasmic Ig, CD19, CD20, CD79, CD22, CD79, ±CD10, CD5 (rare), ±bcl-2 Negative: cyclin D1
Marginal zone lymphoma	Positive: CD20, ±CD43, surface Ig Negative: CD5, CD10, CD23
Hairy cell leukemia	Positive: CD20, surface Ig, CD11c, CD25, CD103, CD123 Negative: CD5, CD10, CD23
Burkitt lymphoma	Positive: CD20, surface Ig, cytoplasmic Ig, CD10, bcl-6 Negative: CD5, CD23, TdT, cyclin D1

(continued on following page)

What are some of the applications of flow cytometry in the evaluation

(continued from previous page)

Lymphoplasmacytic lymphoma	Positive: CD20, surface Ig, cytoplasmic Ig Negative: CD5, CD10, CD23, cyclin D1
B cell prolymphocytic leukemia	Positive: CD20, surface Ig, ±CD5 Negative: CD23, cyclin D1
Myeloma	Positive: cytoplasmic Ig, CD56, CD45, CD43, CD38, CD138 Negative: CD19, CD20, CD22, surface Ig
T CELL AND NATURAL KILLER (NK) CELL NEOPLASMS	
T cell prolymphocytic leukemia	Positive: surface CD3, cytoplasmic CD3, CD7, CD56 Negative: CD5, CD30, CD16
T cell large granular lymphocyte leukemia	Positive: surface CD3, cytoplasmic CD3, CD7, CD8, CD16 Negative: CD5, CD4, CD30, CD56
NK cell leukemia	Positive: ±CD7, ±CD8, CD56 Negative: surface CD3, cytoplasmic CD3, CD5, CD4, CD30, CD16
Hepatosplenic T cell lymphoma	Positive: surface CD3, cytoplasmic CD3, CD7, CD16, ±CD56 Negative: CD5, CD4, CD8, CD30

	Peripheral T cell lymphoma not otherwise specified	Positive: surface CD3, ± CD7, ± CD4, ± CD8, ± CD30, CD56 Negative: cytoplasmic CD3, CD16
	Angioimmunoblastic T cell lymphoma	Positive: surface CD3, cytoplasmic CD3, CD5, CD7, ± CD4, CD56 Negative: CD8, CD30, CD16
	Anaplastic large cell lymphoma	Positive: surface CD3, ±CD5, ±CD7, ±CD4, ±CD8, CD30 Negative: cytoplasmic CD3, CD30, CD56
	Sezary syndrome	Positive: CD3, CD2, CD5, CD4, ±CD7 Negative: CD8
Pearls	• Flow cytometry can also be used to diagnose paroxysmal nocturnal hemoglobinuria by demonstrating the absence of CD55 and CD59 from the surface of erythrocytes[3] • Flow cytometry can be used to analyze samples of cerebrospinal fluid, lymph node sampling, pleural or pericardial effusions, and ascitic fluid in addition to blood and bone marrow	
References	1. Döhner H, Estey E, Amadori S, et al. Diagnosis and management of acute myeloid leukemia in adults: recommendations from an international expert panel, on behalf of the European LeukemiaNet. Blood 2010;115:453-74. 2. Frater J, Winkler A. Laboratory hematology. *American Society of Hematology Self-Assessment Program.* 6th ed.; 2017:282-6. 3. Yang HS, Yang M, Li X, et al. Diagnosis of paroxysmal nocturnal hemoglobinuria in peripheral blood and bone marrow with six-color flow cytometry. Biomark Med 2013;7(1):99-111.	

What is cytogenetic testing, and what is its role in hematologic malignancies?

Key concept	Cytogenetics is the science that combines the methods and findings of cytology and genetics in the study of abnormal chromosomal structure and numbers in evaluating particular disease states. Cytogenetic studies are used along with morphology, flow cytometry, and immunohistochemistry in the evaluation of particular hematologic and lymphoid neoplasms.
Clinical scenario	A 69-year-old man presents with profound fatigue and easy bruising. A complete blood count shows severe pancytopenia and circulating blasts. A bone marrow aspiration and biopsy is performed. The bone marrow aspirate is evaluated for the presence of cytogenetic abnormalities. Chromosome analysis shows a male karyotype with three related abnormal clones. The first clone (7/20 cells) exhibits the 9;22 translocation that leads to the fusion of the ABL1 and BCR genes (Philadelphia chromosome). The second (2/20 cells) and the third clones (9/20 cells) represent evolved clones with additional aberrations including deletion of 5q, deletion of 7q, structural rearrangement of 9q, deletion of 11q, monosomy 13, and monosomy 20. He receives induction chemotherapy and achieves a minimal residual disease–complete remission. Due to his risk cytogenetics, the patient undergoes an allogeneic stem cell transplantation in consolidation.
Action items	***General indications for cytogenetics***[1] • Diagnosis of non-Hodgkin lymphomas (NHL) with known recurring cytogenetic abnormalities • Diagnosis and prognostication of acute leukemias • Diagnosis of chronic myeloid leukemia (CML) and other myeloproliferative disorders (MPDs) • Diagnosis and prognostication of myelodysplastic syndromes (MDSs) • Monitoring of CML and MDS • Subtyping of lymphoproliferative disorders (eg, double-hit lymphomas) • Prognostication of chronic lymphocytic leukemia (CLL) and multiple myeloma

Discussion

Specific recurring cytogenetic abnormalities occur with a variety of hematologic and lymphoid neoplasms. The absence of these abnormalities does not always exclude a diagnosis, and results should be interpreted along with other diagnostic modalities.

For conventional cytogenetics (karyotyping), cells are cultured, arrested in metaphase using a mitotic inhibitor, and stained (G-banding) to detect numerical or structural chromosomal abnormalities such as translocations, deletions, and inversions.[1] Fluorescence in-situ hybridization (FISH) can be used to detect cytogenetic abnormalities not detected by conventional cytogenetics, such as t(15;17) in acute promyelocytic leukemia, 5% of t(9;22) cases in CML, and t(12;21) in B-acute lymphoblastic leukemia.

Common chromosomal abnormalities in AML and acute lymphoblastic leukemia (ALL) are described in the "Acute Leukemias" chapter.

COMMON CHROMOSOMAL ABNORMALITIES IN NHLS[2]	
Burkitt lymphoma	t(8;14), t(2;8), t(8;22)
Mantle cell lymphoma	t(11;14)
Follicular lymphoma	t(14;18)
Diffuse large B cell lymphoma	t(3;14)
Mucosa-associated lymphoid tissue lymphoma	t(11;18), t(14;18), t(1;14)
Primary nodal lymphoplasmacytic lymphoma	t(9;14)
Anaplastic large cell lymphoma	t(2;5)
CLL	Deletion (del) 13q, trisomy 12, del 11q, del 17p

(continued on following page)

(continued from previous page)

CHROMOSOMAL ABNORMALITIES ASSOCIATED WITH OTHER HEMATOLOGICAL DISORDERS	
MDS[3]	Deletion (−) of chromosomes 7, 5 or 13, del 7q, del 5q, del 13q, del 11q, del 12p, del 9q t(11;16), t(3;21), t(1;3), t(1;22), inversion 3, t(6;9)
MPDs[4]	
CML	t(9;22) (Philadelphia chromosome)
Polycythemia vera	del 20q, trisomy 9, trisomy 8, -Y
Essential thrombocythemia	Trisomy 9
Primary myelofibrosis	del 20q, del 13q, trisomy 9, trisomy 8

Pearls

- Cytogenetics can be performed on bone marrow aspirate, peripheral blood, lymph node tissue, effusion fluid, or other tissue that contains viable cells
- Conventional cytogenetics is less sensitive than FISH or polymerase chain reaction (PCR)
- The cytogenetic abnormalities listed above for MDS in a patient with a refractory cytopenia are adequate for diagnosing MDS in the absence of morphological features of the disease[4] on bone marrow evaluation
- Identifying a JAK2 mutation requires the use of FISH or PCR methods; conventional cytogenetics may identify chromosome 9 abnormalities, in which the JAK2 gene is located

References

1. Frater J, Winkler A. Laboratory hematology. *American Society of Hematology Self-Assessment Program.* 6th ed. 2017:283-6.
2. Kahl B, Nowakowski G, Yang D. Non-Hodgkin lymphoma. *American Society of Hematology Self-Assessment Program.* 6th ed. 2017:531-46.
3. Vardiman JW, Thiele J, Arber DA, et al. The 2008 revision of the World Health Organization (WHO) classification of myeloid neoplasms and acute leukemia: rationale and important changes. Blood 2009;114(5):937-51.
4. Zoi K, Croos N. Genomics of myeloproliferative neoplasms. J Clin Oncol 2016;35(9):947-54.

What is the significance of molecular diagnostics in hematological malignancies?

Key concept	Molecular testing has added another level of understanding of the pathobiology of hematological malignancies and has additionally become a tool for sensitive detection of disease beyond the level of detection of traditional methods. Traditional blotting techniques have largely been replaced by quicker, less labor-intensive and more accurate techniques such as fluorescence in-situ hybridization (FISH), polymerase chain reaction (PCR), and DNA microarray technology.
Clinical scenario	A 51-year-old woman presents with an abnormal complete blood count showing a white blood cell count of 218×10^9 cells/L with an abundance of mature neutrophils and basophilia. A bone marrow karyotype analysis for t(9;22) identifies the translocation in 20/20 cells analyzed, confirmed by FISH analysis, consistent with a diagnosis of chronic myeloid leukemia (CML). A bone marrow quantitative real-time (RT)–PCR for the BCR-ABL1 transcript is found to be 100% on the international scale (IS). The b2a2 fusion gene transcripts are quantified in the peripheral blood as 721.9% on the IS, and e1a2 fusion transcripts as 0.35% on the IS. She starts treatment with nilotinib 300 mg twice daily. Three months after initiation of treatment, bone marrow cytogenetics reveal t(9;22) in 10% of cells analyzed, consistent with a partial cytogenetic response. Peripheral blood quantitative RT-PCR shows the b2a2 fusion gene transcripts measuring 0.082% on the IS, consistent with a major molecular response. Her response is deemed optimal, and she continues treatment with nilotinib.
Action items	• Molecular analysis of hematological malignancies should complement other diagnostic data in guiding therapy and prognostication • Clinicians and hematopathologists should routinely review and update their standard molecular testing panels as advancing technologies continue to unravel actionable molecular markers

Discussion

PCR[1]

A technique in which a target DNA sequence is amplified allowing for identification of mutations and deep sequencing. RT-PCR also allows for quantification of the detected sequence.

Clinical applications

- Can detect specific translocations with a higher sensitivity than other methods, such as PML-RARα in acute promyelocytic leukemia and BCR-ABL1 in CML
- Detection of minimal residual disease in hematological malignancies
- Monitoring disease by exploiting the quantification ability of RT-PCR

SELECT EXAMPLES OF MOLECULAR TESTING IN HEMATOLOGICAL MALIGNANCIES (ABBREVIATIONS)	
AML	CEBP-α, FLT3-ITD*,[2] FLT3-TKD*,[2] IDH1, IDH2*,[3] NPM1
ALL	BCR-ABL1*, CRLF2, JAK2
MDS	ASXL1, JAK2, ETV6, EZH2, P53, RUNX1
Lymphoma	BCL-1 (expresses cyclin D1), BCL-2, BCL-6, IgH, TCR
MPDs[4]	JAK2*, MPL, CALR**,[5] SF3B1, SH2B3, EZH2, TP53, U2AF1, IDH2, ASXL1**,[5] KIT, CEBP-α, RUNX1, SRSF2, CBL, PBGFRA*, PDGFRB*

*Approved molecular targeted therapy[4,5]
**Guides treatment decision in myelofibrosis

(continued on following page)

	(continued from previous page) FISH Described in "Common Heme Questions." Microarray technology[6] An analysis of the whole genome in a single assay using a complementary DNA microarray to detect genomic imbalances. Results have a significantly higher resolution than standard karyotype analysis. *Clinical applications* • Gene expression profiling: the use of microarray technology to detect molecular signatures • Proteomics: the use of microarray technology to detect protein expression profiles
Pearls	• RT-PCR yields a more accurate quantification of a target sequence than DNA microarray analysis • PCR requires the knowledge of the specific nucleotide sequence to be analyzed • Sequencing-based approaches (eg, next generation sequencing) are alternative methods for gene expression profiling[7]

References

1. Frater J, Winkler A. Laboratory hematology. *American Society of Hematology Self-Assessment Program.* 6th ed. 2017:283-6.
2. Stone R, Mandrekar S, Sanford B, et al. Midostaurin plus chemotherapy for acute myeloid leukemia with a FLT3 mutation. N Engl J Med 2017;377:454-64.
3. Stein E, DiNardo C, Pollyea D, et al. Enasidenib in mutant-IDH2 relapsed or refractory acute myeloid leukemia. Blood 2017:blood-2017-04-779405.
4. Tefferi A, Pardanani A. Myeloproliferative neoplasms: a contemporary review. JAMA Oncol 2015;1(1):97-105.
5. Tefferi A. Primary myelofibrosis: 2014 update on diagnosis, risk-stratification, and management. Am J Hematol 2014;89:915-25.
6. Peterson J, Aggarwal N, Smith C, et al. Integration of microarray analysis into the clinical diagnosis of hematological malignancies: how much can we improve cytogenetic testing? Oncotarget 2015;6(22):18845-62.
7. Iqbal J, Liu Z, Deffenbacher K, et al. Gene expression profile in lymphoma diagnosis and management. Best Pract Res Clin Hematol 2009;22(2):191-210.

What is immunohistochemistry (IHC), and how is it used to determine the tumor origin?

Key concept

Immunohistochemistry (IHC), which is the detection of cellular antigens (including enzymes, hormones, or tumor markers) with specific antibodies characteristic of a respective malignancy, is one of the principal methods in which the tumor lineage is determined (ie, carcinoma vs. lymphoma).[1]

Factors such as tissue antigenicity or heterogeneity, interobserver variability, and quality of the biopsy specimen can affect IHC testing.[2]

Clinical scenario

A 52-year-old woman presents with a right axilla mass and undergoes further evaluation with diagnostic mammogram and bilateral ultrasounds of her breasts, which does not show any breast masses but re-demonstrates the 3-cm right axillary lymph node. She undergoes further evaluation with CT scans of chest/abdomen/pelvis, and no other tumors are identified. She undergoes biopsy of the lymph node. What specific IHC stains should be ordered?

Action Items

TUMOR LINEAGE[2]	IHC MARKERS
Carcinoma	Pan-keratin (AE1/AE3, CAM 5.2)
Lymphoma (Figures 2-5 and 2-6)	Leukocyte common antigen, CD20: B cell lineage CD3: T cell lineage

ORGAN-SPECIFIC TUMOR	IHC MARKERS
Breast (Figures 2-7 and 2-8)	ER/PR, CK7+, CK20−
Colorectal	CDX2, CK7±, CK20+
Hepatocellular	Glypican-3, HepPar-1
Germ cell	OCT3/4, SALL4
Lung	Napsin A, TTF-1, CK7+, CK20−
Melanoma	S100, SOX10
Neuroendocrine carcinoma	Chromogranin, synaptophysin, CD56
Prostate	PSA, PSAP
Renal cell carcinoma	PAX2, PAX8, carbonic anhydrase IX
Squamous cell carcinoma	CK5/6, p63, or p40
Urothelial	GATA3, p63 or p40, uroplakin II

(continued on following page)

(continued from previous page)

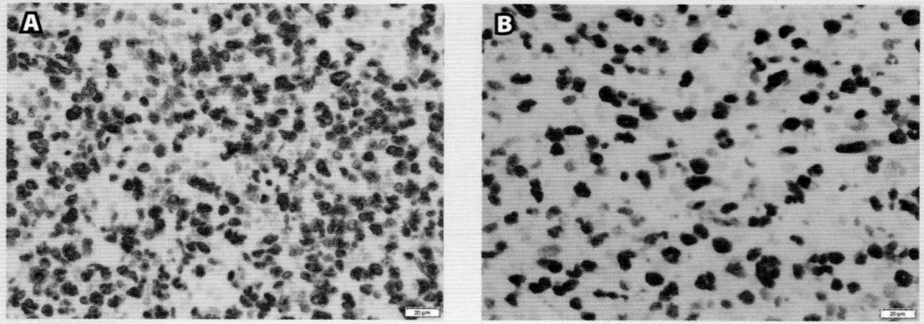

Figure 2-5. Ki-67 staining at 40× magnification. **A.** Diffuse large B cell lymphoma. **B.** Anaplastic large-cell lymphoma. (Reproduced with permission from Jamie M. Everett, MD.)

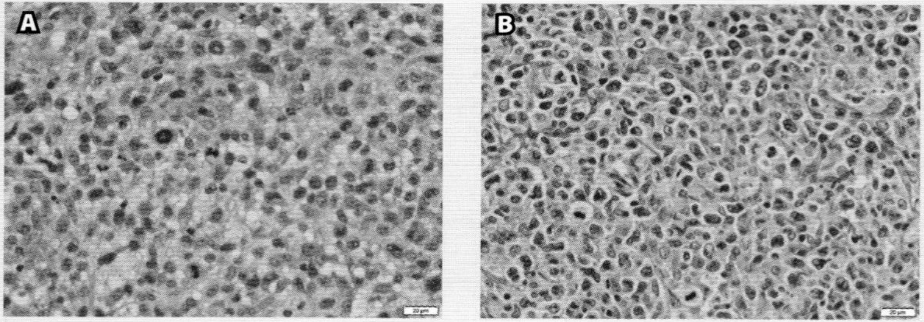

Figure 2-6. **A.** Anaplastic large-cell lymphoma. **B.** Diffuse large B cell lymphoma. Both images at 40× magnification. (Reproduced with permission from Jamie M. Everett, MD.)

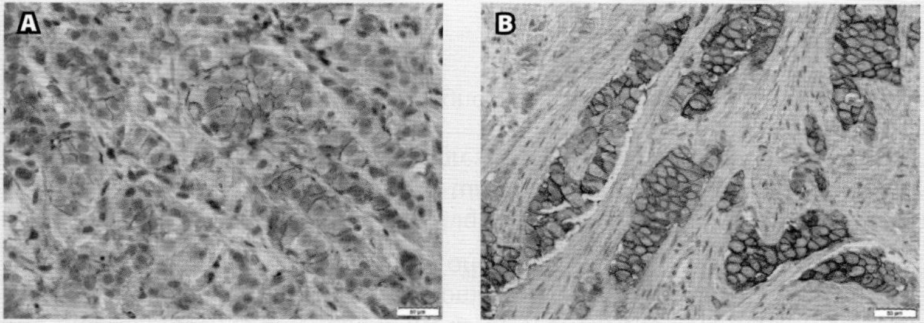

Figure 2-7. Immunohistochemistry staining of HER-2 at 20× magnification. **A.** 2+, defined as circumferential membrane staining that is incomplete and/or weak/moderate and within >10% of tumor cells OR complete and circumferential membrane staining that is intense and within ≤10% of tumor cells. **B.** 3+, defined as circumferential membrane staining that is complete and intense, within >10% of invasive tumor cells. (Reproduced with permission from Jamie M. Everett, MD.)

(continued on following page)

(continued from previous page)

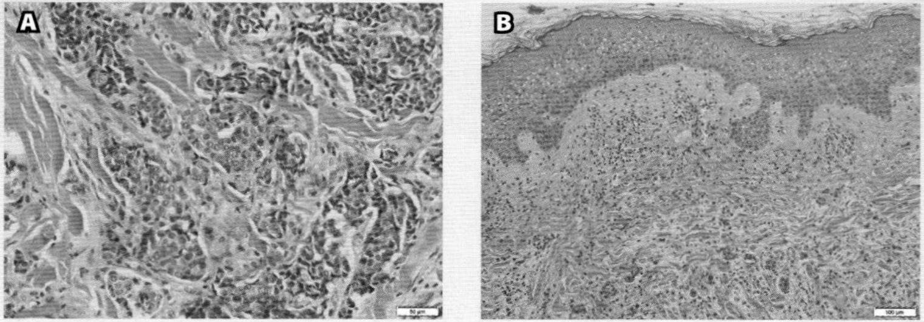

Figure 2-8. Invasive ductal carcinoma of the breast at 20× magnification. **A.** Hemotoxylin and eosin staining of high-grade breast cancer. **B.** Breast cancer cells involving the dermis. (Reproduced with permission from Jamie M. Everett, MD.)

Discussion	The initial approach to determining the tissue of origin is to determine whether the malignancy is a solid (ie, carcinoma) or liquid (ie, lymphoma) tumor. Then the second step is to use organ-specific IHC markers to help determine the tissue of origin.[1,2] Ki-67, a nuclear protein, is expressed at high levels of cell cycles, especially during mitosis. It is used a prognostic factor and is associated with tumor cell proliferation and growth. High Ki-67 is associated with poorly differentiated and more aggressive malignancies, as well as poor prognosis.[3]
Pearl	• Strong diffuse staining with P16 is diagnostic of human papillomavirus–associated carcinoma[2]

References

1. Imam A. Application of immunohistochemical methods in the diagnosis of malignant disease. Cancer Investig 1985;3(4):339-59.
2. National Comprehensive Cancer Network guidelines for occult primary. Version 1.2018. Available at: www.nccn.org.
3. Li LT, Jiang G, Chen Q, et al. Ki67 is a promising molecular target in the diagnosis of cancer. Molec Med Rep 2015;11(3):1566-72.

What are tumor markers, and what malignancies are associated with them?

Key concept

Tumor markers are molecules that are produced either by cancer cells or as a response to cancer cells.[1] Tumor markers can be used for screening and early detection and aid in diagnosis and assessment of response, prognosis, and relapse of disease.[1]

Clinical scenario

A 51-year-old man undergoes his screening colonoscopy and is found to have a circumferential ascending colon mass. What tumor markers are associated with colon cancer?

TYPE OF MALIGNANCY[1,2]	MARKER[1,2]
Breast	• Cancer antigen (CA) 15-3 • CA 27.29 • Estrogen receptor • Her-2-neu receptor • Progesterone receptor
Colorectal cancer	• Carcinoembryonic antigen (CEA) • KRAS mutation • NRAS mutation • BRAF mutation
Gastric cancer	• Gastrin

	Germ cell tumor	• Alpha-feto-protein (AFP) • β-Human chorionic gonadotropin • Lactate dehydrogenase (LDH)
	Hepatocellular	• AFP
	Lung	• ALK gene rearrangements
	Lymphomas	• β-2 microglobulin • LDH
	Pancreas	• CA 19-9
	Prostate	• CEA • Prostate-specific antigen
	Ovarian cancer	• CA-125
	Thyroid cancer	• Thyroglobulin
Pearls	• Tumor markers are specific for certain cancers, but only some are used in conjunction with other diagnostic tests in screening[2] • Tumor markers may be elevated in persons with diseases other than cancer[2]	
References	1. Nagpal M, Singh S, Singh P, et al. Tumor markers: a diagnostic tool. Natl J Maxillofacial Surg 2016;7(1):17. 2. American Association for Clinical Chemistry. Tumor Markers. Labs tests online. Available at: https://labtestsonline.org/understanding/analytes/tumor-markers/start/1.	

What is the difference between genetic polymorphism and mutation?

Key concept	Polymorphisms are DNA sequence variations that commonly occur in the population. A genetic variation is called a "polymorphism" if the frequency in the population is higher than the arbitrary cut-off level of 1%; if it occurs in <1% of the population, it is termed a "mutation."[1] The majority of polymorphisms occur in non-coding regions (intergenic and intronic) of the genome and have no known clinical significances. However, some polymorphisms may be correlated with the risk of developing certain diseases or the efficacy or toxicity of certain drugs.[1] For instance, certain polymorphisms in the *DPYD* gene are known to be associated with decreased dihydropyrimidine dehydrogenase activity and, therefore, a higher risk of adverse drug reaction or even fatal drug toxicity when treated with fluoropyrimidine drugs, such as capecitabine or 5-fluorouracil.[2] Whereas the term "mutation" is used to indicate a disease-causing change, the term "polymorphism" is used to indicate a non–disease-causing alteration. Despite the fact that "mutation" and "polymorphism" terms are still widely used, the Human Genome Variation Society recommends using neutral terms such as sequence variant, sequence alteration, and allelic variant instead, because it is sometimes hard to differentiate polymorphisms from mutations. Additionally, the term "mutation" has developed a negative connotation.
Pearls	Five categories are mostly used to classify sequence variations based on their biological significance (http://www.hgvs.org/mutnomen/recs.html): • affects function • probably affects function • unknown • probably does not affect function (or probably no functional effect) and • no functional effect

References	
	1. Moorcraft SY, Gonzalez D, Walker BA. Understanding next generation sequencing in oncology: a guide for oncologists. Crit Rev Oncol Hematol 2015;96(3):463-74. 2. Caudle KE, Thorn CF, Klein TE, et al. Clinical Pharmacogenetics Implementation Consortium guidelines for dihydropyrimidine dehydrogenase genotype and fluoropyrimidine dosing. Clin Pharmacol Ther 2013;94(6):640-5.

What are the different types of basic genetic variations?

Key concept

To unambiguously report genomic data in molecular diagnostic reports or scientific literature, it is crucial to use a uniform nomenclature system for describing variants detected. The Human Genome Variation Society (HGVS) proposed the sequence variant nomenclature system in 2000, and this has been widely accepted internationally.[1]

HGVS classifies basic DNA sequence variants into various types such as:

Single nucleotide variations (SNVs) or substitution:

DNA sequence change in which one nucleotide is replaced by another one, compared to a reference DNA sequence.[1] Because the sequence of DNA is only altered at a single point, this type of variation is also called a point mutation.[2]

SNVs can be classified as missense (nonsynonymous), silent (synonymous), or nonsense:

- A missense variant leads to a change from one amino acid to another (eg, the gain-of-function c.34G>C *KRAS* mutation results in an amino acid substitution from a glycine [G] to an arginine [R] at position 12 in KRAS protein [p.G12R])
- A silent variant does not alter amino acid/protein and is unlikely to affect protein function (eg, the c.2352G>A variant [reference SNP cluster ID: rs41420046] in the *EGFR* gene that leads to a codon change from GAG to GAA would still result in the introduction of glutamic acid, because both of these codons represent arginine)
- A nonsense mutation results in the introduction of a premature stop codon (eg, the *PTEN* c.31A>T mutation results in the production of the stop codon TGA rather than the AGA codon that represents the amino acid arginine)[2]

	If a variant results in an amino acid alteration in protein, this may or may not have a significant impact on the function of the expressed protein. Some changes may have a minimal effect or no effect at all on the protein, such as the c.1091C>T *EGFR* variant, which results in amino acid substitution of serine for phenylalanine at position 364. Some SNVs lead to impairment in the protein's capability to bind to receptors or other signaling molecules. Mutations in protein-binding sites or essential amino acids in active motifs (eg, tyrosine kinase domains) may produce a significant consequence on a protein's function. For example, the *BRAF* c.1799T>A mutation leads to the amino acid substitution of glutamic acid (E) for valine (V) at amino acid 600. This alteration occurs in the kinase domain of the BRAF protein and results in constitutive activation of this kinase.[2] **Insertions or deletions** are DNA sequence changes that include the addition or deletion of one or more nucleotides, respectively. These variations can lead to frameshift mutations if the number of nucleotides added or removed is not a multiple of 3 (the number of nucleotides in a codon). Frameshift mutations usually introduce premature STOP codons; therefore, in most cases they are classified as deleterious variants. For example, a *PTEN* c.800delA (p. K267fs*9) mutation is a deleterious alteration that results in a frameshift and premature protein translation termination.

(continued on following page)

	(continued from previous page) Deletion or insertion of a number of nucleotides that is a multiple of 3 ("in frame") will lead to deletion or insertion of corresponding codons' amino acid. In-frame variants can decrease or increase protein function, such as in the exon 20 in-frame insertion and exon 19 in-frame deletions in *EGFR* genes.[2] **Deletion-insertion (indel)** is an alteration in the DNA sequence where, compared to a reference DNA, one or more nucleotides are replaced by one or more other nucleotides, if this change is not a substitution, inversion, or conversion. For example, the DNA sequence change from ..AGGCTCATT.. to AGGCGACATT.. is called g.6775delinsGA, since the deletion of nucleotide g.6775 (a T, not described) was replaced by nucleotides GA.[3] **Duplication** is a specific type of insertion in which a copy of one or more nucleotides is inserted downstream of the original copy of that sequence compared to the reference sequence. For instance, the DNA sequence alteration from ACAATTGCC to ACAATTGCTGCC is described as a g.6_8dupTGC variant.[4] **Inversion** is a change in a specific sequence, where, compared to the reference sequence, more than one nucleotide replaces the original sequence and this sequence is the reverse-complement of the original sequence (eg, CTCGA to TCGAG).[5] **Conversion** is a specific type of indel alteration in which a range of nucleotides from the original reference sequence is replaced by a range of nucleotides copied from a homologous sequence present at another site in the genome.[6]
Pearls	The latest edition of sequence variant nomenclature recommendations is available online.[1]

References

1. HGVS. Sequence variant nomenclature. Available at: http://varnomen.hgvs.org/recommendations/DNA/.
2. Moorcraft SY, Gonzalez D, Walker BA. Understanding next generation sequencing in oncology: a guide for oncologists. Crit Rev Oncol Hematol 2015;96(3):463-74.
3. HGVS. Deletion-insertion variant—sequence variant nomenclature. Available at: http://varnomen.hgvs.org/recommendations/DNA/variant/delins/.
4. HGVS. Duplication. Available at: http://varnomen.hgvs.org/recommendations/DNA/variant/duplication/.
5. HGVS. Inversion. Available at: http://varnomen.hgvs.org/recommendations/DNA/variant/inversion/.
6. HGVS. Conversion. Available at: http://varnomen.hgvs.org/recommendations/DNA/variant/conversion/.

What is next generation sequencing (NGS), and what are its advantages in oncology?

Key concept	Cancer genomes acquire a broad spectrum of genetic alterations through clonal evolution, from single-nucleotide variants (SNVs) through insertions/deletions, up to genomic rearrangements and copy number variants. All these types of variants can be detected by deep sequencing of tumor DNA using NGS approaches.[1,2] The genetic alterations detected may provide diagnostic, theranostic, and/or prognostic insights for a particular tumor type.[1] NGS is an umbrella term for technologies capable of sequencing hundreds of genes (targeted gene panels), whole exomes, or even a whole genome from one or more patients in one experiment. The high-throughput feature of NGS is accomplished by a massively parallel sequencing approach that allows scientists to sequence from tens of thousands to more than a billion DNA molecules in a single experiment, depending on the output capacity of the sequencer.[3] In contrast, the traditional approach, focusing on a single gene assay and sometimes single-exon analysis, only detects the most common actionable mutations. Less common mutations are not tested, and therefore not detected, using molecular assays with no or little multiplexing capacity, including but not limited to Sanger sequencing, MALDI-TOF mass spectrometry, and polymerase chain reaction–based assays, due to the design, cost, sample size, and time constraints. For instance, the sample size could be a limiting factor because only a limited number of sections can be obtained from a tumor block. Separate slides are usually required for histopathological evaluations, RNA-, and DNA-based tests. In most cases, if assays with less multiplexing capacity are used, there is simply not sufficient tissue/nucleic acid to test for every alteration that is available. For these reasons, it is reasonable that with the discovery of more molecular markers the "one-drug/one-gene" diagnostic approach is unsustainable. The drive toward precision medicine using more advanced technologies such as NGS is transforming cancer molecular diagnostics practice.[4-6]

	An important characteristic of NGS testing is multiple sequencing of each base in the targeted genomic region. The number of times a given nucleotide or a fragment of DNA is sequenced is called "coverage" or "depth of coverage." Adequate coverage is essential for obtaining NGS data with acceptable quality for both germline and somatic mutation detection. The higher the sequencing depth of a target region, the greater the analytical sensitivity of the NGS assay. Deeper coverage allows for the higher detection sensitivity of genomic alterations, which is particularly crucial for detection of low-allelic fraction mutation in heterogeneous cancer biopsies.[1,7]
References	1. Jennings LJ, Arcila ME, Corless C, et al. Guidelines for validation of next-generation sequencing-based oncology panels: a joint consensus recommendation of the Association for Molecular Pathology and College of American Pathologists. J Mol Diagn 2017;19(3):341-65. 2. Moorcraft SY, Gonzalez D, Walker BA. Understanding next generation sequencing in oncology: a guide for oncologists. Crit Rev Oncol Hematol 2015;96(3):463-74. 3. Moorthie S, Mattocks CJ, Wright CF. Review of massively parallel DNA sequencing technologies. Hugo J 2011;5(1-4):1-12. 4. Rehm HL. Disease-targeted sequencing: a cornerstone in the clinic. Nat Rev Genet 2013;14(4):295-300. 5. Aftimos PG, Barthelemy P, Awada A. Molecular biology in medical oncology: diagnosis, prognosis, and precision medicine. Discov Med 2014;17(92):81-91. 6. Cronin M, Ross JS. Comprehensive next-generation cancer genome sequencing in the era of targeted therapy and personalized oncology. Biomark Med 2011;5(3):293-305. 7. Sims D, Sudbery I, Ilott NE, et al. Sequencing depth and coverage: key considerations in genomic analyses. Nat Rev Genet 2014;15(2):121-32.

CHAPTER 3

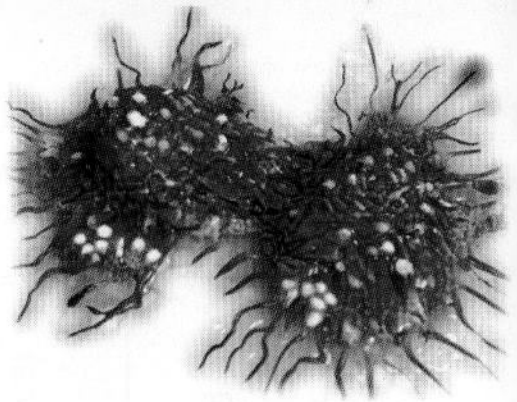

Most Common Hematology Questions

How do I work up my patient with anemia?

Key concept	Anemia is defined in clinical practice as a hemoglobin level <13.5 g/dL in men and <12 g/dL in women. Symptoms of anemia correlate with the degree and rate of development. An underlying abnormality should always be explored in an anemic patient.
Clinical scenario	A 69-year-old man with a history of an *Escherichia coli* urinary tract infection treated 8 days ago with ceftriaxone presents to the emergency room with symptoms of fatigue and jaundice. Physical examination reveals pallor and icteric sclerae. Laboratory evaluation reveals a hemoglobin level of 7.9 g/dL, elevated lactate dehydrogenase (LDH), low haptoglobin, indirect hyperbilirubinemia, and reticulocytosis. Review of the peripheral smear shows increased reticulocytes, anisocytosis, and spherocytic red blood cells (RBCs). A direct antiglobulin test (DAT) is positive for IgG. The patient is managed with supportive measures and recovers spontaneously after 7 days.
Action items	Production of RBCs requires the interaction of several elements and catalysts, including functional bone marrow, erythropoietin, iron, vitamins, and cytokines; deficiency in any of these can lead to anemia. A systematic approach in narrowing down the cause of anemia should be taken to ensure an accurate diagnosis and avoid unnecessary testing.
Discussion	In approaching a patient with anemia, the initial work-up should delineate whether the cause is a result of marrow underproduction or peripheral destruction or sequestration. This should be followed by a focused work-up of the suspected cause. Apparent or occult blood loss should be excluded, after which the pathogenesis can be categorized as follows.

Underproduction anemias

- Anemia plus corrected reticulocyte count <2%
  - Corrected reticulocyte count = reticulocyte % × patient's hematocrit/normal hematocrit[1]

Select examples[1]:

- *Microcytic RBCs:* disorders in heme or globin synthesis (eg, iron deficiency, congenital sideroblastic anemia, thalassemia)
- *Normocytic RBCs:* anemia of chronic disease (can be microcytic), chronic kidney disease, or compound deficiencies (eg, iron and folate deficiency)
- *Macrocytic RBCs:* deficiency of vitamin B12 or folate, or liver disease

Anemia secondary to increased RBC destruction (hemolytic anemia)

- *Intravascular hemolysis*: hemoglobinemia, hemoglobinuria, hemosiderinuria, decreased haptoglobin, or elevated LDH[2]
- *Extravascular hemolysis (spleen, liver):* no release of hemoglobin in the blood; no hemoglobinemia, no hemoglobinuria, no or minimal consumption of haptoglobin, and LDH can be normal
  - Recycled hemoglobin in the spleen or liver can result in indirect hyperbilirubinemia and bilirubinate gallstones[2]

(continued on following page)

(continued from previous page)

Select examples[1,2]

HEMOLYSIS	IMMUNE-MEDIATED	NON–IMMUNE-MEDIATED
Intravascular	Complement-mediated destruction: • Paroxysmal nocturnal hemoglobinuria • Acute hemolytic transfusion reaction (ABO incompatibility) • Paroxysmal cold hemoglobinuria	Examples: • Thrombotic microangiopathy (eg, thrombotic thrombocytopenic purpura, hemolytic uremic syndrome, disseminated intravascular coagulopathy) • Direct trauma (eg, mechanical valve or foot-strike hemolysis)
Extravascular	Removed by macrophages in the reticuloendothelial system: • Drug-immune hemolytic anemia • Autoimmune hemolytic anemia	• RBC defects (eg, membrane defects, hemoglobin defects, or metabolic defects) • Hypersplenism or liver disease • Infections: babesiosis or malaria

Pearls	• Normal RBC life span is ~120 days[1] • Screening tests for hemolysis can direct subsequent investigations; suggested initial work-up includes serum LDH, haptoglobin, indirect bilirubin, free hemoglobin, DAT, and urine hemosiderin • The reticulocyte response should also be evaluated • Features of intravascular and extravascular hemolysis can coexist, especially in cases of severe hemolysis[2] • Anemia of pregnancy results from plasma volume expansion and relative iron, folate, and B12 deficiency • Anemia in the elderly should warrant a work-up; however, the cause may remain unexplained • Folic acid supplementation may improve anemia but worsen neurological deficits of an occult vitamin B12 deficiency; therefore, evaluate vitamin B12 level prior to folic acid replacement[3]
References	1. Keel S, Mohandas N. Acquired underproduction anemias. In: Steensma DP et al., eds. *American Society of Hematology Self-Assessment Program.* 6th ed. Washington, DC: American Society of Hematology; 2017:117-38. 2. Sayani F, Lanzkron S. Hemolytic anemias. In: Steensma DP et al., eds. *American Society of Hematology Self-Assessment Program.* 6th ed. Washington, DC: American Society of Hematology; 2017:139-83. 3. Devalia V, Hamilton MS, et al. Guidelines for the diagnosis and treatment of cobalamin and folate disorders. Br J Haematol 2014;166:496-513.

How do I work up my patient with easy bruisability and a bleeding tendency?

Key concept	Intricate mechanisms come into play to maintain hemostasis, and understanding these factors can help identify causes of bleeding tendencies in individuals. Bleeding disorders range from mild to severe phenotypes—from bleeding disorders suspected on the basis of screening laboratory values at the time of invasive procedures to spontaneous life-threatening bleeding. A proper evaluation of any suspected bleeding tendency could potentially avert complications and identify family members with similar tendencies.
Clinical scenario	A 38-year-old woman with a long-standing history of easy bruisability and menorrhagia presents to the hematology clinic due to prolonged bleeding after a cervical polypectomy. She underwent a lumpectomy for a benign breast mass 5 years prior without bleeding complications. She has no family history of similar symptoms or a bleeding disorder. Electron microscopy shows a deficiency in platelet-dense granules.
Action items	• A systematic approach to diagnosing bleeding disorders allows early identification of the affected pathway, resulting in a focused and thorough evaluation of possible defective mechanisms • As is the case in diagnosing the majority of hematological disorders, a pertinent history can help narrow the differential and avoid irrelevant testing
Discussion	Achieving hemostasis requires complex interactions among 3 systems: the platelet complex, the coagulation system, and the fibrinolytic system. Upon exposure to a hemostatic challenge, platelets form the initial clot (primary hemostasis), followed by stabilization of this clot by fibrin generation via the coagulation system (secondary hemostasis) and removal of the clot via the fibrinolytic system. Bleeding disorders are attributed to quantitative or qualitative defects in any of these mechanisms.

Quantitative platelet disorders[1]

Site of bleeding	Initial laboratory testing	Other laboratory testing
Mucosa and skin	Platelet count	PT/aPTT, ADAMTS13 assay, anti-PF4 antibody, serotonin release assay, peripheral smear review, sequencing of complement inhibitor proteins

Causes

- ***Immune-mediated destruction:*** immune thrombocytopenic purpura, drugs (heparin in heparin-induced thrombocytopenia [HIT]), or post-transfusion purpura
- ***Consumptive:*** disseminated intravascular coagulopathy (DIC), thrombotic thrombocytopenic purpura (TTP), hemolytic uremic syndrome (HUS), after major surgery or blood loss, sepsis, or von Willebrand disease (vWD) type 2B
- ***Underproduction:*** bone marrow failure syndromes and bone marrow infiltration, decreased thrombopoietin production (liver disease), or bone marrow infections (parvovirus B19)
- ***Hemodilution and laboratory artifact (platelet clumping)***
- ***Sequestration:*** hypersplenism or hypothermia

Qualitative platelet disorders[1]

Site of bleeding	Initial laboratory testing	Other laboratory testing
Mucosal and skin	PFA-100 (replaced bleeding time)	Platelet aggregation studies, von Willebrand factor level, activity and multimers, flow cytometry, electron microscopy, genetic testing

(continued on following page)

(continued from previous page)

Causes

- ***Drugs:*** aspirin or NSAIDs
- ***Defective platelet adhesion and aggregation:*** vWD, Bernard-Soulier syndrome, Glanzmann thrombasthenia, or uremia
- ***Deficiency in platelet granules:*** dense granule deficiency, Gray platelet syndrome, Quebec platelet disorder, or Chédiak-Higashi syndrome

Coagulation disorders[2]

Site of bleeding	***Initial laboratory testing***	***Other laboratory testing***
Joints, muscles, deep tissue, and mucocutaneous	PT (extrinsic pathway)/ aPTT (intrinsic pathway)	Mixing studies ± Bethesda assay, clot stability (factor XIII) assay, thrombin time, and fibrinogen activity

Causes

- ***Congenital coagulation factor deficiency:*** hemophilia or factor XI deficiency
- ***Acquired coagulation factor deficiency:*** vitamin K deficiency, liver failure, consumption, or immune-mediated

Fibrinolytic system disorders (hyperfibrinolysis)[2]

Site of bleeding	***Initial laboratory testing***	***Other laboratory testing***
Any, can be delayed	D-dimer, fibrinogen split products, and thromboelastogram	Euglobulin clot lysis time, alfa-1-antiplasmin (α1-AP) level, plasminogen level, and plasminogen activator inhibitor 1 (PAI-1) level

	Causes • ***Congenital:*** α1-AP deficiency or PAI-1 deficiency • ***Acquired:*** liver failure (decreased plasmin clearance), DIC, acute promyelocytic leukemia, post-cardiac surgery, or prostate cancer
Pearls	• Do not transfuse platelets in patients with suspected TTP, HUS, or HIT, as it may increase thrombosis risk[3,4] • Evaluate the peripheral blood smear under light microscopy to exclude platelet clumping; use an alternative anticoagulant in the collection tube (eg, citrate) • The sensitivity of a PFA-100 test is decreased when the platelet count is <100/μL and/or the hemoglobin is <10 g/dL[1] • The degree of thrombocytopenia aids in the diagnosis[3] • Factor XII deficiency does not result in a bleeding tendency, and factor XIII deficiency does not prolong the PT and aPTT[2]
References	1. Cuker A, Greinacher A. Disorders of platelet number and function. In: Steensma DP et al., eds. *American Society of Hematology Self-Assessment Program.* 6th ed. Washington, DC: American Society of Hematology; 2017:249-76. 2. Kempton C, Di Paola J. Bleeding disorders. In: Steensma DP et al., eds. *American Society of Hematology Self-Assessment Program.* 6th ed. Washington, DC: American Society of Hematology; 2017:219-47. 3. Greinacher A, Selleng K. Thrombocytopenia in the intensive care unit patient. Hematol Am Soc Hematol Educ Program 2010;2010:135-43. 4. Greinacher A. Heparin-induced thrombocytopenia. N Engl J Med 2015;373:252-61.

When and how do I work up a patient for a hypercoagulable state?

Key concept	Select patients with a history suggestive of an inherited thrombophilia should undergo a work-up to advise on proper management of their thromboses and potentially inform the management of other family members. Acquired thrombophilias should be tested for in the proper clinical setting.
Clinical scenario	A 69-year-old man presents to the emergency room with sudden right upper quadrant abdominal pain and bloody urine. Laboratory examination reveals a hemoglobin of 7.9 g/dL, platelets 47/μL, lactate dehydrogenase 3313 U/L, elevated indirect bilirubin, and an undetectable haptoglobin. Urine analysis reveals bilirubinuria and hemoglobinuria. Abdominal imaging reveals the presence of a hepatic vein thrombus. Peripheral blood flow cytometry reveals the absence of CD59 and CD55, indicating the diagnosis of paroxysmal nocturnal hemoglobinuria (PNH).
Action items	• The American Board of Internal Medicine Foundation led a campaign to eliminate costly and potentially harmful overuse of tests called The Choosing Wisely Campaign. • In efforts to champion this initiative, the American Society of Hematology highlighted among its recommendations against thrombophilia testing in patients with venous thromboembolism (VTE) and a major transient risk factor.

Discussion

Patients with an acute thrombosis in the absence of a readily identifiable risk factor should undergo an evaluation for an acquired or hereditary thrombophilic condition.

Acquired thrombophilias

Acquired thrombophilia	***Diagnosis***
Malignancy	Age-appropriate cancer screening, imaging
Myeloproliferative disorders (polycythemia vera and essential thrombocythemia)	Jak2 mutation testing, bone marrow biopsy
PNH	Flow cytometry for CD59 and CD55
Disorders of fibrinolysis (decreased function)	PAI-1 level (elevated), tissue plasminogen activator (reduced)
Antiphospholipid antibody syndrome[1]	Anti–β2-glycoprotein antibodies, anti-cardiolipin antibodies, and lupus anticoagulant (repeat in 12 weeks to confirm); dilute Russell Viper Venom time
Heparin-induced thrombocytopenia (HIT)	History (4 Ts), anti-PF4 antibody, or serotonin release assay
Medications	Oral contraceptive pills or steroids

(continued on following page)

(continued from previous page)

Inherited thrombophilias

Inherited thrombophilia	***Diagnosis***	***Timing of testing***
Factor V Leiden[2]	Genetic testing for the mutation or functional testing with the activated protein C resistance assay (less commonly used)	Any for genetic testing, not affected by thrombosis or anticoagulation
Prothrombin gene mutation	Genetic testing for the mutation	Any, not affected by thrombosis or anticoagulation
Protein C deficiency	Protein C antigen and activity level	≥3 weeks after discontinuing warfarin (vitamin K antagonist)
Protein S deficiency	Free protein S antigen and activity level	≥3 weeks after discontinuing warfarin (vitamin K antagonist). Levels depressed in high-estrogen states, liver disease, disseminated intravascular coagulopathy, and nephrotic syndrome
Antithrombin III deficiency	Antithrombin III functional assay and gene testing	≥3 weeks after unfractionated heparin or acute thrombosis. Repeat testing required.

Pearls	• Factor V Leiden is the most common inherited thrombophilia, followed by prothrombin gene mutation[2] • MTHFR C677T, homozygous TT, and A1298C mutations are not risk factors for thrombosis or pregnancy complications[3] • Consider testing for a thrombophilia in patients with an unprovoked VTE in an unusual location, unexplained arterial thrombosis,[4] VTE with intermediate risk for recurrence, unexplained recurrent pregnancy losses, and family members of an index patient with a "strong hemophilia" • Progesterone-only contraceptive methods have a lower risk of VTEs than combined estrogen/progesterone methods
References	1. Miyakis S, Lockshin MD, Atsumi T, et al. International consensus statement on an update of the classification criteria for definite antiphospholipid syndrome (APS). J Thromb Haemost 2006;4(2):295-306. 2. Koster T, Rosendaal FR, de Ronde H, et al. Venous thrombosis due to poor anticoagulant response to activated protein C: Leiden Thrombophilia Study. Lancet 1993;342(8886-8887):1503-6. 3. Den Heijer M, Lewington S, Clarke R. Homocysteine, MTHFR and risk of venous thrombosis: a meta-analysis of published epidemiological studies. J Thromb Haemost 2005;3(2):292-9. 4. Moll S. Thrombophilia: clinical-practical aspects. J Thromb Thrombolysis 2015;39(3):367-78.

For how long do I give anticoagulants to my patient with a venous thrombosis?

Key concept	Optimal management of a venous thromboembolism entails (1) using the appropriate agent(s) (2) for the appropriate duration after (3) weighing benefits against risks of anticoagulation.
Clinical scenario	A 46-year-old woman who underwent bilateral knee arthroplasty surgery 3 weeks ago presents with right lower extremity swelling and erythema. A duplex ultrasound demonstrates an occlusive thrombus in the femoral vein. She is treated with low-molecular-weight heparin (LMWH) and warfarin followed by warfarin alone for 3 months.
Action items	<u>Non–vitamin K oral anticoagulants (NOACs) and their indications</u> • **Dabigatran:** non-valvular atrial fibrillation, treatment of deep venous thrombosis (DVT) and pulmonary embolism (PE) after lead-in therapy, reduction of recurrence risk in previously treated DVT or PE, or prophylaxis after hip replacement surgery • **Rivaroxaban:** non-valvular atrial fibrillation, treatment of DVT and PE, reduction of risk of recurrent DVT and/or PE after 6 months of treatment, or prophylaxis after knee or hip surgery • **Apixaban:** non-valvular atrial fibrillation, prophylaxis after knee or hip surgery, or treatment of DVT and PE • **Edoxaban:** non-valvular atrial fibrillation or treatment of DVT and/or PE after lead-in therapy

Discussion	***Choosing the anticoagulant:***

Discussion

Choosing the anticoagulant:

Unfractionated heparin (UFH), LMWH, and fondaparinux

- Can be used in the acute setting of a VTE or for lead-in therapy
- Unfractionated heparin potentiates the effects of antithrombin III; LMWH and fondaparinux inhibit factor Xa
- Hold LMWH for 24 hours before a procedure; hold fondaparinux for 36–48 hours before a procedure
- UFH: liver elimination; LMWN, fondaparinux: renal elimination
- Antidote for UFH is protamine sulfate

Vitamin K antagonist (eg, warfarin)

- Hepatic elimination
- Monitor with prothrombin time (PT) and international normalized ratio (INR)
- Hypercoagulable state within 24 hours of warfarin administration requires lead-in therapy
- Prothrombin complex concentrate (PCC) or fresh frozen plasma[1]

IV direct thrombin inhibitors (eg, argatroban and bivalirudin)

- Used in suspected or proven heparin-induced thrombocytopenia
- Argatroban is metabolized in the liver; bivalirudin is eliminated renally
- Short half-lives; stop in case of bleeding

(continued on following page)

(continued from previous page)

NOACs[2]

<u>Oral anti-Xa anticoagulants (eg, rivaroxaban and apixaban)</u>

- Rapid onset of action, no lead-in therapy required
- Compared to warfarin, lower rates of intracranial bleeding[3] and higher rates of GI bleeding; overall bleeding higher with rivaroxaban than apixaban
- Monitoring, if indicated, with factor Xa levels
- Renal clearance: hold for 48 hours prior to procedures, longer in patients with renal impairment
- Not recommended in patients with hepatic dysfunction and severe renal impairment (no restrictions on apixaban in severe renal impairment)
- Edoxaban was found to be non-inferior to subcutaneous dalteparin in treating cancer-associated venous thromboembolism with regard to risk of recurrence or major bleeding[4]
- Andexanet alfa can be used for the reversal of the effects of anti-Xa inhibitors rivaroxaban and apixaban[5]

<u>Oral direct thrombin inhibitors (eg, dabigatran)</u>

- Requires lead-in therapy (bridging)
- Antidote available: idarucizumab
- Not recommended in patients with severe renal impairment
- Compared to warfarin, lower rates of intracranial bleeding and higher rates of GI bleeding
- Prolongs PT/PTT and thrombin time
- Hold for 48 hours prior to a procedure, longer in patients with renal impairment; monitor thrombin time before a procedure

Choosing the optimal duration of therapy for VTE

- **Provoked proximal leg DVT or provoked PE:** 3 months
- ***Unprovoked proximal leg DVT or unprovoked PE:** at least 3 months; strongly consider extended anticoagulation
- **Recurrent:** increase target INR or LMWH dose, switch to alternative anticoagulant; investigate for secondary causes of thrombosis
- **Cancer-related:** at least 6 months with LMWH monotherapy[6]
- **APLA syndrome:** indefinite
- **Upper extremity or catheter-related:** at least 3 months, can keep catheter if functional
- **Portal vein thrombosis:** 3–6 months then weigh risks/benefits of long-term anticoagulation; stigmata of liver failure may prohibit initial anticoagulation

*Individualizing duration of anticoagulation in this population

(continued on following page)

(continued from previous page)

FAVORS EXTENDED ANTICOAGULATION	FAVORS LIMITED ANTICOAGULATION
Recurrent VTE	Female sex
Male sex	Distal DVT only
PE	D-dimer negative 4 weeks after discontinuing anticoagulation (applies better to women)
Elevated D-dimer at 3 or 6 months while on anticoagulation	Bleeding complications or high bleeding risk
Elevated D-dimer 4 weeks after discontinuing anticoagulation	Patient's preference
Anticoagulant well-tolerated, little or no impact on lifestyle	
Known thrombophilia	

Choosing the appropriate patient for anticoagulation

- Increased risk of bleeding in older patients, patients on concomitant antiplatelet therapy, uncontrolled hypertension, or history of bleeding and polypharmacy
- Bleeding risk tools: HEMORR2HAGES risk index and HAS-BLED risk score

Pearls	• PCC has been shown to reverse the effects of rivaroxaban but not dabigatran • Edoxaban should not be used in non-valvular atrial fibrillation in patients with a CrCl >95 mL/minute • Counseling on weight reduction should be provided to obese patients with a VTE • Role of anticoagulation in prevention of recurrent pregnancy losses in women with inherited thrombophilias is controversial[7]
References	1. Chai-Adisaksopha C, Hillis C, Siegal DM, et al. Prothrombin complex concentrates versus fresh frozen plasma for warfarin reversal. A systematic review and meta-analysis. Thromb Haemost 2016;116(5):879-90. 2. Mega J, Simon T. Pharmacology of antithrombotic drugs: an assessment of oral antiplatelet and anticoagulant treatments. Lancet 2015;386(9990):281-91. 3. Van Es N, Coppens M, Schulman S, et al. Direct oral anticoagulants compared with vitamin K antagonists for acute venous thromboembolism: evidence from phase 3 trials. Blood 2014;124(12):1968-75. 4. Raskob G, Van Es N, Verhamme P, et al. Edoxaban for the treatment of Cancer-associated venous thromboembolism. N Engl J Med 2018;378:615-24. 5. Siegal DM, Curnutte J, Connolly S, et al. Andexanet alfa for the reversal of factor Xa inhibitor activity. N Engl J Med 2015;373:2413-24. 6. National Comprehensive Cancer Network Practice Guidelines in Oncology for cancer-associated venous thromboembolic disease. Version 1.2017. Available at: www.nccn.org. 7. Middledorp S. Anticoagulation in pregnancy complications. Hematol Am Soc Hematol Educ Program 2014;393-9.

How do I work up my patient with isolated leukocytosis?

Key concept	Leukocytes exhibit dynamic kinetics in response to external stimuli, creating a variation in levels at any specific point in time. The majority of cases of leukocytosis are benign. A systematic approach should be used to reach a diagnosis.
Clinical scenario	A 61-year-old man who is a 70 pack-year smoker presents to the hematology clinic due to a persistently elevated white blood cell count ranging from 11.7 to 13.1×10^9/L with neutrophilia. Reviewing his records revealed this degree of neutrophilia dating back to 4 years prior. Red blood cell and platelet levels are within normal range. Peripheral smear review shows no immature forms. After careful history and physical examination, he is diagnosed with neutrophilia secondary to tobacco use.
Action items	• Neutrophilia, lymphocytosis, eosinophilia, monocytosis, and basophilia can be seen in a myriad of underlying conditions with different diagnostic considerations for each • The degree and pace of leukocytosis should be assessed by serial testing
Discussion	A sequential approach in diagnosing causes of leukocytosis should begin with thorough history-taking to eliminate obvious causes. Often, repeat testing is warranted after resolution of an acute event to confirm the abnormality. Testing with flow cytometry can help identify clonal disorders, and a bone marrow biopsy is sought if other clues to a hematological disorder are found.[1,2] Select examples of etiologies for leukocytosis according to the lineage affected are listed below.

Neutrophilia (absolute neutrophil count >7700/µL)

Non-clonal:

- Inflammation (eg, rheumatological conditions, infections, other inflammatory conditions)
- Stressors: physical or emotional (eg, trauma, burns, or panic)
- Malignancy (eg, underlying occult malignancy)
- Thyrotoxicosis
- Cigarette smoking
- Medication (eg, lithium, beta-agonists, or steroids)
- Asplenia

Clonal

- Myeloproliferative disorders

Lymphocytosis (absolute lymphocyte count [ALC] >3000/µL or upper limit of normal)

Non-clonal:

- Infections: viral, tuberculosis, pertussis, other infections
- Asplenia
- Hypersensitivity drug reaction

Clonal:

- Monoclonal B cell lymphocytosis (MBL)[3]
- Hematological malignancies (eg, chronic lymphocytic leukemia [CLL], acute lymphoblastic leukemia, hairy cell leukemia, prolymphocytic leukemia, other lymphoproliferative disorders, or large granular lymphocytosis)

(continued on following page)

(continued from previous page)

Monocytosis (absolute monocyte count >8000/μL)

Non-clonal:

- Chronic infections (eg, tuberculosis syphilis, other infections)
- Steroids
- Asplenia
- Pregnancy

Clonal:

- Leukemia

Eosinophilia (absolute eosinophil count >500/μL, hypereosinophilia if >1500/μL)

Non-clonal:

- Allergic reactions (eg, asthma, drug reactions, other allergic reactions)
- Infections (eg, parasitic, aspergillosis, HIV, other infections)
- Adrenal insufficiency
- Vasculitides
- Occult malignancy
- Bone marrow recovery

Clonal

- Primary hypereosinophilic syndrome
- Chronic eosinophilic leukemia

	Basophilia (absolute basophil count >3000/μL) Non-clonal • Allergic reactions • Parasitic infections Clonal • Hematological malignancies (eg, chronic or acute myeloid leukemia)
Pearls	• Screen for an underlying malignancy in a patient with otherwise unexplained neutrophilia • MBL is a premalignant condition characterized by an ALC <5000/μL and no systemic features of CLL/small lymphocytic lymphoma (eg, lymphadenopathy or hepatosplenomegaly) • Flow cytometry is the most widely used method to detect clonality • Monocytosis can be an early sign of bone marrow recovery after myelosuppressive chemotherapy • Hypereosinophilia can lead to organ infiltration and damage regardless of the cause (primary or secondary) • Basophilia is associated with hematological malignancies and should prompt further investigations[4]
References	1. George T. Malignant or benign leukocytosis. Hematol Am Soc Hematol Educ Program 2012;2012:475-84. 2. Neunert C, Rajasekhar A, et al. Consultative hematology I: Hospital-based and Selected Outpatient Topics. In: Steensma DP et al., eds. *American Society of Hematology Self-Assessment Program.* 6th ed. Washington, DC: American Society of Hematology; 2017:23-52. 3. Strati P, Shanafelt T. Monoclonal B-cell lymphocytosis and early-stage chronic lymphocytic leukemia: diagnosis, natural history, and risk stratification. Blood 2015;126:454-62. 4. Wimazal F, Germing U, Kundi M, et al. Evaluation of the prognostic significance of eosinophilia and basophilia in a larger cohort of patients with myelodysplastic syndromes. Cancer 2010;116(10):2372-81.

What are the potential complications when transfusing blood products?

Key concept	Transfusion of blood products could be a seemingly benign procedure, yet complications are observed and require the correct characterization to guide the appropriate course of action.
Clinical scenario	A 39-year-old man is undergoing a preoperative evaluation. His last prior surgery was 10 years ago, when he had a tonsillectomy. He required one unit of packed red blood cells (PRBCs) at that time. His blood type is O positive, and his antibody screen reveals no antibodies. He receives 2 units of PRBCs during surgery. One week later, he presents with fevers, fatigue, and jaundice; laboratory findings include an elevated lactate dehydrogenase, indirect hyperbilirubinemia, and a low haptoglobin level. A direct antiglobulin test shows IgG, and a repeat antibody screen detected a new antibody.
Action items	Understanding the potential complications of transfusions in the recipient patient can allow for blood product processing in the blood bank prior to delivering the product.[1] • ***Leukoreduction by filtration:*** reduces febrile reactions, cytomegalovirus (CMV) transmission,[2] and HLA alloimmunization; used in immunocompromised patients, transplant patients, and CMV-seronegative pregnant women • ***Irradiation:*** prevents replication of T lymphocytes; used in stem cell transplant patients and severely immunocompromised patients to prevent transfusion-associated graft-versus-host disease (TA-GVHD), as well as transfusions from a relative donor • ***Washing:*** can prevent allergic reactions, including anaphylaxis in IgA-deficient recipients

Discussion	Acute versus delayed, immune-mediated versus non–immune-mediated <u>Acute, immune-mediated transfusion reactions:</u> ***minutes to hours*** ***Acute hemolytic transfusion reaction*** • Complement-mediated intravascular hemolysis • ABO mismatch or clerical errors • Fever, hematuria, flank pain, and "feeling of impending doom" • Supportive management ***Acute febrile non-hemolytic reaction*** • Most common reaction • Antibodies against white blood cells in blood product or accumulated cytokines in stored units • Often seen in multiparous women or patients with a history of multiple transfusions • Fevers, chills ± rigors within a few hours • Leukoreduction can be preventative • Stop transfusion and exclude hemolysis • Supportive measures; resume when symptoms resolve if no hemolysis ***Allergic reaction*** • Minor urticarial reactions are common and treated with antihistamines • Recipient antibody reacts to donor proteins or vice versa • Stop transfusion and resume at slower rate when symptoms resolve • Anaphylactic reactions can occur in IgA-deficient recipients

(continued on following page)

What are the potential complications when transfusing blood products?

(continued from previous page)

Transfusion-related acute lung injury (TRALI)

- Donor antibody reacts to recipient's WBCs; other factors may be involved
- Leading cause of transfusion-related death in the United States
- Rapid hypoxemia, bilateral chest infiltrates, and no circulatory overload
- Stop transfusion and give aggressive support; most patients improve in 2–4 days
- Use only blood from male donors in the future

Acute, non–immune-mediated transfusion reactions

Transfusion-associated circulatory overload (TACO)

- High volume or rate of transfusion
- Stop transfusion and give diuretics

Bacterial contamination

- Platelets more than PRBCs; platelets stored at room temperature
- Gm+ cocci (eg, coagulase-negative *Staphylococcus* in platelets) or Gm− bacteria (eg, *Yersinia* in PRBCs)
- Supportive measures
- Notify blood bank to culture product

Delayed, immune-mediated transfusion reactions: ***days to weeks***

Delayed hemolytic transfusion reaction

- Mismatch in other RBC antigens; prior sensitization required
- IgG alloantibody-mediated extravascular hemolysis
- Pre-transfusion antibody screen may be negative if levels sub-detectable due to remote exposure
- Antigens are in the Rh, Kidd, Kell, Duffy, and MNS systems

HLA alloimmunization

- Recipient antibodies to donor leukocyte HLA antigens
- Results in platelet refractoriness due to anti-HLA platelet antibodies
- Transfuse ABO, HLA-matched platelets

TA-GVHD

- Transfer of T lymphocytes from donor to immunosuppressed recipient
- T lymphocytes target host organs: GI, skin, and liver
- Nearly 100% mortality

Post-transfusion purpura[3]

- Recipient antibodies to donor platelet antigens (anti-HPA antibodies)
- Effects extend to recipient's own platelets; results in severe thrombocytopenia
- Treat with intravenous immunoglobulin (IVIG) and plasmapheresis

(continued on following page)

	(continued from previous page) <u>Delayed, non–immune-mediated transfusion reactions</u> ***Infections*** • Available donor testing for: West Nile virus, Zika virus, HTLV-1/2, HIV, and hepatitis B/C • No testing available for: Creutzfeldt-Jakob disease prions, malaria, *Babesia*, or *Borrelia burgdorferi* (Lyme disease) <u>Miscellaneous</u> ***Massive transfusion*** • Defined as replacement of one blood volume (~10 units of PRBCs) within a 24-hour period • Can result in dilutional coagulopathy and bleeding, hypocalcemia, acidosis, and hypothermia • Treat with transfusions of platelets, cryoprecipitate, and fresh frozen plasma[4]
Pearls	• Target a hemoglobin of 7–9 g/dL in critically ill patients (TRICC Trial)[5] • PRBC washing and irradiation shorten the shelf life of the unit • *Allo*-antibodies are antibodies against non-self-antigen; *auto*-antibodies are antibodies against self-antigens

References

1. Savage W, Bakdash S. Transfusion medicine. In: Steensma DP et al., eds. *American Society of Hematology Self-Assessment Program.* 6th ed. Washington, DC: American Society of Hematology; 2017;303-37.
2. Nichols WG, Price TH, Gooley T, et al. Transfusion-transmitted cytomegalovirus infection after receipt of leukoreduced blood products. Blood 2003;101:4195-200.
3. Heddle NM, Klama L, Singer J, et al. The role of the plasma from platelet concentrates in transfusion reactions. N Engl J Med 1994;331:625-8.
4. Holcomb J, Tilley B, Baraniuk S, et al. Transfusion of plasma, platelets, and red blood cells in a 1:1:1 vs a 1:1:2 ratio and mortality in patients with severe trauma: the PROPPR randomized clinical trial. JAMA 2015;313(5):471-82.
5. Hébert PC, Wells G, Blajchman MA, et al. A multicenter, randomized, controlled clinical trial of transfusion requirements in critical care. N Engl J Med 1999;340:409-17.

When should I transfuse my patient with blood products?

Key concept	Whole blood is collected from random donors and separated into various products. Each separated blood component has different storage requirements and a defined shelf life. Evidence-based guidelines should be implemented across institutions to regulate the use of these finite blood bank resources.
Clinical scenario	A 29-year-old woman diagnosed with acute lymphoblastic leukemia undergoes induction therapy with an asparaginase-containing regimen. Fibrinogen levels are monitored daily and show a gradual decline as a result of asparaginase use. She requires a prophylactic transfusion of cryoprecipitate to avoid coagulopathy complications of hypofibrinogenemia.
Action items	Whole blood is centrifuged to separate packed red blood cells (PRBCs; hematocrit 60%) and platelet-rich plasma (PRP). PRP in turn is centrifuged to separate platelets and plasma, which is stored as fresh frozen plasma (FFP). FFP is thawed and centrifuged to separate cryo-poor plasma and cryoprecipitate.
Discussion	Whole blood is collected from volunteer donors at American Red Cross and other centers and used in many conditions in clinical practice. A summary of blood products, in order of separation from whole blood, and their clinical use is reviewed here. PRBCs **Storage and shelf life:** 42 days at 4°C, ≥10 years if frozen (rare blood types) **Volume:** 250–300 mL (with additive solution) **Clinical indication:** Improve oxygen delivery; anticipated hemoglobin (Hgb) increase of 1 g/dL per unit transfused

Recommendations for transfusion:

- Hgb <7–8 g/dL, symptomatic (higher cut-off in patients with comorbidities)
- Hgb <7 g/dL in hemodynamically stable ICU patients (TRICC Trial)[1]
- Hgb <8 g/dL non-inferior to Hgb <10 g/dL trigger after cardiac surgery (TRACS Trial)[2]
- Sickle cell anemia: simple or exchange transfusion

<u>Platelets</u>

Storage and shelf life: 5 days at room temperature, collected by apheresis or pooling

Volume: 50 mL

Clinical indication: Thrombocytopenia or platelet dysfunction; 1 unit increases platelet count by 20,000–50,000/μL

Recommendations for transfusion[3,4]:

- Prophylaxis if platelets <10,000/μL
- Prophylaxis if platelets <20,000/μL in patients with coagulopathy, fever, hypertension, uremic platelet dysfunction, or other co-occurring conditions
- Active non–central nervous system (CNS) bleeding or prophylaxis for major surgery if platelets <50,000/μL
- CNS bleeding or prophylaxis in neurosurgical or ophthalmologic procedure if platelets <100,000/μL

<u>Plasma</u>

Storage and shelf life: 1 year at −18°C

Volume: 200 mL

Clinical indication: Replenish plasma proteins (eg, clotting factors or ADAMTS13); each 1 mL contains 1 IU of each clotting factor, dose typically 10–20 mL/kg

(continued on following page)

(continued from previous page)

Recommendations for transfusion:

- PT/PTT >1.5× upper limit of normal and active bleeding
- Multiple factor deficiency and active bleeding (eg, liver disease, vitamin K deficiency, warfarin overdose, massive transfusion [relative deficiency], or DIC)
- TTP
- Prophylactic use controversial

Prothrombin complex concentrate (PCC)

Storage and shelf life: Can be stored at room temperature; more readily available than FFP

Volume: Small volume, can be transfused over 10 minutes; higher concentration of clotting factors than FFP

Clinical indication: Replace vitamin K–dependent clotting factors (II, VII, IX, X ± protein C, S); 3-factor PCC does not contain factor VII

Recommendations for transfusion:

- Urgent reversal of vitamin K antagonist effect and active bleeding[5]

Cryoprecipitate

Storage and shelf life: 1 year at −18°C

Volume: 1 unit is ~25 mL, usual dosing is 1 unit per 5 kg body weight

Clinical indication: Replace fibrinogen, factor VIII, vWF, factor XIII, and fibronectin; 10 units increase fibrinogen by ~100 mg/dL

	Recommendations for transfusion: • Fibrinogen <100 mg/dL or dysfibrinogenemia • Uremic platelet dysfunction and active bleeding • vWD and hemophilia A if recombinant factor unavailable • TTP; equivalent to FFP • Factor XIII deficiency
Pearls	• Do not eliminate clinical judgment when following PRBC transfusion guidelines, taking into account rate of hemoglobin decrease, comorbidities, and the overall clinical picture • Patients with splenomegaly may not demonstrate proper platelet level increments due to sequestration • Cost of PCC is ~20 times that of FFP • Plasmapheresis is indicated in cryoglobulinemia, TTP, leukostasis, chronic inflammatory demyelinating polyneuropathy, and familial hypercholesterolemia, among other conditions[6] • Platelet units can be collected by apheresis from a single donor or pooled with other donors and have comparable platelet contents
References	1. Hébert PC, Wells G, Blajchman MA, et al. A multicenter, randomized, controlled clinical trial of transfusion requirements in critical care. N Engl J Med 1999;340:409-17. 2. Hajjar LA, Vincent JL, Galas FR, et al. Transfusion requirements after cardiac surgery: the TRACS randomized controlled trial. JAMA 2010; 304(14):1559-67. 3. Schiffer C, Anderson K, Bennett CL, et al. Platelet transfusion for patients with cancer: clinical practice guidelines of the American Society of Clinical Oncology. J Clin Oncol 2001;19(5):1519-38. 4. Stanworth S, Estcourt L, Powter G, et al. A no-prophylaxis platelet-transfusion strategy for hematologic cancers. N Engl J Med 2013;368:1771-80. 5. Guyatt G, Akl E, Crowther M, et al. Antithrombotic therapy and prevention of thrombosis, 9th ed: American College of Chest Physicians Evidence-Based Clinical Practice Guidelines. Chest 2012;141;48S-52S. 6. Schwartz J, Winters J, Padmanabhan A, et al. Guidelines on the use of therapeutic apheresis in clinical practice—evidence-based approach from the Writing Committee of the American Society for Apheresis: the sixth special issue. J Clin Apher 2013;28:145-284.

How do I treat my patient with iron overload?

Key concept	Under normal circumstances, the human body regulates its iron content to maintain a steady state; the amount of iron intake equals the amount lost. However, mechanisms to eliminate supraphysiologic levels of iron do not exist, resulting in iron overload states and deposition of iron in organ tissues, leading to organ damage.
Clinical scenario	A 72-year-old man with myelodysplastic syndrome is being managed with packed red blood cell (PRBC) transfusions averaging 1 unit every 2 weeks for the past 6 years. He presents with fatigue and hepatomegaly and is found to have mild transaminitis, a transferrin saturation of 70%, and a ferritin level of 1200 µg/L.
Action items	• Hepcidin is an iron-regulating hormone that plays a central role in iron metabolism and balance states; through its interaction with ferroportin, the iron exporter, iron absorption is either increased or decreased • In iron overload states, hepcidin is up-regulated, leading to down-regulation of ferroportin and vice versa in iron-deficient states[1]
Discussion	Removal of excess iron can be achieved by therapeutic phlebotomies or chelating agents. The triggering ferritin level depends on the underlying etiology for iron overload as described below.

Hereditary hemochromatosis (HH)[2]

- Includes HFE (human factors engineering) hemochromatosis (most common), TFR2 (transferrin receptor) hemochromatosis, hemojuvelin hemochromatosis, hepcidin hemochromatosis, and ferroportin disease
- Iron predominantly accumulates in hepatocytes
- Diagnosed incidentally or later in life (by age 60, earlier in hemojuvelin variant); may manifest later in women due to menstrual iron losses
- Homozygous C282Y mutation results in the phenotype; however, homozygous H63D or heterozygous C282Y or H63D rarely manifest
- Liver dysfunction (most common), endocrinopathies, joint pain, cardiac arrhythmias, and dysfunction
- HFE gene mutation testing, role for liver biopsy or MRI if unavailable
- Weekly phlebotomies to a goal of ferritin <50 μg/L, chelation if cannot tolerate phlebotomies (eg, hypotension)

(continued on following page)

	(continued from previous page) <u>Transfusional iron overload</u>[3] • One unit of PRBCs contains 100× the daily dietary amount absorbed • Iron predominantly accumulates in macrophages-monocytes • More prominent in patients with hemoglobinopathies due to ineffective erythropoiesis and increased iron absorption • Initiate chelation once ferritin >1000 µg/L, or after 10–20 transfusions; higher levels are accepted than in HH <u>Other causes</u> • Ineffective erythropoiesis (eg, thalassemia or sickle cell disease) • Iatrogenic • Aceruloplasminemia • Chronic liver disease • Porphyria cutanea tarda
Pearls	• Ferritin can hold up to 4500 iron atoms • A transferrin saturation >50% in men or >45% in women should warrant a work-up for iron overload • Ferritin is an acute phase reactant and its level can be affected by other conditions

	• A liver biopsy should be obtained in HH patients with a ferritin level >1000 μg/L to evaluate for cirrhosis • A liver and cardiac MRI can assess organ iron content and guide therapy[3] • Avoidance of alcohol and iron-containing foods should be advised • Patients with iron overload should avoid raw seafood due to increased risk of *Vibrio* and *Yersinia* infections; also at risk for mucormycosis
References	1. Ganz T. Hepcidin and iron regulation, 10 years later. Blood 2011;117:4425-33. 2. Hoffman R, Benz EJ, Silberstein LE, et al. *Hematology: Basic Principles and Practice*, 6th ed. London: Churchill Livingstone: 2013. 3. Hoffbrand A, Taher A, Cappellini MD. How I treat transfusional iron overload. Blood 2012;120:3657-69.

How do I evaluate a patient with leukocytopenia?

Key concept	Patients can present with varying degrees of leukocytopenia and a proportionate risk for infections. In the majority of cases of leukocytopenia, neutropenia is the predominately affected subtype.
Clinical scenario	A 37-year-old man who recently immigrated from Nigeria presents to his primary care physician for an initial visit. He is found to have a white blood cell count of 2.9/μL and an absolute neutrophil count (ANC) of 1100/μL. Other cell lines are intact. He reports no history of recurrent infections. After reviewing past neutrophil counts, he is diagnosed with benign ethnic neutropenia (BEN).
Action items	• Mature neutrophils exit the bone marrow into the systemic circulation, where they have a short life span of 6–8 hours on average before being cleared by the reticuloendothelial system (spleen, liver, and bone marrow) or undergo apoptosis[1] • On a routine complete blood count, the neutrophil count reflects <5% of the total body neutrophils, and neutropenia reflects either a decrease in the circulating neutrophil pool or both a decreased circulating pool *and* bone marrow (BM) neutrophil reserve, the latter often demonstrating a higher degree of neutropenia and risk of infections
Discussion	**Neutropenia:** (mild: ANC 1000–1500/μL, moderate: ANC 500–1000/μL, severe: ANC <500/μL) In evaluating cases of neutropenia, the classification approach is similar to that of anemia and thrombocytopenia: classify the etiology as either neutrophil underproduction or increased peripheral clearance. The table below also identifies the neutrophil compartment affected, whether the circulating neutrophils or both the circulating neutrophils and the BM pool.

CAUSES	CIRCULATING POOL	BM POOL (RESERVE)
Neutrophil underproduction Congenital disorders* Aplastic anemia Myelodysplastic syndrome Acute leukemias Myelophthisic conditions Vitamin B12, folate, or copper deficiency	Low	Low
Neutrophil clearance Autoimmune neutropenia Infections Drug-induced neutropenia T cell large granular lymphocyte leukemia (T-LGL)	Low	Severe forms of infection, primary or secondary autoimmune neutropenia, or drug-induced neutropenia (eg, agranulocytosis) can result in clearance of BM neutrophil precursors
Sequestration, margination, and decreased chemotaxis Hypersplenism Hemodialysis BEN	Low	Normal or high

*Congenital disorders not discussed here

(continued on following page)

(continued from previous page)

Lymphocytopenia[3]

- Most cases are reversible
- A persistent absolute lymphocyte count (ALC) <1000/μL should warrant further testing, including testing for HIV
- Lymphopenia is common in the elderly, if ALC >500/μL without infectious complications consider observation only

Primary	Congenital immunodeficiency disorders (eg, severe combined immunodeficiency or common variable immune deficiency)
Secondary	Infections: HIV (moderate-severe), bacterial or fungal sepsis, or other viral infections such as hepatitis, influenza Drugs: corticosteroids, methotrexate, rituximab, fludarabine, and cladribine Autoimmune diseases: inflammatory bowel disease, lupus, rheumatoid arthritis, or sarcoidosis Malignancy: lymphoproliferative diseases and solid organ malignancies Other: recent surgery, cardiac failure, renal failure, malnutrition, or alcohol abuse

Pearls

- A careful review of the peripheral blood smear may provide evidence of an underlying marrow dysfunction (eg, tear drop cells, nucleated red blood cells, or pseudo-Pelger-Huët cells)
- Other cell lines are often affected in patients with underproduction neutropenias

	• Secondary autoimmune neutropenias occur in the setting of other autoimmune conditions (eg, systemic lupus erythematosus or rheumatoid arthritis)[2] • Clozapine, NSAIDs, β-lactams, ticlopidine, anti-thyroid drugs, and sulfasalazine are among medications that can cause agranulocytosis • Neutropenia secondary to sequestration or margination or decreased chemotaxis confers a low to no increased risk of infections • Fevers in a patient with severe neutropenia should be managed with intravenous antibiotics as an inpatient • Patients with a sudden severe neutropenia are at the highest risk of infections, such as in drug-induced agranulocytosis and chemotherapy-induced neutropenia • T-LGL can result in neutropenia through several mechanisms • Granulocyte colony-stimulating factor administration in neutropenic patients may shorten the duration of neutropenia, however, without a clear impact on mortality; its use is justified in agranulocytosis • Patients with chronic severe lymphopenia (ALC <500/μL) are predisposed to opportunistic infections such as *Pneumocystis jiroveci* pneumonia infections, systemic cytomegalovirus infections, esophageal candidiasis, and herpes zoster infections
References	1. Summers C, Rankin S, Condliffe AM, et al. Neutrophil kinetics in health and disease. Trends Immunol 2010;31(8):318-24. 2. Bux J, Kissel K, Nowak K, et al. Autoimmune neutropenia: clinical and laboratory studies in 143 patients. Ann Hematol 1991;63:249-52. 3. Brass D, McKay P, Scott F. Investigating an incidental finding of lymphopenia. BMJ 2014;348:g1721.

How do I treat my patient with iron-deficiency anemia?

Key concept	The total body iron content is determined by the balance between iron absorption in the upper GI tract and iron losses. Feedback mechanisms regulate iron absorption to increase in the setting of iron deficiency and decrease in iron overload. Pharmacologic replacement of iron losses may be warranted to maintain iron homeostasis.
Clinical scenario	A 36-year-old woman who underwent bariatric surgery presents with progressive fatigue and shortness of breath. She is found to have a hemoglobin level of 8.1 g/dL and a mean corpuscular volume of 73 fL. Iron studies reveal low serum iron, low ferritin, and elevated total iron binding capacity (TIBC) and red blood cell (RBC) distribution width. She has a total iron deficit of 1005 mg. She receives 8 weekly doses of intravenous ferric gluconate (125 mg) with normalization of her iron and RBC indices.
Action items	<u>Recommendations in managing iron deficiency</u> • Always investigate the underlying cause • Transfuse blood in cases of severe anemia or hemodynamic instability • Begin with oral iron if able • Consider adding docusate sodium 100 mg orally twice daily to prevent constipation when using oral iron • Monitor iron and RBC indices monthly while on replacement therapy • Initiate oral iron with once- or twice-daily dosing and increase as tolerated to a goal of 100–200 mg of elemental iron daily. For example, ferrous sulfate 325 mg contains 65 mg of elemental iron
Discussion	Body iron exists in 3 forms, measured by different surrogate markers: *storage iron* (ferritin and serum transferrin receptor), *transport iron* (serum iron, TIBC, and % saturation), and *functional iron* (hemoglobin, RBC indices, and reticulocyte count). Lack of iron depletes storage iron, followed by transport iron, then functional iron, with the end result of a microcytic anemia, and successful iron supplementation replenishes in reverse order (functional→transport→storage).

	In repleting iron stores with oral iron, we aim to deliver 100–200 of elemental iron daily in one or divided doses. Failure to achieve a hemoglobin increment of 1 g/dL in 4 weeks with this dose is generally considered iron-refractory.[1] Once iron and RBC indices normalize, continue supplementation for 3 months to replete iron stores.[2] Parenteral iron can be given in cases of oral iron refractoriness or intolerance. Total parenteral iron dosing is based on the following calculation to estimate total body iron deficit: $\text{Total iron deficit} = \text{Hemoglobin iron deficit} + \text{Storage iron deficit}$ $\text{Total iron deficit (mg)} = [\text{Wt (kg)} \times (14 - \text{Hgb}) \times 2.145] + [\text{Wt (kg)} \times 5]$
Pearls	• Oral iron can result in GI upset and constipation, which are common causes for medication nonadherence • An early sign of successful iron supplementation is reticulocytosis in 1–2 weeks • Various parenteral iron preparations are available; take into account institution availability and cost, risks of anaphylaxis, infusion time, and number of doses required for each preparation • Iron absorption can be impaired by concomitant antacids[3] widely used and can be enhanced by taking with orange juice or vitamin C • Iron-refractory patients should be evaluated for celiac disease and *Helicobacter pylori* gastritis • Iron-refractory iron-deficiency anemia (IRIDA) is an inherited iron-deficiency anemia refractory to oral iron[4]
References	1. Hershko C, Camaschella C. How I treat unexplained refractory iron deficiency anemia. Blood 2014;123:326-33. 2. Lopez A, Cacoub P, Macdougall IC, et al. Iron deficiency anaemia. Lancet 2016;387(10021):907-16. 3. Goodnough LT, Nemeth E, Ganz T. Detection, evaluation, and management of iron-restricted erythropoiesis. Blood 2010;116(23):4754-61. 4. Heeney MM, Finberg KE. Iron-refractory iron deficiency anemia (IRIDA). Hematol Oncol Clin North Am 2014;28(4):637-52.

CHAPTER 4

Screening

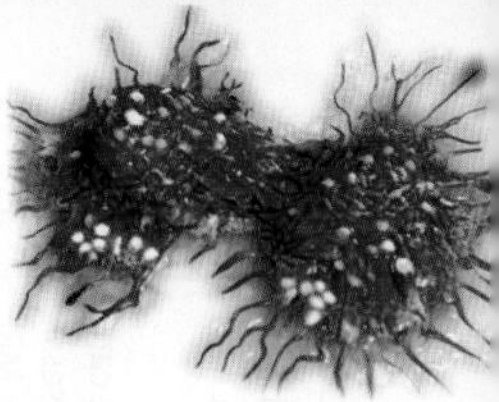

What are the recommendations for breast cancer screening?

Key concept	The average lifetime risk of breast cancer for a woman in the United States is estimated to be 12.3%. The mortality rate from breast cancer has decreased 38% from 1989 through 2014. This decrease has been partly attributed to mammographic screening. The components of a breast screening evaluation depend on age and on medical and family history. These can include breast awareness (patient familiarity with her breasts), clinical encounters (eg, breast cancer risk assessment and clinical breast exam), breast imaging with screening mammography, and, in selected cases, breast MRI. Patients are stratified into average or high risk groups (those with >20% lifetime risk) based on history and risk prediction tools.
Clinical scenario	A 31-year-old woman presents to establish her care with a primary care physician. She is worried about her risk of breast cancer due to her mother having had breast cancer at age 38 and her maternal aunt at age 42. She wants to know if she should do increased screening for breast cancer.
Action items	Major factors used to determine a risk category, based on a patient's history, are: • Personal history of ovarian, peritoneal (including tubal), or breast cancer • Family history of breast, ovarian, or peritoneal cancer with lifetime risk of >20% as defined by models based on that history • Genetic predisposition (if the patient's *BRCA* or other genetic marker status is known) • Radiotherapy to the chest between ages 10 and 30 years • 5-year risk of invasive breast cancer >1.7% in women ≥35 years old, or • ≥20% lifetime risk if personal history of lobular carcinoma in situ or breast abnormalities such as atypical ductal hyperplasia and atypical lobular hyperplasia Patients with any of the above factors are considered to be at increased lifetime risk for breast cancer.

	Patients with a family pedigree suggestive of a known genetic predisposition should be referred for genetic counseling and testing. If testing is negative, prediction models can be used to estimate lifetime risk and guide screening recommendations and start age.

Discussion	Average-risk screening recommendations per NCCN guidelines:
	• Age 25–40: clinical encounter every 1–3 years and breast awareness
	• Age >40: annual clinical encounter and screening mammogram with consideration of tomosynthesis and breast awareness
	
	Increased-risk screening recommendations:
	• Depending on patient-specific risk factors, start age recommendations vary
	• For family history–related risk, screening mammogram recommended to start 10 years younger than the youngest relative diagnosed with breast cancer (but not before age 30) and screening may include:
	  • More frequent clinical encounters every 6–12 months
	  • Consideration of yearly MRI in addition to screening mammogram (this can start as young as age 25, depending on the risk factor)
	  • Breast awareness
	• Some patients with increased risk are candidates for risk reduction strategies (including risk-reducing agents and surgery)

Pearls	• Only patients at very high risk, such as those with *BRCA* mutations, are considered for risk-reducing mastectomies and/or risk-reducing bilateral salpingoophorectomy
References	1. Siegel RL, Miller KD, Jemal A. Cancer statistics, 2017. CA Cancer J Clin 2017;67(1):7-30. 2. Humphrey LL, Helfand M, Chan BK, et al. Breast cancer screening: a summary of the evidence for the U.S. Preventative Services Task Force. Ann Intern Med 2002;137:347-60. 3. NCCN guidelines for breast cancer screening. Available at: http://www.nccn.org

What are the guidelines for cervical cancer screening?

Key concept	Screening with Papanicolaou (PAP) testing with cytology has decreased the mortality for squamous cell cervical cancer by 50%.[1,2] Early screening for cervical cancer for pre-invasive lesions has reduced the overall incidence of invasive cancer and improved the 5-year survival rate to around 92%.[2] Human papillomavirus (HPV) types 16 and 18 are the high-risk HPV genotypes associated with cervical cancer. HPV-16 and HPV-18 account for 55%–60% and 10%–15% of cervical cancers, respectively.[2]
Clinical scenario	A 24-year-old woman is here for follow-up for well-woman exam and asks about her risk for HPV and what kind of screening tests should she undergo. What are the recommended screening methods for women for cervical cancer?

Cervical Cancer Screening Based on Patient Population[1,3]

PATIENT POPULATION	SCREENING METHOD	MANAGEMENT OF SCREEN RESULTS
<21 years old	No screening • Women and girls <21 years old should not be screened for cervical cancer regardless of sexual intercourse status	Not applicable

21–29 years old	Cytology alone every 3 years
	• HPV testing should not be done to screen women for cervical cancer due to the high prevalence of HPV infection
		• If cytology negative or HPV-negative ASC-US, rescreen with cytology in 3 years
		• If ASC-US, then:
		  • HPV DNA testing (preferred if liquid-based cytology or co-collection)
		  • Repeat cytology at 6 and 12 months
		  • Colposcopy
		• If cytology of LSIL, then will need colposcopy

30–65 years old	HPV and cytology co-testing every 5 years
	• Co-testing has increased sensitivity of detecting CIN3+
		• If co-testing is negative or HPV-negative ASC-US, then repeat co-testing in 5 years
		• If ASC-US, then three options:
		  • HPV DNA testing (preferred if liquid-based cytology or co-collection)
		  • Repeat cytology at 6 and 12 months
		  • Colposcopy
		• If cytology of LSIL, then will need colposcopy
		• If HPV+, cytology negative, options include:
		  • 12 month follow-up with co-testing
		  • Test for HPV-16 or -18 genotypes, if HPV16+ or HPV16/18+, then refer for colposcopy
		  • Test for HPV 16 or 18 genotypes, if negative, then repeat co-testing in 12 months

(continued on following page)

(continued from previous page)

	Cytology alone every 3 years	• If cytology negative or HPV negative ASC-US, then rescreen with cytology in 3 years
		• If ASC-US, then three options:
		  • HPV DNA testing (preferred if liquid-based cytology or co-collection)
		  • Repeat cytology at 6 and 12 months
		  • Colposcopy
		• If cytology of LSIL, then will need colposcopy

>65 years old	No screening if adequate prior negative screening	If history of CIN-2+ severe, then will need to continue routine screening for at least 20 years
Following hysterectomy	No screening	

ASC-US, atypical squamous cells of undetermined significance; CIN, cervical intraepithelial neoplasia; LSIL, low-grade squamous intraepithelial lesion

References

1. Saslow D, Solomon D, Lawson, et al. American Cancer Society, American Society for Colposcopy and Cervical Pathology, and American Society for Clinical Pathology screening guidelines for the prevention and early detection of cervical cancer. CA Cancer J Clin 2012;62(3):147-72.
2. Cancer facts and figures 2017. Available at: https://www.cancer.org/content/dam/cancer-org/research/cancer-facts-and-statistics/annual-cancer-facts-and-figures/2017/cancer-facts-and-figures-2017.pdf.
3. Wright TC Jr, Massad LS, Dunton CJ, et al. 2006 consensus guidelines for the management of women with abnormal cervical screening tests. J Low Genit Tract Dis 2007;11:201-22.

Is prostate cancer screening necessary?

Key concept	Prostate cancer is the most common malignancy in the United States. Although a man in the United States has a 16% chance to develop prostate cancer during his lifetime, the risk of mortality from prostate cancer is $<3\%$. Today, many controversies exist around the role of prostate cancer screening on overall outcomes. The potential benefit of screening should be weighed against the risks, including overdiagnosis, overtreatment, risk of biopsy, and cost.[1]
Clinical scenario	A 56-year-old African-American man with no past medical history presents to discuss the role of prostate cancer screening. His father died of prostate cancer at the age of 65. Is prostate cancer screening necessary?
Action items	• A thorough discussion with the patient about the risks, benefits, and supporting evidence is important in making an informed individualized decision about whether to proceed with screening; recommendations in terms of when to start and stop screening, how often to screen vary between different medical societies in the field[1] • Prostate-specific antigen (PSA) remains the tumor marker of choice for screening; the role of digital rectal exam is controversial[1,2] • The age to begin the screening is undefined; NCCN guidelines[2] support starting the discussion about screening at age 45, but it is reasonable to start this process earlier in patients at higher risk to develop prostate cancer, such as African-Americans, those at risk for BRCA1/2 mutations, and those with a family history of prostate cancer at age <65[1,2] • Whenever prostate cancer screening is pursued, PSA level is usually checked at intervals of 1–4 years, depending on the PSA level; screening is also continued up to the age of 69–75 • For patients with a life expectancy of <10 years, prostate cancer screening is not recommended[1,2] • Men with a PSA level >3 ng/mL (for men age <75) or >4 ng/mL (for men age ≥ 75) or very suspicious digital rectal exam results should be evaluated for prostate biopsy[2]

Discussion	Whereas screening PSA may reduce the chance of death from prostate cancer, the overall survival benefit is mixed, and at best the absolute benefit is small, according to multiple randomized studies.[1-5] The European Randomized Study of Screening for Prostate Cancer (ERSPC) showed that PSA screening reduces the rate of death from prostate cancer by 20% after 9 years of follow-up, although 1410 men need to be screened and 48 diagnosed with prostate cancer in order to prevent one prostate cancer–related death. Moreover, the benefit was observed only among the subgroup of patients between the ages of 55 and 69.[3] By contrast, another randomized controlled trial, the United States Prostate, Lung, Colorectal and Ovarian Cancer (PLCO) trial, showed no significant reduction in prostate cancer mortality with screening after 15 years of follow-up.[4] A meta-analysis of 6 randomized controlled trials, including the ERSPC and PLCO trials, showed that screening with PSA with or without digital rectal exam does not decrease prostate cancer–related mortality.[5]
References	1. Up-to-date. Screening for prostate cancer. Available at: https://www.uptodate.com/contents/screening-for-prostate-cancer. 2. National Comprehensive Cancer Network. Guidelines for prostate cancer. Version 2.2017. Available at: https://www.nccn.org/. 3. Schröder FH, Hugosson J, Roobol MJ, et al. Screening and prostate-cancer mortality in a randomized European study. N Engl J Med 2009;360(13):1320-8. 4. Pinsky PF, Prorok PC, Yu K, et al. Extended mortality results for prostate cancer screening in the PLCO trial with median follow-up of 15 years. Cancer 2017;123(4):592-9. 5. Djulbegovic M, Beyth RJ, Neuberger MM, et al. Screening for prostate cancer: systematic review and meta-analysis of randomised controlled trials. BMJ 2010;341:c4543.

Does my patient need lung cancer screening?

Key concept	Lung cancer is the leading cause of cancer-related death. Most patients (>50%) have stage IV disease at the time of diagnosis. Screening for lung cancer can help reduce lung cancer mortality.[1,2]

Clinical scenario	<u>Screening recommended</u>
	• Age 55–74 years and
	  • ≥30 packs/year history of smoking and
	  • if current non-smoker, smoking cessation <15 years ago
	• Age >50
	  • ≥20 packs/year history of smoking and
	  • additional risk factors such as: chronic obstructive pulmonary disease, first-degree relative with lung cancer, radon exposure, occupational exposure to carcinogens
	<u>Screening not recommended</u>
	• Age <50 years
	• <20 packs/year history of smoking

Action items	• Shared decision-making between clinician and patient about benefits and risks of lung cancer screening • Annual low-dose CT scan (LDCT) for screening (without IV contrast) • Optimal duration of screening is unknown

Discussion	The National Lung Cancer Screening Trial (NLST), published in 2011, showed that annual low-dose CT scans in the high-risk population (age 55–74 years; ≥30 packs/year history of smoking) reduced lung cancer mortality by 20%. Patients undergoing screening should be counseled about the benefits of quitting smoking.
Pearls	• Patients in NLST undergoing low-dose CT scans had a very high rate (96.4%) of detecting false-positive lesions • These were followed up with CT scans, PET scans, bronchoscopy, and biopsy
References	1. The National Lung Cancer Screening Trial Research Team. Reduced lung cancer mortality with low-dose computed tomography screening. N Engl J Med 2011;365(5):395-409. 2. National Comprehensive Cancer Network guidelines for lung cancer screening. Available at: www.nccn.org.

What are the guidelines for "average risk" colon cancer (CRC) screening?

Key concept	The age at CRC screening depends on individual risk assessment, which includes medical history significant for inflammatory bowel disease (IBD; ie, ulcerative colitis or Crohn disease), family history of CRC, and personal history of adenomas or polyps. The subsequent schedule and frequency after initial screening depends on clinical findings.
Clinical scenario	During a primary care physician (PCP) visit, a 51-year-old woman with no family history of cancer asks her PCP about what type of colon cancer screening should she have done.
Action items	• For average risk, CRC screening can start at age 50 and include the following four modalities: • **Stool based studies** including fecal occult blood test (FOBT) or fecal immunochemical-based testing (FIT) and DNA-based testing. If any test is positive, then further testing is indicated. • FOBT identifies blood through peroxidase reaction of heme; FIT detects human globulin within hemoglobin. DNA-based stool testing detects DNA mutations (ie, *KRAS* mutations, aberrant *NDRG4* and *BMP3* methylation, or β-actin) associated with carcinogenesis of CRC • FOBT and FIT are repeated yearly versus DNA-based stool testing, which is done every 3 years • The disadvantages of FOBT are that it may miss tumors that bleed smaller amounts or intermittently and that it requires certain dietary restriction to prevent false-positive results; FIT does not require dietary restrictions • **Flexible sigmoidoscopy** ± stool based studies: repeat every 5–10 years • **Colonoscopy:** repeat every 10 years

	• **CT colonography:** repeat every 5 years • Limitations include that ≤5 mm lesions cannot be identified, no intervention can be done at the initial screening, radiation exposure is involved with CT scans, and bowel prep is still required • If any lesions ≥6 mm are found, follow-up colonoscopy is recommended • Repeat every 5 years
Pearls	• Patients with a personal history of IBD should undergo screening 8–10 years after onset of symptoms of IBD • In IBD patients, colonoscopies should begin when primary sclerosing cholangitis (PSC) is first diagnosed and performed yearly regardless of colonoscopy findings, because PSC is a risk factor for dysplasia
References	1. National Comprehensive Cancer Network guidelines for colorectal cancer screening. Version 2.2016. Available at: www.nccn.org.

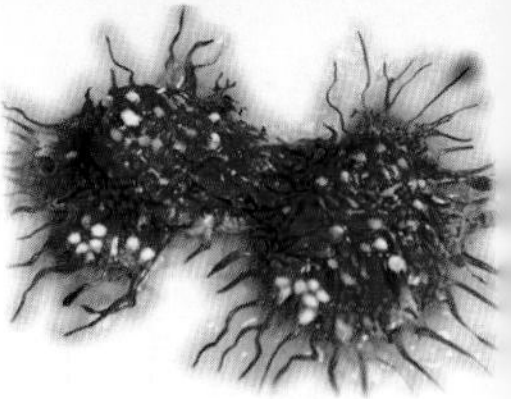

CHAPTER 5

Breast Cancer

What are the receptors tested in breast cancer?

Key concept	Breast cancer is composed of several biological subtypes. Newly diagnosed breast cancers must be tested for estrogen receptor (ER) and progesterone receptor (PR) expression and for overexpression of human epidermal growth factor 2 (HER2) receptors. This information is critical for both prognostic and therapeutic purposes.[1]
Clinical scenario	A 51-year-old woman with stage I breast cancer presents after lumpectomy and sentinel lymph node biopsy surgery for discussion of systemic therapy. The ER/PR and HER2 neu status are pending.
Action items	The proportions of breast cancers with different receptor phenotypes were evaluated in one study and showed the following case distribution[2]: • Hormone receptor (ER and/or PR)–positive cancers: 80% of cases • HER2 overexpression: 23% of cases • Of these, 67% and 32% were hormone receptor–positive and –negative, respectively • ER, PR, and HER2–negative (triple-negative) cancers: 13% of cases The frequency of subtypes varies according to race. Compared with white women, African-American women are less likely to have hormone receptor (ER/PR)–positive, HER2-negative disease (48% vs. 64%, respectively) and more likely to have ER/PR/HER2-negative disease (22% vs. 11%, respectively).[3]

Discussion	ER and PR expression are prognostic factors for invasive breast cancer, particularly in the first 5 years after the initial diagnosis. In addition, patients who are ER- and/or PR-positive are candidates for endocrine therapy as neoadjuvant or adjuvant treatment. ER positivity is defined by immunohistochemistry (IHC) for ER and PR in $>1\%$ of tumor cells.[1] HER2 overexpression is present in 20% of patients and predicts those who will benefit from HER2-directed therapy. HER2 overexpression is detected by uniform intense membrane staining of $>30\%$ of invasive tumor cells (IHC 3+) or the presence of HER2 gene amplification by fluorescence in-situ hybridization (FISH) defined as a ratio of HER2/CEP17 (centromeric probe to chromosome 17) ratio ≥ 2.0.[1] Assays for tumor expression of ER, PR, and HER2 neu have well-established utility in the clinical management of patients with both early stage and advanced breast cancer. They identify tumors for which endocrine and/or anti-HER2 therapies are valuable therapeutic options, and they should be routinely obtained on all tumor specimens.
Pearls	• IHC has rapidly become the predominant method for measuring ER and PR in clinical practice[4] • Due to variability in ER and PR IHC assay caused by a variety of factors, national guidelines for testing have been developed[4]
References	1. NCCN Clinical Practice Guidelines in Oncology for breast cancer. Available at: http://www.nccn.org. 2. Parise CA, Bauer KR, Brown MM, et al. Breast cancer subtypes as defined by the estrogen receptor (ER), progesterone receptor (PR), and the human epidermal growth factor receptor 2 (HER2) among women with invasive breast cancer in California, 1999-2004. Breast J 2009; 15:593-602. 3. O'Brien KM, Cole SR, Tse CK, et al. Intrinsic breast tumor subtypes, race, and long-term survival in the Carolina Breast Cancer Study. Clin Cancer Res 2010; 16:6100-10. 4. Hammond ME, Hayes DF, Dowsett M, et al. American Society of Clinical Oncology/College of American Pathologists guideline recommendations for immunohistochemical testing of estrogen and progesterone receptors in breast cancer. Arch Pathol Lab Med 2010;134(7):e48-72.

What is the staging scheme used in breast cancer?

Key concept	The Tumor, Node, Metastasis (TNM) staging system for breast cancer is an internationally accepted system used to determine the disease stage. This disease stage is used to determine prognosis and guide management. The eighth edition of the TNM staging system, effective as of January 1, 2018, includes anatomic stage groups as well as, for the first time, prognostic stage groups, which incorporate biomarker testing.[1]
Clinical scenario	A 50-year-old woman with ER/PR-positive, HER2 neu–negative breast cancer presents after surgery for discussion of systemic therapy. The final pathology showed a 2.5-cm invasive ductal carcinoma, grade 1 tumor with negative sentinel lymph node biopsy. An Oncotype DX test (a multigene reverse transcription polymerase chain reaction [RT-PCR] assay) is performed and gives a score of 10 with a risk of systemic recurrence in 10 years of 7%.
Action items	• According to the TNM staging system, the above patient has stage IIA breast cancer (T2N0) • According to the prognostic stage group, the stage is IA due to being ER/PR-positive HER2 neu–negative and having a low grade and low recurrence score on the Oncotype DX test
Discussion	The following biological factors have been incorporated into the prognostic staging system in the 8th edition of the American Joint Committee on Cancer (AJCC) staging manual: • **Estrogen receptor (ER) and progesterone receptor (PR) expression:** A tumor is considered ER or PR positive if $\geq$1% of tumor cells stain for the respective protein • **Human epidermal growth factor receptor 2 (HER2):** HER2 is assayed using either immunohistochemistry to assess protein levels or fluorescent in-situ hybridization (FISH) to quantify gene copy number • **Histological grade:** The grade of a tumor is determined by assessing morphological features (ie, formation of tubules, mitotic count, and variability and the size and shape of cellular nuclei), assigning a score between 1 (most favorable) and 3 (least favorable) for each feature and totaling the scores • Grade 1 corresponds to combined scores between 3 and 5, grade 2 to a combined score of 6 or 7, and grade 3 to a combined score of 8 or 9

	• **Recurrence score (RS):** The results of a multigene assay should be incorporated into the prognostic staging for patients with hormone receptor–positive, HER2-negative, node-negative tumors that are <5 cm
	  • Specifically, for such patients, an RS <11 on Oncotype DX denotes a prognosis similar to those with T1a to b N0M0 tumors, and they are assigned a prognostic stage of IA
	  • The Oncotype DX is a genomic assay of 21 genes assessed by RT-PCR
	  • A score <11 denotes a favorable prognosis; the TAILORx trial demonstrated a 5-year distant recurrence-free survival of 99.3% for such patients with endocrine therapy alone[2]
	• **Clinical vs. pathological staging:** Each characteristic of a tumor (size, nodal involvement, metastases) can be evaluated and reported either clinically, using physical exam, with or without imaging; or pathologically after surgery
	  • Pathological staging is generally considered to be more accurate than clinical staging
	  • Clinical staging is useful for making initial treatment recommendations for neoadjuvant therapy (systemic treatment given prior to surgical management)
	  • Subsequent pathology results may alter the clinical TNM classification

Pearls	• The 8th edition of the AJCC staging manual outlines a new prognostic staging system that relies not only on the anatomic extent of disease, but also on prognostic biomarkers • Although the prognostic staging system provides refined information regarding outcomes, the anatomic staging was retained to allow a common staging for patients treated worldwide who may not have access to biomarker testing • Periodic revisions are necessary because advanced imaging techniques and treatments evolve and impact survival
References	1. Amin MB, Edge SB, Greene FL, et al., eds. American Joint Committee on Cancer Cancer Staging Manual, 8th ed. Chicago: Springer; 2017. 2. Sparano JA, Gray RJ, Makower DF, et al. Prospective validation of a 21-gene expression assay in breast cancer. N Engl J Med 2015;373:2005-14.

What are the different surgical options for breast cancer?

Key concept	Surgical treatment of breast cancer includes addressing the breast and the axilla. Breast surgical therapy includes: • Breast conservation, also called lumpectomy, segmentectomy, quadrantectomy, and/or partial mastectomy • Breast conservation is the goal and standard if oncological principles can be maintained and good cosmesis can be achieved • Mastectomy is indicated for a large tumor/breast ratio, multicentric cancers, patient preference, or inflammatory breast cancer • There is no survival benefit for mastectomy over breast conservation[1] • External beam radiotherapy (EBRT) reduces the risk of local recurrence
Clinical scenario	A 56-year-old woman with a history of hypertension underwent screening mammography and was found to have a 2-cm area of calcifications in the upper outer portion of the left breast. No palpable mass on physical exam. Core needle biopsy demonstrates invasive ductal carcinoma with DCIS, grade 2, ER+, PR+, Her2−. She has no suspicious lymphadenopathy on exam or imaging. What treatment options can be offered?
Action items	• Breast conservation would be the option of choice if there is no cancer involving the nipple areola complex and there is enough breast tissue that cosmesis would not be hindered • For larger lesions, consider neoadjuvant therapy to downstage the tumor and allow for breast conservation[2] • When feasible, oncoplastic techniques have been shown to be safe and demonstrate increased patient satisfaction with cosmesis[3,4]

Pearls	• Early stage breast cancer is generally treated with surgery first, but neoadjuvant chemotherapy can be used to downstage a tumor to make the patient a candidate for breast conservation • Surgical excision margins need to be clear of tumor and are considered negative when there is no invasive breast cancer on the inked margin of the surgical specimen[5] • Recommendations for surgical excision margins for DCIS are 2 mm to reduce local recurrence[6] • Skin- and/or nipple-sparing mastectomy is safe in selected patients[7,8]
References	1. Fisher B, Montague E, Redmond, et al. Comparison of radical mastectomy with alternative treatments for primary breast cancer: A first report of results from a prospective randomized clinical trial. Cancer 1977; 39(6):2827-39. 2. Schwartz G, Birchansky C, Kormanicky L, et al. Induction chemotherapy followed by breast conservation for locally advanced carcinoma of the breast. Cancer 1994;73(2):362-9. 3. Kaur N, Petit JY, Rietjens M, et al. Comparative study of surgical margins in oncoplastic surgery and quadrantectomy in breast cancer. Ann Surg Oncol 2005;12(7):539-45. 4. Loskin A, Dugal C, Styblo T, et al. A meta-analysis comparing breast conservation therapy alone to the oncoplastic technique. Ann Plast Surg 2014;72(2):145-9. 5. Buchholz T, Somerfield M, Griggs J, et al. Margins for breast-conserving surgery with whole-breast irradiation in stage I and II invasive breast cancer: American Society of Clinical Oncology Endorsement of the Society of Surgical Oncology/American Society for Radiation Oncology Consensus Guideline. J Clin Oncol 2014;32(14):1502-6. 6. Dunne C, Burke J, Morrow M, et al. Effect on margin status on local recurrence after breast conservation and radiation therapy for ductal carcinoma in situ. J Clin Oncol 2009;27(10):1615-20. 7. Filho P, Capko D, Barry JM, et al. Nipple-sparing mastectomy for breast cancer and risk-reducing surgery: the Memorial Sloan-Kettering Cancer Center experience. Ann Surg Oncol 2011;18:3117. 8. National Comprehensive Cancer Network guidelines for breast cancer. Version 2.2017. Available at: www.nccn.org.

What are the different surgical options for the axilla management for breast cancer?

Key concept	Surgical treatment of the axilla in breast cancer includes sentinel lymph node biopsy and axillary dissection. Axillary surgical therapy should be considered as follows: • **Axilla preservation** is achieved by reducing unnecessary axillary dissections • **Sentinel lymph node biopsy** is the standard for assessing lymph node involvement in a clinically negative axilla (normal lymph node evaluation on physical exam and imaging) • **Axillary dissection** is indicated for known lymph node metastasis based on needle biopsy or sentinel lymph node biopsy • **There are some clinical scenarios when axillary dissection can be avoided even in lymph node–positive disease**
Clinical scenario	A 56-year-old woman with a history of hypotension felt a palpable mass in the upper outer portion of the left breast. She underwent screening and diagnostic mammography as well as a complete breast ultrasound and was found to have a 3-cm suspicious mass. She has a suspicious lymph node on exam which is confirmed by ultrasound. Core needle biopsy is performed on the mass and the lymph node as well, and clips are placed in both. The pathology on the breast mass demonstrates invasive ductal carcinoma with DCIS, grade 2, ER+/PR+/Her2−. The pathology on the lymph node demonstrates invasive carcinoma. What treatment options can be offered?
Action items	• Sentinel lymph node biopsy is performed on invasive breast cancer when axilla is clinically negative[1] • For early-stage breast cancer patients undergoing segmental mastectomy, axillary dissection can be avoided if <3 nodes are positive on sentinel lymph node biopsy[2] • After a clinically good response to neoadjuvant chemotherapy, if the axilla was node positive before chemotherapy and is negative on exam and ultrasound after chemotherapy, sentinel lymph node biopsy can be performed to assess whether the axilla remains positive or has downstaged[3-6]

	• Do not routinely perform a sentinel lymph node biopsy on clinically node-negative women >70 years old with hormone-positive invasive breast cancer[7] • This is a consensus statement by the Society of Surgical Oncology to avoid unnecessary axilla surgery and part of the Choosing Wisely Campaign[8]
Pearls	• Early-stage breast cancer is generally treated with surgery first • Neoadjuvant chemotherapy can be used to downstage a breast tumor to make the patient a candidate for breast conservation as well as to downstage the axilla[3,4] • If the axilla remains positive after neoadjuvant chemotherapy, on exam, ultrasound, or with sentinel lymph node biopsy, a complete axillary dissection is performed[3-6] • The false-negative rate decreases with >2 positive nodes and if the original clipped node is removed[3-6]
References	1. Lyman G, Giuliano A, Somerfield M, et al. American Society of Clinical Oncology Guideline Recommendations for sentinel lymph node biopsy in early-stage breast cancer. J Clin Oncol 2005;23(30):7703-20. 2. Giuliano A, Hunt K, Ballman K. Axillary dissection vs no axillary dissection in women with invasive breast cancer and sentinel node metastasis: a randomized clinical trial. JAMA 2011;305(6):569-75. 3. Kuehn T, Bauerfield I, Fehm T, et al. Sentinel-lymph-node biopsy in patients with breast cancer before and after neoadjuvant chemotherapy (SENTINA): a prospective, multicentre cohort study. Lancet Oncol 2013;14(7):609-18. 4. Boughey J, Suman V, Mittendorf E, et al. Sentinel lymph node surgery after neoadjuvant chemotherapy in patients with node-positive breast cancer: the ACOSOG Z1071 (Alliance) Clinical Trial. JAMA 2013;310(14):1455-61. 5. Caudle A, Yang W, Krishnamurthy S, et al. Improved axillary evaluation following neoadjuvant therapy for patients with node-positive breast cancer using selective evaluation of clipped nodes: implementation of targeted axillary dissection. J Clin Oncol 2016;34(10):1072-8. 6. National Comprehensive Cancer Network guidelines for breast cancer. Version 2.2017. Available at: www.nccn.org. 7. Martelli G, Miceli R, Daidone MG, et al. Axillary dissection versus no axillary dissection in elderly patients with breast cancer and no palpable axillary nodes: results after 15 years of follow-up. Ann Surg Oncol 2011;18(1):125-33. 8. Choosing Wisely Campaign. Available at: http://www.choosingwisely.org/clinician-lists/sso-sentinel-node-biopsy-in-node-negative-women-70-and-over/.

What is the current role of radiation treatment in breast cancer?

Key concept	Breast cancer is a leading cause of morbidity and mortality among women, with an estimated 252,710 cases of invasive cancer expected in 2017.[1] Given mammographic screening, most women will present with localized or regional breast cancer at diagnosis, for which the 5-year survival rates range from 75% to 99%.[2] The historical (Halstedian) treatment paradigm focused on complete mastectomy. This was supplanted by well-conducted randomized trials demonstrating no survival difference between breast-conserving and mastectomy approaches for stage 1–2 cancers[3] and DCIS,[4] respectively. A recent meta-analysis quantifies the effects of radiation as a reduction in first relapse by 15.7%, with reduction of breast cancer mortality by 3.8% for breast-conserving surgery.[5]
Clinical scenario	A 57-year-old patient without a personal history of cancer presents with a new palpable mass in her left breast upper outer quadrant. Mammogram and ultrasound corroborate the findings, without additional lesions detected. Nodal basins are radiographically normal. Stereotactic biopsy confirms infiltrating ductal carcinoma, ER+/PR+/Her-2-Neu−. The patient opts for breast-conserving surgery and undergoes needle localization lumpectomy with findings of a 0.9-cm residual tumor and 1 negative sentinel node. Margins are negative at 2 mm minimum using the shave margin technique. The postoperative course is uncomplicated. She receives consultation under a medical oncologist. Her Oncotype DX score is 10. Adjuvant radiation therapy and endocrine therapy are recommended. The patient is simulated in the prone position to achieve maximal cardiac clearance. Treatment planning ensues and results in good cardiac sparing and excellent coverage of the breast target volume. The axilla is not irradiated due to pathological stage IA disease. The patient is prescribed a hypo-fractionated course of 42.4 Gy in 16 fractions. Radiation treatment is completed without adverse events, other than mild erythema without desquamation.

Pearls

- Adjuvant radiation is recommended for women with breast cancer after breast-conserving surgery
- For women ≥65 years old with node-negative stage 1 and early node-negative stage 2 (with primary tumors up to 3 cm), hormone receptor-positive breast cancer who are treated with endocrine therapy, radiation therapy (RT) may reasonably be excluded. The risk of an in-breast recurrence is quite low for this population, such that RT may not provide a clinically meaningful benefit[6]
- For women with node-positive disease, postmastectomy RT results in improved breast cancer–specific survival (54.7% vs. 60.1% with no RT) and reduced local recurrence at 15 years (7.8% vs. 29% with no RT)[7]

Discussion

Breast-conserving treatment with radiation has become an oncological mainstay due to long-term proven tumor control outcomes, low overall toxicity with modern heart-sparing techniques, and given that it allows organ-preserving treatment.[3-5,8] With modern techniques, 10-year failure rates of <10% are expected, and the traditional 6-week radiation therapy courses have been replaced by hypofractionated 3–4-week schedules.[8]

References

1. U.S. breast cancer statistics. Available at: http://www.breastcancer.org/symptoms/understand_bc/statistics.
2. Breast cancer facts & figures 2015–2016. Available at: https://www.cancer.org/content/dam/cancer-org/research/cancer-facts-and-statistics/breast-cancer-facts-and-figures/breast-cancer-facts-and-figures-2015-2016.pdf.
3. Fisher B, Anderson S, Bryant J, et al. Twenty-year follow-up of a randomized trial comparing total mastectomy, lumpectomy, and lumpectomy plus irradiation for the treatment of invasive breast cancer. N Engl J Med 2002;347(16):1233-41.
4. Fisher B, Dignam J, Wolmark N, et al. Tamoxifen in treatment of intraductal breast cancer: National Surgical Adjuvant Breast and Bowel Project B-24 randomised controlled trial. Lancet 1999;353(9169):1993-2000.
5. Early Breast Cancer Trialists' Collaborative Group. Effect of radiotherapy after breast-conserving surgery on 10-year recurrence and 15-year breast cancer death: meta-analysis of individual patient data for 10 801 women in 17 randomised trials. Lancet 2011;378(9804):1707-16.
6. Kunkler IH, Williams LJ, Jack WJ, et al. Breast-conserving surgery with or without irradiation in women aged 65 years or older with early breast cancer (PRIME II): a randomised controlled trial. Lancet Oncol 2015;16(3):266-73.
7. Clarke M, Collins R, Darby S, et al. Effects of radiotherapy and of differences in the extent of surgery for early breast cancer on local recurrence and 15-year survival: an overview of the randomised trials. Lancet 2005;366(9503):2087-106.
8. Whelan TJ, Pignol JP, Levine MN, et al. Long-term results of hypofractionated radiation therapy for breast cancer. N Engl J Med 2010;362(6):513-20.

What is the role of adjuvant chemotherapy and anti–human epidermal growth factor receptor 2 (HER2) targeted therapy in breast cancer?

Key concept	The use of adjuvant systemic therapy is responsible for much of the reduction in cause-specific mortality from breast cancer.[1] The goal of cytotoxic chemotherapy after breast cancer surgery is to eradicate microscopic foci of cancer cells that could grow and recur as metastatic cancer. Similar regimens are used regardless of estrogen (ER) or progesterone (PR) receptor status. Treatment targeting HER2 is added for those patients with HER2 overexpression.[2]
Clinical scenario	A 45-year-old woman with stage IIB ER/PR-positive, HER2 neu–negative breast cancer presents after surgery for discussion of systemic therapy. The final pathology showed a 2.5-cm invasive ductal carcinoma, and 3/18 axillary lymph nodes with metastatic disease were identified.

Action items	• **Triple negative breast cancer (ER/PR/HER2 neu negative):** Adjuvant chemotherapy is standard for tumors >0.6 cm in size or pathologically involved lymph nodes (regardless of tumor size)
	  • This is the only form of adjuvant treatment available to this subtype, and studies have suggested a significant risk of recurrence if left untreated[2]
	• **Hormone receptor–positive breast cancer:** Chemotherapy treatment decision-making for women with ER-positive, HER2-negative breast cancers is more complicated
	  • The decision is based on an assessment of the risk of recurrence and likely benefit of treatment based on patient age; tumor type, size, and grade; lymph node status; lymphovascular invasion; or the results of a gene expression profile such as the Recurrence Score (RS)[2,3]
	• **HER2-positive breast cancers:** Adjuvant chemotherapy plus HER2-directed treatment is recommended for all HER2-positive, node-positive breast cancer and for women with HER2-positive, node-negative tumors >0.6 cm in size
	  • The monoclonal antibody trastuzumab is administered concomitantly with chemotherapy; following completion of chemotherapy, it is continued as a single agent (ie, maintenance treatment) for total of 1 year[4]
	  • For those with node-positive disease or tumors >2 cm, pertuzumab, another monoclonal antibody, can be considered concomitantly with trastuzumab for 1 year[5]

	Endocrine therapy is given for patients with ER- and/or PR-positive breast cancer concurrently with trastuzumab during maintenance treatment (following completion of adjuvant chemotherapy) and thereafter for 5–10 years total, depending on the perceived risk of recurrence.
Discussion	In patients with ER/PR-positive breast cancer, decisions regarding the addition of chemotherapy to adjuvant endocrine therapy should be individualized, and gene expression profiles can facilitate this process. Among the gene expression profiles, the 21-gene RS is well-validated, providing a prognostic signature for outcome with endocrine therapy alone. The RS is the only assay shown to predict the benefit from chemotherapy for women with ER-positive breast cancer and either limited or no nodal involvement. Patients with ER-positive cancers that are node negative derive substantial benefit from chemotherapy if the 21-gene RS is high (typically, >24). By contrast, if the score is low (<18), there is no marginal benefit to adding chemotherapy to endocrine treatment.[3]
Pearls	• Chemotherapy can reduce the risk of recurrence in women with early-stage breast cancer • The absolute benefits can reduce and not worth added toxicity among women with a baseline low risk of recurrence • The general approach to treatment in early-stage breast cancer is using a risk-stratified approach based on the presence of factors associated with an increased risk of recurrence
References	1. Berry DA, Cronin KA, Plevritis SK, et al. Effect of screening and adjuvant therapy on mortality from breast cancer. N Engl J Med 2005;353:1784-92. 2. Henry NL, Somerfield MR, Abramson VG, et al. Role of patient and disease factors in adjuvant systemic therapy decision making for early-stage, operable breast cancer: American Society of Clinical Oncology Endorsement of Cancer Care Ontario Guideline Recommendations. J Clin Oncol 2016;34:2303-11. 3. Paik S, Tang G, Shak S, et al. Gene expression and benefit of chemotherapy in women with node-negative, estrogen receptor-positive breast cancer. J Clin Oncol 2006;24:3726-34. 4. Romond EH, Perez EA, Bryant J, et al. Trastuzumab plus adjuvant chemotherapy for operable HER2-positive breast cancer. N Engl J Med 2005;353:1673-84. 5. von Minckwitz G, Procter M, de Azambuja E, et al. Adjuvant pertuzumab and trastuzumab in early HER2-positive breast cancer. N Engl J Med 2017;377:122-31.

What is the role of adjuvant hormone therapy in breast cancer?

Key concept	Breast cancer is composed of several biological subtypes. Hormone receptor–positive (ie, estrogen receptor [ER]– and/or progesterone receptor [PR]–positive) are the most common types of breast cancer, accounting for 75% of all cases. Patients with non-metastatic, hormone receptor–positive breast cancer are candidates for endocrine therapy.[1]
Clinical scenario	A 51-year-old woman with stage I ER/PR-positive HER2 neu–negative breast cancer presents after surgery for discussion about systemic therapy. The breast tumor is sent for 21-gene testing by polymerase chain reaction, and the score is 10, giving her a 7% risk of systemic recurrence in the next 10 years (low-risk group). Endocrine therapy alone is recommended.
Action items	• For pre-menopausal women of average risk (no chemotherapy indicated, low risk-recurrence risk score, >35 years old), tamoxifen is recommended[1] • For pre-menopausal women with high-risk breast cancer (requiring adjuvant chemotherapy, high risk-recurrence score [>31 on the 21-gene recurrence assay], <35 years old), ovarian suppression plus exemestane is recommended[2] • For postmenopausal women, aromatase inhibitors (AIs) are indicated[3] • For women who wish to discontinue an AI due to side effects, changing to tamoxifen therapy is reasonable[4] • Duration of endocrine therapy is a minimum of 5 years: data suggest that longer durations improve disease-free survival, with a greater magnitude of benefit for patients at a higher risk for recurrence; however, decisions must be made based on the original prognosis, the presence of ongoing side effects, and the potential for toxicity[5] • Patients with higher-risk features (eg, those with ≥T3 or node-positive disease) are the most likely to benefit from extended therapy, particularly tamoxifen[5] • For patients with lower-risk disease who are tolerating treatment well and wish to minimize their risk of recurrent or new breast cancers, extended endocrine therapy is also an appropriate option[5]

Discussion	Tamoxifen is a selective estrogen receptor modulator (SERM) that inhibits the growth of breast cancer cells by competitive antagonism of the ER. Side effects include: • A significantly increased risk of thromboembolic disease (by 2%–3%) • Increased the risk of uterine cancer (4% vs. 1% in placebo for women >55 years old) • Increased fatty liver disease, hot flashes, vaginal discharge, sexual dysfunction, and menstrual irregularities[1] AIs suppress plasma estrogen levels by inhibiting or inactivating aromatase, the enzyme responsible for the peripheral conversion of androgens to estrogens. Side effects include: • AI-associated musculoskeletal syndrome (AIMSS), characterized by joint pain and stiffness in 20%–70% of women in studies • Carpal tunnel syndrome • Increased risk of osteoporosis[4]

Pearls	Definitions of menopause are[1]:
	• Women ≥60 years old
	• Women <60 years old if one of the following:
	  • Previous bilateral oophorectomy
	  • No menstrual periods for ≥12 months in the absence of tamoxifen, chemotherapy, or ovarian suppression, and serum estradiol is in the postmenopausal range

References	1. NCCN Clinical Practice Guidelines for breast cancer. Available at: http://www.nccn.org. 2. Francis PA, Regan MM, Fleming GF, et al. Adjuvant ovarian suppression in premenopausal breast cancer. N Engl J Med 2015;372:436-46. 3. Smith IE, Dowsett M. Aromatase inhibitors in breast cancer. N Engl J Med 2003;348:2431-42. 4. Kidwell KM, Harte SE, Hayes DF, et al. Patient-reported symptoms and discontinuation of adjuvant aromatase inhibitor therapy. Cancer 2014;120:2403-11. 5. Davies C, Pan H, Godwin J, et al. Long-term effects of continuing adjuvant tamoxifen to 10 years versus stopping at 5 years after diagnosis of oestrogen receptor-positive breast cancer: ATLAS, a randomised trial. Lancet 2013;381:805-16.

How do I approach a patient with metastatic breast cancer?

Key concept	Patients with relapsed/metastatic breast cancer are categorized according to local vs. systemic recurrence, metastatic sites (bone only vs. visceral disease), and estrogen receptor (ER), progesterone receptor (PR), and HER2 neu receptor status. Performance status and previous treatment are important for therapy selection, as well as tumor burden and palliative symptom management.[1]
Clinical scenario	A 54-year-old woman with a previous history of stage 1 right breast cancer 4 years previously presents with worsening back pain. Lumbar X-rays show lesions in L2–L5 suspicious for metastatic disease. MRI of the spine without contrast confirms findings and reveals evidence of cord compression.
Action items	• **For local relapse only:** Treatment depends on whether the patient underwent mastectomy or breast-conserving therapy including radiation: • For those who had initial breast-conserving therapy, consider mastectomy followed by adjuvant chemotherapy • For those who underwent prior mastectomy, consider surgical resection (if feasible) followed by local radiation • **For distant metastasis:** Depends on site of metastatic disease and receptor status • **Staging evaluation:** CT scan of the chest, abdomen, and pelvis and bone scan; routine PET/CT scan is not recommended • **Repeat biopsy:** To confirm histology and receptor status: there can be discordance in receptor status between primary and metastatic disease, which can impact available therapeutic options

	• **Bone metastasis:** Bisphosphonates such as zoledronic acid or denosumab, which target the RANK ligand, should be used to prevent skeletal-related events such as fracture and cord compression even though they do not improve overall survival • Patients should also be on calcium/vitamin D supplementation • Osteonecrosis of the jaw is a significant risk factor for these patients • Interventions that improve quality of life should be offered, such as radiation therapy for bone pain, impending fractures in weight-bearing areas, and cord compression
Discussion	For patients with ER-positive disease, endocrine therapies can be used sequentially. Combinations with new targeted agents such as CDK4/6 inhibitors and mTOR inhibitors can improve progression-free survival (PFS) and overcome endocrine resistance. For triple-negative breast cancer, chemotherapy is the only systemic treatment available, and the overall prognosis is worse than that of other subtypes. For HER2-positive breast cancer, there are several approved agents in the metastatic setting that improve PFS over trastuzumab/chemotherapy combinations alone: TDM1 (an antibody-drug conjugate), lapatinib, and pertuzumab.
Pearls	• Metastatic breast cancer patients with intact primary may require surgery for palliative reasons (eg, ulceration or bleeding); however, it does not impact overall survival • Less-toxic therapy such as sequential endocrine therapy is recommended for ER-positive breast cancers • Patients with visceral disease or rapidly progressing cancer are offered systemic chemotherapy upfront
References	1. National Comprehensive Cancer Network guidelines for breast cancer. Version 3.2017. Available at: www.nccn.org.

What is the treatment for hormone receptor–positive metastatic breast cancer?

Key concept	Patients with metastatic breast cancer positive for hormone receptors (the estrogen receptor [ER] or progesterone receptor [PR]) should receive upfront endocrine therapy. The choice of therapy depends on menopausal status and prior exposure to these agents. Sequential use of endocrine therapy at disease progression should be considered in patients with prior clinical benefit to first-line endocrine therapy.[1,2]
Clinical scenario	A 48-year-old woman with a previous history of breast cancer stage IIB ER/PR-positive and HER2 neu–negative 3 years ago. She was treated with lumpectomy, axillary lymph node dissection, chemotherapy, and radiation therapy. She is currently taking tamoxifen and presents with 2 months of low back pain. Imaging reveals evidence of pathological compression fracture but no cord compression. Biopsy reveals metastatic invasive ductal carcinoma that is ER/PR-positive and HER 2 neu–negative. What is the appropriate treatment?
Action items	• Repeat biopsy to document the hormonal status of metastatic lesions should be performed when clinically feasible • Up to 15% of metastatic cancers may have ER results discordant with that of the primary tumor
Discussion	**For pre-menopausal patients:** If there is no prior exposure to endocrine therapy, these patients can be treated with a selective ER modulator such as tamoxifen. Another option is ovarian suppression/ablation plus an aromatase inhibitor (AI). Patients with prior exposure to tamoxifen within the preceding 12 months should be treated with ovarian suppression/ablation and AIs. The addition of CDK4/6 inhibitors can be considered for pre-menopausal patients receiving ovarian suppression plus fulvestrant for second-line therapy.

	For post-menopausal patients: These patients have several options available: • Letrozole plus a CDk4/6 inhibitor (palbociclib, ribociclib, or abemaciclib)[3-5] **or** • Non-steroidal AI: single-agent anastrozole or letrozole • Steroidal AI: exemestane • ER down-regulator: fulvestrant • Exemestane plus everolimus (an mTOR inhibitor) after initial endocrine therapy resistance • Fulvestrant plus CDk4/6 inhibitor (in patients who progressed on initial AI therapy) • Selective ER modulators: tamoxifen
Pearls	• Patients with ER-positive breast cancer have several endocrine therapy options • After patients progress to 3 lines of therapy, or for rapidly progressing visceral disease, chemotherapy remains an option
References	1. National Comprehensive Cancer Network guidelines for metastatic breast cancer. Version 2.2017. Available at: www.nccn.org. 2. Lindström LS, Karlsson E, Wilking UM, et al. Clinically used breast cancer markers such as estrogen receptor, progesterone receptor, and human epidermal growth factor receptor 2 are unstable throughout tumor progression. J Clin Oncol 2012;30:2601-8. 3. Finn RS, Martin M, Rugo HS, et al. Palbociclib and letrozole in advanced breast cancer. N Engl J Med 2016;375:1925-36. 4. Hortobagyi GN, Stemmer SM, Burris HA, et al. Ribociclib as first-line therapy for HR-positive, advanced breast cancer. N Engl J Med 2016;375:1738-48. 5. Goetz MP, Toi M, Campone M, et al. MONARCH 3: abemaciclib as initial therapy for advanced breast cancer. J Clin Oncol 2017;35:3638-46.

When do I use chemotherapy in metastatic breast cancer, and what is the role of anti–HER2 neu therapy?

Key concept	Cytotoxic chemotherapy is used for patients with metastatic breast cancer who are refractory to endocrine therapy or those with symptomatic, rapidly progressing visceral metastasis. Single or combination chemotherapy can be used: there is no proven benefit of combination chemotherapy over single agent. HER2 neu–positive patients should be treated with HER2-targeted therapy ± chemotherapy or endocrine therapy, depending on tumor receptors, previous treatment, and performance status.[1]
Clinical scenario	A 65-year-old woman with ER/PR-positive, HER2 neu–negative metastatic breast cancer that has metastasized to bones and who has previously received endocrine therapy presents with increasing right upper quadrant pain and is found to have a new liver metastasis.
Action items	• Sequential chemotherapy can be used with various agents, including anthracyclines, taxanes, and anti-metabolites such as capecitabine, eribulin, and ixabepilone • There is no survival advantage of adding bevacizumab to chemotherapy in metastatic breast cancer[1]
Discussion	Several options are available to treat HER2 neu–positive patients: • Pertuzumab plus trastuzumab in combination with taxanes is the preferred first choice; side effects include rash, diarrhea, and febrile neutropenia[2] • T-DM1 (an antibody drug conjugate) can be used as a single agent in first-line therapy for patients who cannot tolerate the preferred therapy or as second-line therapy[3] • Trastuzumab can be used as a single agent or in combination with chemotherapy such as taxanes and capecitabine • For ER-positive breast cancer, it can be used as first- or second-line therapy in combination with endocrine therapy[4]

	• Lapatinib plus capecitabine (both oral agents) can also be used after initial progression on other regimens[5] • Dual anti-HER2 therapy can be used, such as trastuzumab/lapatinib or trastuzumab/pertuzumab
Pearl	• Patients who progress on trastuzumab-containing regimens should be continued on HER2 blockade after progression
References	1. National Comprehensive Cancer Network guidelines for breast cancer. Version 2.2017. Available at: www.nccn.org. 2. Swain SM, Baselga J, Kim SB, et al. Pertuzumab, trastuzumab, and docetaxel in HER2-positive metastatic breast cancer. N Engl J Med 2015;372:724-34. 3. Verma S, Miles D, Gianni L, et al. Trastuzumab emtansine for HER2-positive advanced breast cancer. N Engl J Med 2012;367:1783-91. 4. Kaufman B, Mackey JR, Clemens MR, et al. Trastuzumab plus anastrozole versus anastrozole alone for the treatment of post-menopausal women with human epidermal growth factor receptor 2-positive, hormone receptor-positive metastatic breast cancer: results from the randomized phase III TAnDEM study. J Clin Oncol 2009;27:5529-37. 5. Geyer CE, Forster J, Lindquist D, et al. Lapatinib plus capecitabine for HER2-positive advanced breast cancer. N Engl J Med 2006;355:2733-43.

How do I treat a patient with inflammatory breast cancer (IBC)?

Key concept	IBC is an aggressive form of breast cancer characterized by skin erythema and dermal edema (peau d'orange; Figure 5-1) of the involved breast. It accounts for 0.5%–2% of invasive breast cancers diagnosed in the United States.[1] They are often hormone receptor negative and HER2-positive. Irrespective of the size of primary tumor, they are considered locally advanced and classified as T4d. 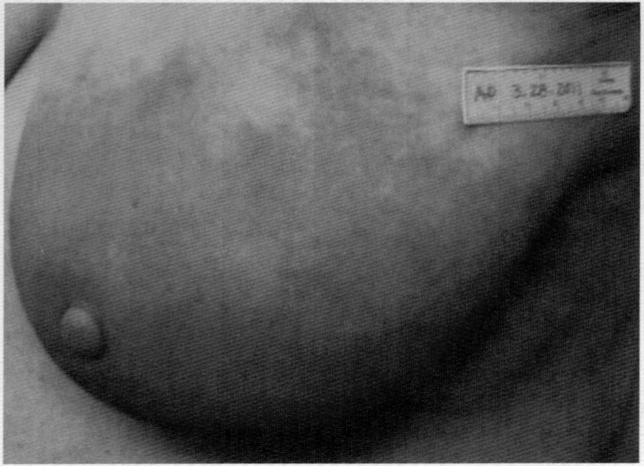 **Figure 5-1.** Inflammatory breast cancer: peau d'orange. (Reproduced with permission from Dr. Anneliese Gonzalez.)

Clinical scenario	A 54-year-old woman presents with redness and thickening of the skin in her left breast. This developed over 3 weeks, with no pain or fever. On exam, there is peau d'orange present with no palpable mass.
Action items	Initial work-up should include mammogram and ultrasound of the breast with core biopsy of suspicious masses and/or axillary lymph nodes and referral to a surgeon for full-thickness skin biopsy. All of the following criteria must be met for diagnosis of IBC[2]: • Rapid onset of breast erythema, edema, and/or peau d'orange, and/or warm breast, with or without an underlying palpable mass • Duration of history <6 months • Erythema occupying at least one-third of the breast • Pathological confirmation of invasive carcinoma Patients should undergo staging studies, CT scans of the chest, abdomen, and pelvis, and bone scan, as this is already locally advanced disease due to the skin involvement with a high probability of metastatic disease. *(continued on following page)*

(continued from previous page)

Discussion	Patients are treated with neoadjuvant (preoperative) chemotherapy including anthracyclines and taxanes for maximal clinical benefit. The addition of anti–human epidermal growth factor receptor 2 (HER2) therapy (trastuzumab/pertuzumab) and/or endocrine therapy is based on ER/PR and HER2 neu status. Patients should undergo mastectomy and axillary lymph node dissection following neoadjuvant chemotherapy. Breast-conserving therapy and sentinel lymph node dissection are not recommended due to skin involvement, causing a high risk of local recurrence. Patients should receive post-mastectomy radiation.[3,4] IBC is associated with a particularly poor prognosis and a high risk of early recurrence, although with proper primary and adjuvant therapies, the survival rate is much higher than in the past. Poor prognostic features include triple-negative receptor status, hormone receptor-positive/HER2-negative status, $\geq$4 involved lymph nodes prior to therapy, and lack of response to neoadjuvant chemotherapy.[5]
Pearls	• Diagnosis of IBC is clinically based on characteristics mentioned above • Skin erythema/peau d'orange is caused by dermal lymphatic invasion by tumor cells on pathological review of skin biopsy (although its presence is not necessary to make a diagnosis of IBC)

References

1. Hance KW, Anderson WF, Devesa SS, et al. Trends in inflammatory breast carcinoma incidence and survival: the surveillance, epidemiology, and end results program at the National Cancer Institute. J Natl Cancer Inst 2005;97:966-75.
2. Dawood S, Merajver SD, Viens P, et al. International expert panel on inflammatory breast cancer: consensus statement for standardized diagnosis and treatment. Ann Oncol 2011;22:515-23.
3. Yang CH, Cristofanilli M. Systemic treatments for inflammatory breast cancer. Breast Dis 2005-2006;22:55-65.
4. Lyman GH, Somerfield MR, Bosserman LD, et al. Sentinel lymph node biopsy for patients with early-stage breast cancer: American Society of Clinical Oncology Clinical Practice Guideline update. J Clin Oncol 2017;35(5):561-4.
5. Liu J, Chen K, Jiang W, et al. Chemotherapy response and survival of inflammatory breast cancer by hormone receptor- and HER2-defined molecular subtypes approximation: an analysis from the National Cancer Database. J Cancer Res Clin Oncol 2017;143:161-8.

What are phyllodes tumors, and how are they managed?

Key concept	Phyllodes tumors are uncommon fibroepithelial breast tumors that exhibit a diverse range of biological behaviors. They can behave like benign fibroadenomas, with a propensity to recur locally after excision without wide margins. Other phyllodes tumors can metastasize distantly and can degenerate histologically into sarcomatous lesions. They usually present as a breast mass or an abnormal mammographic or sonographic finding.[1]
Clinical scenario	A 45-year-old woman presents with a new, rapidly enlarging breast mass. On examination, she has a 4-cm multinodular, well-defined, firm mass that is mobile and painless on the left breast. On mammogram she has a mass that is smooth and lobulated, consistent with a fibroadenoma. What are the next steps?
Action items	• Phyllodes tumors should be suspected on palpable, large (>3 cm), rapidly growing breast masses • Imaging features can be suggestive of fibroadenoma, but rapidly enlarging lesions should undergo core biopsy, and, if inconclusive, surgical excision • Microscopically, the spectrum ranges from resembling a benign fibroadenoma to a high-grade sarcoma • Histologically, phyllodes tumors are classified as benign, borderline, or malignant based on the assessment of four features: (1) the degree of stromal cellular atypia, (2) mitotic activity, (3) infiltrative or circumscribed tumor margins, and (4) the presence or absence of stromal overgrowth (ie, the presence of pure stroma devoid of epithelium) • >50% of phyllodes tumors are classified as benign and 25% as malignant; stromal overgrowth is most consistently associated with aggressive (metastatic) behavior

Discussion

The typical appearance on mammography is a smooth, polylobulated mass resembling a fibroadenoma.

Phyllodes tumors should be completely excised; axillary lymph node dissection is not necessary. Surgical margins ≥1 cm have been associated with a lower local recurrence rate in borderline and malignant phyllodes. If adequate margins can be achieved, breast-conserving surgery and mastectomy are equally effective.[2]

Adjuvant radiation therapy (RT) may benefit borderline or malignant, but not benign, tumors. If adequate surgical margins cannot be achieved, adjuvant RT is recommended. Adjuvant RT reduces local recurrence of borderline or malignant phyllodes tumors but has no effect on overall or disease-free survival.[3]

Chemotherapy is reserved for patients with large, high-risk, or recurrent malignant phyllodes tumors. Hormone therapy is not used.

Phyllodes tumors metastasize most often to the lungs. Tumors that metastasize are typically large (≥5 cm) or have malignant histological features. Pulmonary metastases of phyllodes tumors should be resected when technically feasible.[4]

Pearls

- Phyllodes tumors have been associated with Li-Fraumeni syndrome, a rare autosomal-dominant condition that is characterized by the development of multiple tumors in childhood and early adulthood
- Metastatic disease has been reported in 13%–40% of patients with phyllodes tumors
- The mean overall survival is 30 months in patients who develop metastatic disease
- The majority of patients with benign and borderline phyllodes tumors are cured by surgery
- The survival rate for malignant phyllodes tumors is ~60%–80% at 5 years

References

1. National Comprehensive Cancer Network guidelines for breast cancer. Version 3.2017. Available at: www.nccn.org.
2. Pezner RD, Schultheiss TE, Paz IB. Malignant phyllodes tumor of the breast: local control rates with surgery alone. Int J Radiat Oncol Biol Phys 2008;71:710-3.
3. Zeng S, Zhang X, Yang D, et al. Effects of adjuvant radiotherapy on borderline and malignant phyllodes tumors: a systematic review and meta-analysis. Mol Clin Oncol 2015;3:663-71.
4. Grabowski J, Salzstein SL, Sadler GR, et al. Malignant phyllodes tumors: a review of 752 cases. Am Surg 2007;73:967-9.

CHAPTER 6

Head and Neck Cancer

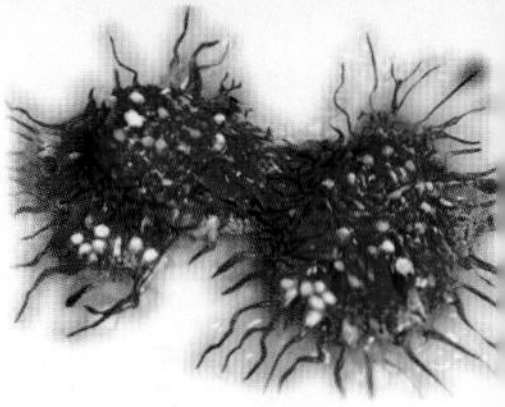

When should I add chemotherapy concurrently to radiation therapy in resected advanced head and neck squamous cell carcinoma (HNSCC)?

Key concept	Disease recurrence is a major problem in resected advanced head and neck cancer. The addition of radiation treatment after surgical resection can reduce the risk of locoregional relapse. The addition of chemotherapy may further reduce that risk and improve outcomes in specific settings.
Clinical scenario	A 53-year-old man is post laryngectomy and left neck dissection for locally advanced laryngeal squamous cell carcinoma. His surgical pathology revealed positive margins, and 2 of 16 lymph nodes were positive for metastatic disease with presence of extracapsular extension (ECE). What adjuvant treatment should he receive?
Action items	Cisplatin is the drug of choice in the adjuvant setting. Cisplatin can be administered either weekly (40 mg/m^2) or every 3 weeks (100 mg/m^2), concurrently with adjuvant radiation. The role of cetuximab in the adjuvant setting remains investigational. Chemotherapy strongly recommended • Positive surgical margin • ECE of nodal disease Chemotherapy to be considered • Pathologic N2/N3 disease • Pathologic T3/T4 disease • Presence of perineural invasion • Presence of lympho-vascular invasion

Discussion	The RTOG95-01 trial, a randomized controlled study comparing adjuvant radiation to combined adjuvant cisplatin and radiation in patients with resected locally advanced HNSCC, revealed that in subgroups of patients with ECE or positive surgical margins, the locoregional failure rate (LRF) and disease-free survival at 10 years were significantly in favor of the chemoradiation arm. There were a trend toward improvement in overall survival (OS) in that study arm as well.[1] Similarly, the EORTC-22931 study enrolled patients with resected HNSCC with high-risk features, including positive surgical margins, ECE, pathologic N2/N3 or T3/T4 stage, perineural involvement, and vascular tumor embolism. Concurrent high-dose cisplatin and radiation improved progression-free survival and OS and lowered LRF compared with adjuvant radiation only.[2]
Pearls	The addition of cisplatin concurrently with radiation improves clinical outcome in patients with high-risk features (and is strongly recommended in patients with ECE or positive margins), at the expense of increased toxicities.
References	1. Cooper JS, Zhang Q, Pajak, TF, et al. Long-term follow-up of the RTOG 9501/intergroup phase III trial: postoperative concurrent radiation therapy and chemotherapy in high-risk squamous cell carcinoma of the head and neck. Int J Radiat Oncol Biol Phys 2012;84(5):1198-205. 2. Bernier J, Domenge C, Ozsahin M, et al. Postoperative irradiation with or without concomitant chemotherapy for locally advanced head and neck cancer. N Engl J Med 2004;350(19):1945-52.

When should I recommend the placement of a feeding tube in a head and neck cancer (HNSCC) patient receiving radiation treatment?

Key concept	Treatment with radiation with or without chemotherapy has improved the outcome of HNSCC patients. However, development of mucosal toxicities is common in these patients and often leads to weight loss. The question is whether a feeding tube should be added prophylactically prior to treatment initiation vs. as needed during or after treatment. Another question arises regarding the optimal method of nutritional support (feeding tube vs. nasogastric tube).
Clinical scenario	A 55-year-old man with no significant history of smoking or alcohol is found to have left neck swelling. Biopsy of the swelling confirms p16-positive squamous cell carcinoma with a left tonsil primary. Patient is recommended to have concurrent chemoradiation. Due to concern for severe mucositis, the oncologist also recommends a feeding tube to help with nutrition.
Action items	• Prophylactic feeding tube placement should be considered for patients with[1]: • Severe weight loss (5% weight loss over 1 month or 10% weight loss over 6 months) • Difficulty swallowing, impairing adequate oral intake • Significant comorbidities that can be worsened with weight loss and reduce calorie intake • Severe aspiration • Anticipation for long-term swallowing disorders, such as in patients expected to receive large-field radiation treatment • Prophylactic feeding tube placement is not recommended in the absence of weight loss, dysphagia, or comorbidities • Gastrostomy and nasogastric tube placement are the options for patients requiring additional enteral feeding support

Discussion	Retrospective data has shown that patients receiving adequate calorie intake support while undergoing radiation with or without chemotherapy are less prone to complication-related hospitalization and treatment interruption.[2] Enteral support with nutritional supplementation can be administered orally or via gastric or nasogastric tube. However, prophylactic feeding tube placement has not been shown to improve outcome and may negatively affect quality of life if used unselectively[3]; it is recommended only in the subgroup of patients at high risk for weight loss or those with swallowing problems. It is important to discuss the risks of gastrostomy tube use, including the procedure-related complications and swallowing muscle disuse, that may lead to feeding tube dependence.[3] Whether the use of a gastrostomy tube is superior to that of a nasogastric tube remains unclear.
Pearls	For patients able to swallow, aggressive oral nutritional support is recommended over prophylactic feeding tube placement. Even patients with a feeding tube in place should be encouraged to continue oral intake if they can swallow without the risk of aspiration. Involvement of a nutritionist and speech therapist is important.
References	1. National Comprehensive Cancer Network guidelines for head and neck cancers. Available at: https://www.nccn.org. 2. Lee JH, Machtay M, Unger LD, et al. Prophylactic gastrostomy tubes in patients undergoing intensive irradiation for cancer of the head and neck. Arch Otolaryngol Head Neck Surg 1998;124(8):871. 3. Hardy S, Haas K, Vanston VJ, Angelo M. Prophylactic feeding tubes in head and neck cancers. J Palliat Med 2016;19(12):1343-4.

What is the role of induction chemotherapy in advanced head and neck squamous cell carcinoma (HNSCC)?

Key concept	The role of induction chemotherapy in locally advanced HNSCC prior to definitive therapy and its impact on overall outcome remain a matter of debate. Induction chemotherapy has the potential benefits of reducing the tumor volume and improving function prior to definitive chemoradiation. It could treat micrometastasis without delay and provide prognostic information to select chemoradiation intensity. By contrast, it can be associated with increased toxicity and can delay or prevent the completion of local definitive therapy.
Clinical scenario	A 53-year-old man presents with severe dysphagia and bulky neck lymph nodes bilaterally. Endoscopy reveals a large hypopharyngeal mass for which the biopsy is positive for squamous cell carcinoma. The patient's calcium level is 13 mg/dL. Would he benefit from induction chemotherapy?

Action items	• Induction chemotherapy may be considered in selected situations such as:
	  • Patients with symptomatic disease for whom a delay in radiation initiation is anticipated for different reasons (eg, logistics or an inability to lie flat on radiation machine)
	  • Patients at high risk for distant metastasis, such as those with bulky cervical lymph nodes, lower neck disease, or questionable distant metastasis on imaging
	• A taxane-containing regimen such as docetaxel, cisplatin, and 5-fluorouracil (DCF) is recommended. Other regimens that are easier to administer and appear to have a good safety profile (such as a weekly carboplatin, paclitaxel, and cetuximab [PCC] regimen) are decent alternatives

Discussion	In two randomized controlled trials, TAX-323 and TAX-324, the addition of docetaxel to induction chemotherapy with cisplatin and 5-fluorouracil was associated with improved overall survival.[1,2] While the Paradigm[3] and Spanish Head and Neck Cooperative group[4] studies showed no survival advantage to adding induction chemotherapy prior to definitive concurrent chemoradiation therapy, an Italian study presented at ASCO2014 revealed a survival advantage with DCF induction chemotherapy regardless of the radiosensitizer used concurrently with definitive radiotherapy (either cisplatin or cetuximab).[5] In a meta-analysis that included randomized controlled trials comparing induction chemotherapy followed by concurrent chemoradiation vs. definitive chemoradiation upfront, induction chemotherapy was associated with higher rate of complete response and lower rate of distant metastasis, but no effect on 2-year overall survival and an increased risk of neutropenic fever.[6]

	A phase 2 trial showed that an alternative regimen consisting of 6 cycles of weekly PCC was associated with an objective response rate of 96%, a 3-year overall survival rate of 91%, and that it was relatively well tolerated.[7]
Pearls	The role of induction chemotherapy in locally advanced HNSCC remains to be defined. Although it is associated with prompt disease control and a lower rate of distant metastasis, its impact on long-term survival has not been confirmed, and can be associated with high toxicity. Whenever used, a taxane-based regimen is recommended (such as DCF or weekly PCC). Further research is needed to define the patients most likely to benefit from this treatment.
References	1. Vermorken J, Remenar E, van Herpen C, et al. Cisplatin, fluorouracil and docetaxel in unresectable head and neck cancer. N Engl J Med 2007;357(17):1695-704. 2. Lorch JH, Goloubeva O, Haddad RI, et al. Induction chemotherapy with cisplatin and fluorouracil alone or in combination with docetaxel in locally advanced squamous-cell cancer of the head and neck: long-term results of the TAX 324 randomised phase 3 trial. Lancet Oncol 2011;12(2):153-9. 3. Haddad R, O'Neill A, Rabinowits G, et al. Induction chemotherapy followed by concurrent chemoradiotherapy (sequential chemoradiotherapy) versus concurrent chemoradiotherapy alone in locally advanced head and neck cancer (PARADIGM): a randomised phase 3 trial. Lancet Oncol 2013;14(3):257-64. 4. Hitt R, Grau JJ, López-Pousa A, et al. A randomized phase III trial comparing induction chemotherapy followed by chemoradiotherapy versus chemoradiotherapy alone as treatment of unresectable head and neck cancer. Ann Oncol 2014;25(1):216-25. 5. Ghi MG, Paccagnella A, Ferrari D, et al. Concomitant chemoradiation (CRT) or cetuximab/RT (CET/RT) versus induction docetaxel/cisplatin/5-fluorouracil (TPF) followed by CRT or CET/RT in patients with locally advanced squamous cell carcinoma of head and neck (LASCCHN). A randomized phase III factorial study. 2014 ASCO annual meeting, abstract #6001. J Clin Oncol 2014;32(15 suppl):6004. 6. Zhang L, Jiang N, Shi Y, et al. Induction chemotherapy with concurrent chemoradiotherapy versus concurrent chemoradiotherapy for locally advanced squamous cell carcinoma of head and neck: a meta-analysis. Sci Rep 2015;5:10798. 7. Kies MS, Holsinger FC, Lee JJ, et al. Induction chemotherapy and cetuximab for locally advanced squamous cell carcinoma of the head and neck: results from a phase II prospective trial. J Clin Oncol 2010;28(1):8-14.

When is the organ preservation approach not considered equivalent to the surgical approach in head and neck cancer?

Key concept	The VA Laryngeal Cancer Study Group study established the larynx preservation approach using chemotherapy and radiotherapy as an alternative to total laryngectomy followed by adjuvant radiotherapy in locally advanced resectable laryngeal cancer.[1] However, in certain clinical scenarios, the organ-preservation modality is not considered equivalent to surgery.
Clinical scenario	A 64-year-old man with a history of smoking presents with remarkable voice changes. Ear, nose, and throat (ENT) exam reveals a large right glottic mass of which the biopsy was positive for squamous cell carcinoma. The mass is eroding through the outer cortex of the thyroid cartilage on CT scan of the neck. A PET/CT shows absence of nodal and distant metastasis. Total laryngectomy is recommended. The patient asks whether he is a good candidate for less-invasive treatment.
Action items	• This patient has T4aN0M0 larynx cancer. In this case, total laryngectomy followed by adjuvant treatment is considered the standard of care • An organ preservation approach using definitive concurrent chemoradiation should not be considered equivalent • In oral cavity and maxillary sinus squamous cell carcinoma, upfront surgery is the preferred treatment approach, followed by adjuvant treatment depending on final staging

Discussion	Previous clinical trials only infrequently included T4a laryngeal cancer, oral cavity cancer, and maxillary sinus cancer. Analysis of the National Cancer Database[1] demonstrated that patients with T4a laryngeal cancer who have undergone total laryngectomy followed by adjuvant radiotherapy have better overall survival (OS) than patients treated with larynx preservation chemoradiation.[1] In another retrospective study, the outcome of patients with locally advanced oral cavity cancers was analyzed. Treatment with surgery and adjuvant radiation therapy yielded a better OS than treatment with concurrent chemoradiation.[2] In a clinical trial conducted in Singapore, patients with resectable, locally advanced head and neck cancer were randomized to undergo primary surgery followed by adjuvant radiotherapy or to receive definitive concurrent chemoradiation. Subgroup analysis revealed a significant superiority of primary surgery in maxillary sinus and oral cavity cancer.[3]
Pearls	In T4a laryngeal cancer, oral cavity, and maxillary sinus squamous cell carcinoma, the organ preservation approach with concurrent chemotherapy and radiation are not considered equivalent to surgery.
References	1. Grover S, Swisher-McClure S, Mitra N, et al. Total laryngectomy versus larynx preservation for T4a larynx cancer: patterns of care and survival outcomes. Int J Radiat Oncol Biol Phys 2015;92(3):594-601. 2. Gore SM, Crombie AK, Batstone MD, Clark JR. Concurrent chemoradiotherapy compared with surgery and adjuvant radiotherapy for oral cavity squamous cell carcinoma. Head Neck 2015;37(4):518-23. 3. Iyer NG, Tan DS, Tan VK, et al. Randomized trial comparing surgery and adjuvant radiotherapy versus concurrent chemoradio-therapy in patients with advanced, nonmetastatic squamous cell carcinoma of the head and neck: 10-year update and subset analysis. Cancer 2015;121(10):1599-607.

What are the systemic treatment options for metastatic head and neck cancer?

Key concept	The treatment of metastatic or recurrent head and neck cancer is affected by different factors, including prior local or systemic therapy (in the adjuvant, definitive, or metastatic setting), timing of the relapse, performance status, organ function, disease symptoms, tumor burden, and site of the disease recurrence. Decisions regarding treatment planning should be based on multidisciplinary evaluation.
Clinical scenario	A 62-year-old man with a history of locally advanced head and neck squamous cell carcinoma (HNSCC) who completed concurrent chemotherapy and radiotherapy 1 year previously presents with multiple lung and liver lesions for which the biopsy is positive for metastatic basaloid squamous cell carcinoma of head and neck origin. The patient remains active and wonders what treatment he should receive.
Action items	• Treatment depends on different clinical scenarios and is influenced by the clinical factors mentioned above[1,2]: • Locally recurrent disease: may consider salvage therapy with curative intent consisting of surgery and/or re-irradiation ± chemotherapy if the patient is a suitable candidate • Oligometastatic disease: surgical resection or stereotactic radiation therapy if the patient is a suitable candidate • Prior recent systemic therapy (within 6 months): treatment with second-line treatment. Pembrolizumab and nivolumab are the agents of choice. An alternative to immunotherapy is single-agent chemotherapy (such as methotrexate, a taxane, or cetuximab) • No prior recent systemic therapy: platinum-based combination therapy (ie, platinum/fluorouracil [5-FU]/cetuximab, platinum/taxane). If the patient is not a candidate for multidrug therapy, single-agent chemotherapy or best supportive care are options • Enrollment in a clinical trial should be encouraged

Discussion

In a SWOG trial,[3] patients with metastatic/recurrent HNSCC were randomized to receive 1 of 3 regimens: cisplatin/5-FU, carboplatin/5-FU, or single-agent methotrexate. Although the overall response rate (ORR) was superior for both combination regimens, no statistically significant difference in overall survival (OS) was noticed among all 3 regimens. Cisplatin/5-FU was associated with more grade 3-4 toxicities than the other 2 regimens. In another ECOG phase 3 trial,[4] combined cisplatin/5-FU was compared to cisplatin/paclitaxel. There was no difference in OS or ORR, and toxicity rates were lower in the cisplatin/paclitaxel arm.

In the EXTREME trial,[5] patients with recurrent or metastatic HNSCC were randomized to receive platinum-5FU or platinum-5FU plus cetuximab. Patients were treated with up to 6 cycles of chemotherapy. Cetuximab could be continued as maintenance in the second arm. The addition of cetuximab was associated with significant improvement in OS (10.1 vs. 7.4 months, $p < 0.05$) as well as in progression-free survival and response rate. Of note, 36% of patients enrolled in this trial had received prior chemotherapy as a part of definitive treatment at least 6 months prior to randomization. These patients benefited from the addition of cetuximab to a similar extent relative to previously untreated patients.

Pearls

Patients with locoregional recurrence should be evaluated by a multidisciplinary team to determine whether the disease is amenable to definitive curative treatment. Combination chemotherapy in the palliative first-line setting increases response rate and disease control at the expense of increased toxicity. The addition of cetuximab to platinum-based chemotherapy improves survival. In the second-line setting, checkpoint inhibitors (pembrolizumab or nivolumab) are the treatment of choice.

References

1. Up-to-date. Available at: https://www.uptodate.com.
2. National Comprehensive Cancer Network guidelines for head and neck cancers. Available at: https://www.nccn.org.
3. Forastiere AA, Metch B, Schuller DE, et al. Randomized comparison of cisplatin plus fluorouracil and carboplatin plus fluorouracil versus methotrexate in advanced squamous-cell carcinoma of the head and neck: a Southwest Oncology Group study. J Clin Oncol 1992;10(8):1245-51.
4. Gibson MK, Li Y, Murphy B, et al. Randomized phase III evaluation of cisplatin plus fluorouracil versus cisplatin plus paclitaxel in advanced head and neck cancer (E1395): an intergroup trial of the Eastern Cooperative Oncology Group. J Clin Oncol 2005;23(15):3562-7.
5. Vermorken JB, Mesia R, Rivera F, et al. Platinum-based chemotherapy plus cetuximab in head and neck cancer. N Engl J Med 2008;359(11):1116-27.

When can I use immunotherapy in the treatment of advanced head and neck cancer?

Key concept	The prognosis of patients with recurrent or metastatic HNSCC who have progressed on platinum-based chemotherapy is generally poor. Prior to the approval of PD1 inhibitors, the standard of care second-line treatment for metastatic HSNCC consisted mainly of single-agent drugs such as methotrexate, docetaxel, and cetuximab. These agents are associated with modest response.
Clinical scenario	A 65-year-old man is undergoing palliative chemotherapy for relapsed head and neck squamous cell cancer. After completion of 4 cycles of carbo-5FU-cetuximab, a repeat CT scan shows progression of disease with new metastasis bilaterally in lungs. The oncologist recommends immunotherapy.
Action items	• Administer pembrolizumab 200 mg IV every 3 weeks for up to 24 months if no disease progression • Administer nivolumab 3 mg/kg or 240 mg every 2 weeks
Discussion	In a phase IB trial, 174 patients with recurrent or metastatic HNSCC who had progressed on or after platinum-based chemotherapy as a part of recurrent or metastatic disease treatment, or as part of induction, concurrent, or adjuvant therapy, were treated with pembrolizumab 10 mg/kg every 2 weeks or 200 mg every 3 weeks. The overall response rate was 16%; the CR rate was 5%. Among responders, 82% had responses of ≥6 months.[1] In the CheckMate-141 trial, 361 patients with recurrent or metastatic HNSCC who progressed within 6 months of platinum-based chemotherapy were randomized to receive nivolumab 3 mg/kg every 2 weeks or investigator chemotherapy of choice (docetaxel, methotrexate, or cetuximab). The median overall survival (OS) and 1 year OS were significantly superior for nivolumab (7.5 vs. 5.1 months, $p = 0.01$; 36.0% vs. 16.6%). Subgroup analysis revealed that OS was superior with nivolumab in p16- or PD-L1–positive patients. Nivolumab was better tolerated than chemotherapy.[2]

Pearls	The PD1 inhibitors pembrolizumab and nivolumab are FDA-approved as standard-of care second-line treatment for patients with recurrent or metastatic HNSCC who have progressed on or after platinum-based therapy. Other checkpoint inhibitors are currently being tested.
References	1. Seiwert TY, Burtness B, Mehra R, et al. Safety and clinical activity of pembrolizumab for treatment of recurrent or metastatic squamous cell carcinoma of the head and neck (KEYNOTE-012): an open-label, multicentre, phase 1b trial. Lancet Oncol 2016;17(7):956-65. 2. Ferris R, Blumenschein G Jr, Fayette J, et al. Nivolumab for recurrent squamous-cell carcinoma of the head and neck. N Engl J Med 2016;375:1856-67.

CHAPTER 7

Gastrointestinal Cancers

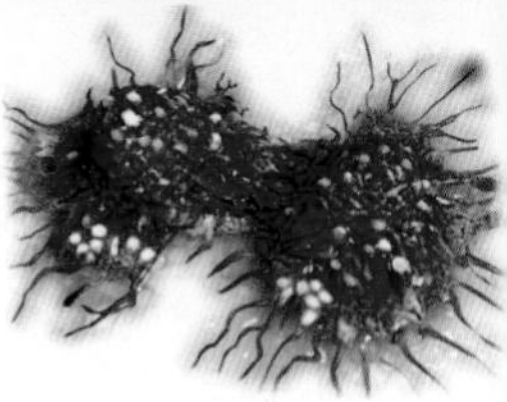

How is anal cancer (AC) treated?

Key concept	AC is a rare cancer with an estimated 8200 new cases diagnosed in 2017; however, there has been a recent increase in the incidence. Some 86%–97% of ACs are associated with human papillomavirus (HPV) infection; HPV-16 and HPV-18 are the high-risk forms associated with AC. Other risk factors associated with AC include history of receptive anal intercourse, immunosuppression after solid-organ transplantation or HIV infection, or other autoimmune disorders.[1] Most patients with AC will present with non-metastatic disease, which is treated with combined modality with chemotherapy and radiation. Metastatic AC represents around 10%–20% of cases, which are treated with systemic chemotherapy.[1]
Clinical scenario	A 48-year-old woman undergoes evaluation by her primary care physician for rectal bleeding. Digital rectal examination revealed a 2-cm mobile mass 2 cm from the anal verge. She undergoes biopsy of the mobile mass, and results are consistent with squamous cell carcinoma of the anus. HIV test is negative, and PET scan is negative for any distant metastasis. MRI of the pelvis demonstrates sub-centimeter inguinal lymph nodes but no other pathologically enlarged lymph nodes. What are her treatment options?
Discussion	Clinical trials has investigated the role of radiation therapy (RT) alone versus combined modality with chemoradiation.[2-4] The landmark UKCCCR** Anal Cancer Trial demonstrated chemoradiation as the standard treatment for AC, compared with RT alone, with lower local failure rates and improvements in recurrence-free survival.[2]

	The RTOG/ECOG[#] conducted a subsequent trial comparing 5-fluorouracil (5FU)/radiation therapy with 5FU-mitomycin-RT and found improved colostomy-free survival and disease-free survival with the 5FU-mitomycin arm, which then became the standard of care.[2,3] One phase 2 study has evaluated capecitabine, which has been used interchangeably with 5FU in colorectal trials, along with mitomycin C. Results showed a tolerable side effect profile and comparable efficacy, with 77% with complete clinical response and 16% partial response.[4]
Pearl	In an HIV-positive patient presenting with AC as their HIV/AIDS-defining illness and a CD4 count >200, consider a chemotherapy regimen similar to 5FU and mitomycin as for an HIV-negative patient.[5,6]
References	1. National Comprehensive Cancer Network guidelines for anal carcinoma. Version 2.2017. Available at: www.nccn.org. 2. Flam M, John M, Pajak TF, et al. Role of mitomycin in combination with fluorouracil and radiotherapy, and of salvage chemo-radiation in the definitive nonsurgical treatment of epidermoid carcinoma of the anal canal: results of a phase III randomized intergroup study. J Clin Oncol 1996;14(9):2527-39. 3. Northover J, Glynne-Jones R, Sebag-Montefiore D, et al. Chemoradiation for the treatment of epidermoid anal cancer: 13-year follow-up of the first randomised UKCCCR Anal Cancer Trial (ACT I). Br J Cancer 2010;102(7):1123-8. 4. Glynne-Jones R, Meadows H, Wan S, et al. EXTRA—a multicenter phase II study of chemoradiation using a 5 day per week oral regimen of capecitabine and intravenous mitomycin C in anal cancer. Int J Radiat Oncol Biol Phys 2008;72(1):119-26. 5. Fraunholz I, Weiss C, Eberlein K, et al. Concurrent chemoradiotherapy with 5-fluorouracil and mitomycin C for invasive anal carcinoma in human immunodeficiency virus-positive patients receiving highly active antiretroviral therapy. Int J Radiat Oncol Biol Phys 2010;76(5):1425-32. 6. Hoffman R, Welton ML, Klencke B, et al. The significance of pretreatment CD4 count on the outcome and treatment tolerance of HIV-positive patients with anal cancer. Int J Radiat Oncol Biol Phys 1999;44(1):127-31.

**United Kingdom Coordinating Committee for Cancer Research.
#Radiation Therapy Oncology Group (RTOG)/Eastern Cooperative Oncology Group (ECOG).

What are the epidemiology and risk factors for esophageal cancer (EC)?

Key concept	EC is the sixth most common cancer worldwide.[1] EC is classified either as squamous cell carcinoma (SCC) or adenocarcinoma (AC).[2] In Eastern Europe and Asia, SCC is the most common type of EC versus AC in the United States and Western Europe.[2]
Clinical scenario	A 64-year-old obese man with body mass index (BMI) >40 and a history of Barrett esophagus undergoes surveillance endoscopy, and biopsy demonstrates esophageal adenocarcinoma. What are his risk factors for developing esophageal cancer?
Action items	See risk factors table below

RISK FACTORS	
EC-SCC[1,2]	**EC-AC[1,2]**
• Male sex • Alcohol* • Tobacco use* • Intake of nitrosamines in salted vegetables and fish	• Male sex • Gastroesophageal reflux • Barrett esophagus • Obesity (specifically abdominal distribution) • Higher BMI • Tobacco

*Synergistic effect of alcohol and tobacco

Pearl	The incidence of EC and the type of histology varies based on geography and ethnicity as well as exposure to risk factors.[1,2]
References	1. National Comprehensive Cancer Network guidelines for esophageal and esophagogastric junction adenocarcinoma. Version 2.2017. Available at: www.nccn.org. 2. Napier KJ, Scheerer M, Misra S. Esophageal cancer: a review of epidemiology, pathogenesis, staging work-up and treatment modalities. World J Gastrointest Oncol 2014;6(5):112-20.

What is the staging work-up for esophagogastric and pancreatic malignancies?

Key concept	Evaluation of esophagogastric[#] and pancreatic malignancies involves a multidisciplinary approach that should include medical oncologists, surgical oncologists, gastroenterologists, radiation oncologists, and pathologists.[1-5]
Clinical scenario	A 63-year-old obese man with a history of Barrett esophagus undergoes endoscopy and is found to have an esophageal mass. What further staging work-up should he undergo?
Action items	

	ESOPHAGOGASTRIC	PANCREATIC
T STAGE	• Tumor (T) staging work-up includes upper GI endoscopy and endoscopic ultrasound (EUS) with biopsy of the primary tumor, and will define the depth of tumor invasion.[1-3]	• If a pancreatic tumor is identified, a multidisciplinary review on approach to biopsy should be done.[4,5] • If no pancreatic mass identified on imaging, then evaluation with EUS, endoscopic retrograde cholangiopancreatography (ERCP), or magnetic resonance cholangiopancreatography (MRCP) is needed.[4,5]
N STAGE	• CT of the chest/abdomen with oral and intravenous contrast can evaluate for nodal disease and any distant metastasis.[3] • EUS provides a more accurate T and N stage in more advanced stage lesions but is limited in T1-T2 lesions.[3]	• Pancreas protocol CT involves triphasic (ie, arterial, late, and venous phases) imaging, which provides improved enhancement between the parenchyma and adenocarcinoma. This imaging will help determine resectability of the cancer by visualizing important arteries including the celiac axis, superior mesenteric artery and vein, splenic vein, and portal vein.[4,5]

	M STAGE	• PET scans are more sensitive in detecting distant metastasis. Up to 15%–20% of patients will be found to have distant metastasis based on PET scan, which can be ordered if all staging work-up has been negative.[1-3]	• If imaging studies are negative for distant metastasis, a diagnostic staging laparoscopy can be considered to detect occult peritoneal metastases.[5] • PET scans are not routinely included in staging but can be considered in high-risk populations, including those with borderline resectable disease, markedly elevated CA19-9 levels, and large pancreatic masses and positive regional lymph nodes.[4]
	OTHER STAGING TESTS	• If staging work-up demonstrates metastatic disease, then pathologic evaluation for deficient mismatch repair or microsatellite instability, human epidermal growth factor receptor 2, and programmed death ligand-1 testing can lead to potential use of either immunotherapy or targeted therapy such as pembrolizumab or trastuzumab, respectively.[1,2]	• CA19-9 is a tumor marker with sensitivity of 50%–81% and specificity of 80%–85%. However, CA19-9 can be elevated in other conditions, such as pancreatitis or biliary obstruction.[4,5] • Studies have shown that an elevated CA19-9 level >100–215 U/mL has been associated with increased likelihood of advanced metastatic disease.[5]
References	1. National Comprehensive Cancer Network (NCCN) guidelines for esophageal and esophagogastric junction cancer. Version 4.2017. Available at: www.nccn.org. 2. National Comprehensive Cancer Network (NCCN) guidelines for gastric adenocarcinoma. Version 5.2017. Available at: www.nccn.org. 3. Berry MF. Esophageal cancer: staging system and guidelines for staging and treatment. J Thoracic Dis 2014;6(Suppl 3):S289. 4. National Comprehensive Cancer Network (NCCN) guidelines for pancreatic adenocarcinoma. Version 3.2017. Available at: www.nccn.org. 5. De La Cruz MS, Young AP, Ruffin MT. Diagnosis and management of pancreatic cancer. Am Fam Physician 2014;89(8):626-32.		

#Esophagogastric malignancies include esophageal, esophagogastric, and gastric malignancies. The above evaluation can be considered for these tumor sites.

What are the risk factors for pancreatic ductal adenocarcinomas, and who should undergo pancreatic cancer (PC) screening?

Key concept	In 2017, although PC was not among the cancers with leading incidence, PC was the fourth leading cause of cancer death in both men and women.[1] Risk factors for PC include family history of PC; hereditary cancer syndromes, including BRCA 1 and 2, Lynch syndrome, and familial malignant melanoma syndrome; chronic pancreatitis; diabetes; and lifestyle factors such as smoking, heavy alcohol consumption, and obesity.[1-3]
Clinical scenario	During a primary care visit, a 60-year-old woman with a history of diabetes and family history, whose father was diagnosed with PC, asks her primary care physician about her risk factors for pancreatic cancer and whether she should undergo PC screening.
Action items	

RISK FACTORS FOR PANCREATIC CANCER

HEREDITARY	**NON-HEREDITARY**
Family history of PC Hereditary cancer syndromes with germline mutations[2]: • BRCA1, 2 • Lynch-DNA mismatch repair genes (MLH1, MSH2, MSH6, or PMS2) • Peutz-Jeghers (STK11 gene) • Familial pancreatitis (PRSS1, SPINK1, or CFTR) • Familial malignant melanoma syndrome (CDKN2A)	• Cigarette smoking • Heavy alcohol consumption • Exposure to chemical and heavy metals (ie, benzenes, pesticides, and chlorinated hydrocarbons) • Obesity or increased body mass index • Long-standing diabetes • Chronic pancreatitis

Discussion	Patients with a family history suspicious of hereditary cancer syndrome should undergo a detailed family history and genetic counseling.[2,4] An international consortium of Cancer of the Pancreas Screening (CAPS) in 2011 developed consensus guidelines for high-risk pancreas cancer screening that include endoscopic ultrasound and/or magnetic resonance imaging/cholangiopancreatography for high-risk individuals[2,4]: • First-degree relatives (FDRs) of patients with PC with at least two affected FDRs • BRCA2 or p16 mutation carriers or Lynch with an affected FDR • Peutz-Jeghers syndrome
Pearl	At the CAPS consortium, there was no consensus on the age to start or stop surveillance, although prior familial studies evaluating PC screening started at age 50.[2,4]
References	1. American Cancer Society. Cancer Facts & Figures 2017. Available at: https://www.cancer.org/research/cancer-facts-statistics/all-cancer-facts-figures/cancer-facts-figures-2017.html. 2. National Comprehensive Cancer Network guidelines for pancreatic adenocarcinoma. Version 3.2017. Available at: www.nccn.org. 3. De La Cruz MS, Young AP, Ruffin MT. Diagnosis and management of pancreatic cancer. Am Fam Physician 2014;89(8):626-32. 4. Canto MI, Harinck F, Hruban RH, et al. International Cancer of the Pancreas screening (CAPS) Consortium summit on the management of patients with increased risk of familial pancreatic cancer. Gut 2013;62:339-47.

What defines resectability for localized pancreatic adenocarcinoma?

Key concept	A multiphase, contrast-enhanced CT including arterial, portal, and venous phase should be ordered to determine the resectability of pancreatic cancer.[1,2] An endoscopic ultrasound (EUS) and endoscopic retrograde cholangiopancreatography (ERCP) can facilitate the pathologic diagnosis of pancreatic cancer.[1,2] Resectability depends on the proximity of vasculature, including the celiac axis (CA), superior mesenteric artery (SMA), common hepatic artery (CHA), superior mesenteric vein (SMV), and portal vein (PV).[1,2]
Clinical scenario	A 63-year-old woman with back pain is found to have a pancreatic mass. She undergoes EUS/ERCP and biopsy of mass shows pancreatic ductal adenocarcinoma. Multiphase CT scan demonstrates a mass at the head of the pancreas with abutment of the common hepatic artery and <90° abutment of superior mesenteric artery. Is she is considered a candidate for resection?
Action items	

RESECTABILITY STATUS[1,2]	**ARTERIAL**	**VENOUS**
Resectable	No arterial contact around the CA, SMA, or CHA	No venous contact with ≤180° SMV or PV
Borderline resectable	<u>Pancreatic head/uncinate process:</u> • Solid tumor contact with CHA without extension to celiac axis or SMA ≤180°	Solid tumor contact with SMV or PV >180° and inferior vena cava
	<u>Pancreatic body/tail:</u> • Solid tumor contact with CA ≤180° and >180° without involvement of aorta or gastroduodenal artery	

Discussion	The type of surgical resection depends on the location of the pancreatic mass. If the tumor is located in the head of the pancreas, then a pancreaticoduodenectomy, also known as a Whipple procedure, is performed, which involves resection of the gallbladder, common bile duct, and the second portion of the duodenum.[2] The hospital mortality following a Whipple procedure is $<2\%$; however, the morbidity of the procedure is around 60%, which is often due to postoperative complications such as delayed gastric emptying, infections, and pancreatic fistulas. Improved long-term survival is associated with an uncomplicated postoperative course.[3]
Pearl	Lymph node involvement and positive margins are poor prognostic factors.[2]
References	1. National Comprehensive Cancer Network guidelines for pancreatic adenocarcinoma. Version 2.2017. Available at: www.nccn.org. 2. De La Cruz MS, Young AP, Ruffin MT. Diagnosis and management of pancreatic cancer. Am Fam Physician 2014;89(8):626-32. 3. Ansari D, Gustafsson A, Andersson R. Update on the management of pancreatic cancer: surgery is not enough. World J Gastroenterol WJG 2015;21(11):3157-65.

What are systemic treatment options for metastatic pancreatic adenocarcinoma?

Key concept

The diagnosis of pancreatic cancer (PC) can be difficult due to nonspecific signs and symptoms and a lack of useful screening tests. If patients present with symptoms such as jaundice (due to biliary obstruction from a pancreatic mass), weight loss, or abdominal pain, PC is likely in more advanced stages, in which >80% of patients presenting have unresectable disease.[1,2]

Systemic therapy for PC has evolved over the years. Since 1997, gemcitabine had been the primary treatment for advanced PC, until the recent development of combination of cytotoxic agents, FOLFIRINOX (5-fluorouracil [5FU], oxaliplatin, irinotecan, and leucovorin) and gemcitabine/nab-paclitaxel. Improvement of quality of life (QOL) has been noted with these novel therapies.[3–5]

Clinical scenario

A 59-year-old woman with weight loss presents to her primary care physician and is found to have elevated liver enzymes with bilirubin of 4.5. She undergoes further imaging and is found to have a pancreatic head mass with involvement of the celiac axis and superior mesenteric vein and 3 hypodense liver lesions consistent with metastasis. CA19-9 is elevated to ~3145. She is a previously healthy female who exercises 3–4 times per week. What are the potential treatment options for this patient?

Action items

TRIAL	TREATMENT ARMS	OUTCOMES	ADVERSE EFFECTS
PRODIGE	FOLFIRINOX vs. Gemcitabine (Gem)	**MEDIAN OVERALL SURVIVAL (OS):** FOLFIRINOX 11.1 vs. Gem 6.8 mo **OBJECTIVE RESPONSE RATE (ORR):** FOLFIRINOX 31.6% vs. Gem 9.4%	5.4% incidence rate of febrile neutropenia in the FOLFIRINOX arm Higher incidence of grade 3–4 neutropenia**, thrombocytopenia, diarrhea, and sensory neuropathy in the FOLFIRINOX arm

	MPACT	Gem/nab-paclitaxel (GA) vs. Gem	**MEDIAN OVERALL SURVIVAL (OS):** GA 8.5 vs. Gem 6.7 mo **OBJECTIVE RESPONSE RATE (ORR):** GA 23% vs. Gem 7%	Peripheral neuropathy is the most common side effect and cumulative but reversible once nab-paclitaxel is discontinued or dose reduced
Pearl	Due to a higher incidence of adverse effects of FOLFIRINOX, a modified FOLFIRINOX regimen (no 5FU bolus) has been evaluated with improved safety profile while maintaining efficacy.[6] Although FOLFIRINOX is a good option for patients with metastatic pancreatic cancer, careful evaluation of comorbidities and patients with good performance (ECOG 0–1) and serum bilirubin <1.5 the upper limit of normal can be considered for this intensive chemotherapy regimen due to high risk of infections.[2]			
References	1. National Comprehensive Cancer Network guidelines for pancreatic adenocarcinoma. Version 3.2017. Available at: www.nccn.org. 2. De La Cruz MS, Young AP, Ruffin MT. Diagnosis and management of pancreatic cancer. Am Fam Physician 2014;89(8):626-32. 3. Conroy T, Desseigne F, Ychou M, et al. FOLFIRINOX versus gemcitabine for metastatic pancreatic cancer. N Engl J Med 2011;364(19):1817-25. 4. Von Hoff DD, Ervin T, Arena FP, et al. Increased survival in pancreatic cancer with nab-paclitaxel plus gemcitabine. N Engl J Med 2013;369(18):1691-703. 5. Gourgou-Bourgade S, Bascoul-Molevi C, Desseigne F, et al. Impact of FOLFIRINOX compared with gemcitabine on quality of life in patients with metastatic pancreatic cancer: results from the PRODIGE 4/ACCORD 11 randomized trial. J Clin Oncol 2013;31(1):23-9. 6. Mahaseth H, Brutcher E, Kauh J, et al. Modified FOLFIRINOX regimen with improved safety and maintained efficacy in pancreatic adenocarcinoma. Pancreas 2013;42(8):1311-5.			

**Based on Common Terminology Criteria for Adverse Events Version 4.0, grade 3 is defined as <1000–500/mm^3 and grade 4 is defined as <500/mm^3.

What are the different biliary tract cancers and their risk factors?

Key concept	Biliary tract cancers include gallbladder (GB) cancers and cholangiocarcinomas.[1] Cholangiocarcinomas are divided anatomically as either intrahepatic or extrahepatic and histologically as mass-forming, periductal-infiltrating, or intraductal-growing. Extrahepatic cholangiocarcinomas are further subdivided into hilar (also known as Klatskin) tumors, which occur at or near the junction of the right and left hepatic ducts, or distal tumors, which arise in the extrahepatic biliary tree above the ampulla of Vater (Figure 7-1).[1] The common risk factor for biliary tract cancers includes chronic inflammation.[1] Evaluation of a cholangiocarcinoma includes cross-sectional imaging with either CT or MRI and sometimes magnetic resonance cholangiography (MRC), which can delineate bile duct dilatation or strictures.[2] Treatment options for biliary tract cancers vary depending on whether the patient presents with resectable disease or metastatic disease.[1]

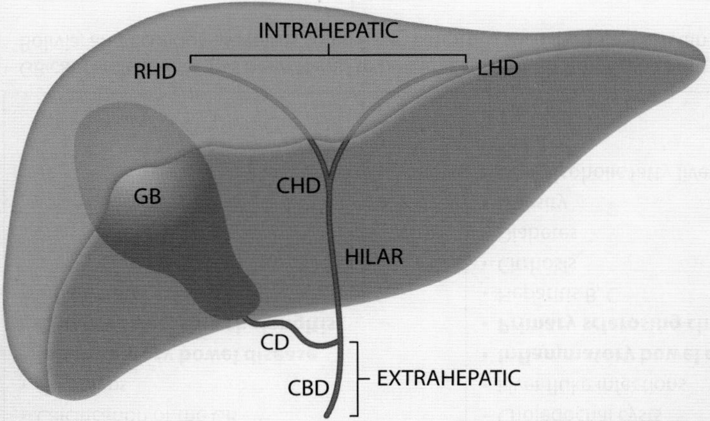

Figure 7-1. Subtypes of Cholangiocarcinoma. GB: gallbladder, RHD: right hepatic duct, LHD: left hepatic duct, CHD: common hepatic duct, CD: cystic duct, CBD: common bile duct.

(continued on following page)

(continued from previous page)

Clinical scenario

A 63-year-old man from Chile with a past medical history of gallstones was admitted for gallstone attack. He underwent laparoscopic cholecystectomy of the GB, and the pathology demonstrated gallbladder adenocarcinoma. What are his risk factors, and what is the next step in management?

Action items

RISK FACTORS	
GB CANCER	**CHOLANGIOCARCINOMA**
• Cholelithiasis • Calcification of the GB • GB polyps • **Inflammatory bowel disease** • **Primary sclerosing cholangitis** • Inflammatory disease	• Chronic calculi of bile duct • Choledochal cysts • Liver fluke infections • **Inflammatory bowel disease** • **Primary sclerosing cholangitis** • Hepatitis B, C • Cirrhosis • Diabetes • Obesity • Non-alcoholic fatty liver disease • Tobacco • Alcohol

- GB cancer incidence has been found to be highest in South American countries, particularly Chile, Bolivia, and Ecuador, as well as some Asian countries such as India, Pakistan, Japan, and Korea[3,4]

Pearls	• For any patient who undergoes cholecystectomy and pathology shows an incidental finding of gallbladder adenocarcinoma, a subsequent surgical resection should include hepatic resection (usually involving the hepatic segments IVb and V) and portal lymphadenectomy involving the lymph nodes in the porta hepatis, gastrohepatic ligament, and retroduodenal regions with the goal to obtain negative margins[1] • Neoadjuvant chemoradiation and liver transplantation can be considered in a patient with hilar cholangiocarcinoma with the tumor size <3 cm in diameter and no evidence of intrahepatic or extrahepatic metastases[2]
References	1. National Comprehensive Cancer Network guidelines for hepatobiliary cancers. Version 3.2017. Available at: www.nccn.org. 2. Razumilava N, Gores GJ. Cholangiocarcinoma. Lancet 2014;383(9935):2168-79. 3. Strom BL, Soloway RD, Rios-Dalenz JL, et al. Risk factors for gallbladder cancer. An international collaborative case–control study. Cancer 1995:76(10);1747-56. 4. Randi G, Franceschi S, La Vecchia C. Gallbladder cancer worldwide: geographical distribution and risk factors. Int J Cancer 2006;118(7):1591-602.

What are the guidelines for hepatocellular carcinoma (HCC) screening?

Key concept	The HCC incidence rate among patients with cirrhosis has been shown to be 2%–4% per year.[1] HCC is associated with several risk factors, most commonly cirrhosis, hepatitis B virus, hepatitis C virus, alcohol, diabetes, nonalcoholic fatty liver disease, and environmental exposures such as aflatoxins B and smoking as well as other less common etiologies such as Wilson disease, hemochromatosis, and alpha-1 antitrypsin deficiency.[1,3]
Clinical scenario	A 58-year-old Hispanic man with BMI >40 and a history of diabetes presents for consultation for elevated liver function tests. An ultrasound of the liver is obtained and demonstrates cirrhosis and no discrete masses found. Should the patient continue HCC surveillance?
Action items	• All patients with risk factors for HCC and/or underlying cirrhotic liver should undergo HCC screening[1,3] • Certain populations of hepatitis B carriers (regardless if not cirrhotic) should undergo HCC screening, including Asian men >40 years old, Asian women >50 years old, patients of African and North African ancestry, and those with a family history of HCC[1]
Discussion	• There are no randomized controlled trials of HCC surveillance in patients; however, there are observational cohort studies that have demonstrated some survival benefit and detection of early-stage HCC[1] • Based on 2017 guidelines by American Association of Liver Diseases, HCC surveillance is generally considered with ultrasound with or without alpha-fetoprotein (AFP) every 6 months[1-3] • If a nodule or lesion >1 cm is found on ultrasound, the next step would be obtaining contrast-enhanced imaging, which could be either triple-phase contrast-enhanced CT or multiphasic MRI[1,2]
Pearl	AFP has not shown adequate sensitivity and specificity for HCC surveillance and should not be used alone for HCC surveillance.[2]

References

1. Heimbach J, Kulik LM, Finn R, et al. AASLD guidelines for the treatment of hepatocellular carcinoma. Hepatology 2018;67(1):358-80.
2. Bruix J, Sherman M. Management of hepatocellular carcinoma: an update. Hepatology 2011;53(3):1020-2.
3. National Comprehensive Cancer Network guidelines for hepatobiliary cancer. Version 2.2017. Available at: www.nccn.org.

What are the criteria for liver transplantation and bridging therapies in hepatocellular carcinoma?

Key concept	Evaluation for liver transplantation for HCC requires a multidisciplinary approach and involves evaluation of the patient's tumor burden and liver function.[1-3]
Clinical scenario	A 65-year-old white man with a history of hepatitis C cirrhosis presents for liver transplant evaluation. His triple-phase CT of abdomen demonstrates two liver lesions measuring 4.5 and 2 cm, and his alpha-fetoprotein (AFP) is approximately 123. What are the therapies to bridge the patient to transplant?

Discussion	• Milan Criteria, which were established by the landmark study by Mazzaferro in 1996,[1] have become the United Network for Organ Sharing (UNOS) transplant criteria and include the following[2]:
	  • Single tumors ≤5 cm in diameter
	  • No more than three nodules ≤3 cm in diameter
	  • No evidence of gross vascular invasion
	  • No regional nodal or extrahepatic distant metastases
	• The University of California at San Francisco (UCSF) criteria expand beyond the Milan/UNOS criteria to include[2]:
	  • Single tumors ≤6.5 cm
	  • Maximum of 3 total tumors with no tumor >4.5 cm
	  • Cumulative tumor size <8 cm
	• The MELD score is a measure of liver function and is used as a measure of pre-transplant mortality[2]
	  • MELD exception points are granted for transplant-eligible HCC patients that reflect the mortality risk due to HCC[1,2]
	• Different locoregional therapies, including transarterial embolization and Y90 ablative therapy, can be used to bridge patients with T2 tumors to liver transplant, in order to decrease disease progression and subsequent dropout from the waiting list; no studies have shown that any strategy appears superior to another[1]

References

1. Mazzaferro V, Regalia E, Doci R, et al. Liver transplantation for the treatment of small hepatocellular carcinomas in patients with cirrhosis. N Engl J Med 1996;334(11):693-700.
2. Heimbach J, Kulik LM, Finn R, et al. AASLD guidelines for the treatment of hepatocellular carcinoma. Hepatology 2018;67(1):358-80.
3. National Comprehensive Cancer Network guidelines for hepatobiliary cancer. Version 2.2017. Available at: www.nccn.org.

What are the different modalities for locoregional therapies for hepatocellular carcinoma (HCC)?

Key concept	Locoregional therapy (LRT) is a common treatment of patients diagnosed with HCC who are *not* considered liver transplant or surgical candidates. LRT includes: • **Ablative techniques** such as radiofrequency, cryotherapy, percutaneous alcohol injection, and microwave • **Arterially directed therapies** such as transarterial embolization or radioembolization with yttrium-90 (y90) microspheres, and • **External beam radiotherapy (EBRT)** Transarterial embolization can be either bland (TAE) or involve the use of chemotherapy agents such as doxorubicin or mitomycin (TACE), or TACE with doxorubicin-eluting embolic beads.[1]
Clinical scenario	A 63-year-old Vietnamese man with a history of hepatitis B underwent HCC surveillance screening and was found to have a 3-cm liver lesion that involves the portal vein with evidence of main portal invasion. He has no history of hepatic encephalopathy, and a physical exam is negative for any ascites. His albumin is 3.8, INR 1.0, and total bilirubin is 1.0. What treatment options can be offered?
Discussion	• Ablative techniques can be considered "curative" for patients with lesions $\leq$3 cm • Lesions >5 cm should be considered for arterially-directed therapies, either TAE, TACE, or y90; multifocal HCC should not be treated with LRT, and patients should undergo evaluation for systemic therapy with sorafenib[1] • A phase 3 randomized, double-blind, placebo-controlled trial (STORM) demonstrated no improvement in recurrence-free survival (RFS) in patients who underwent surgical resection or local ablative therapy with adjuvant sorafenib[2] • Recent trials have demonstrated no improvement in time to progression with adjuvant sorafenib after arterially directed therapies[3,4]

Pearls	• For ablative therapies, the tumor should NOT be near blood vessels, major bile ducts, diaphragm, or other organs, including heart, stomach, or other abdominal organs[1] • Patients with tumors with main portal vein thrombosis, Child-Pugh score C, or total bilirubin >3 mg/dL are NOT considered candidates for arterially directed therapies[1] • EBRT includes advanced techniques such as intensity-modulated radiation therapy and stereotactic body radiation therapy that can be performed on any liver tumor, irrespective of tumor location, but should be considered carefully in patients with Child-Pugh B or worse liver dysfunction (prior EBRT trials consisted of HCC patients with Child-Pugh A liver disease)[1]
References	1. National Comprehensive Cancer Network guidelines for hepatobiliary cancer. Version 2.2017. Available at: www.nccn.org. 2. Bruix J, Takayama T, Mazzaferro V, et al. Adjuvant sorafenib for hepatocellular carcinoma after resection or ablation (STORM): a phase 3, randomised, double-blind, placebo-controlled trial. Lancet Oncol 2015;16(13):1344-54. 3. Pawlik TM, Reyes DK, Cosgrove D, et al. Phase II trial of sorafenib combined with concurrent transarterial chemoembolization with drug-eluting beads for hepatocellular carcinoma. J Clin Oncol 2011;29(30):3960-7. 4. Kudo M, Imanaka K, Chida N, et al. Phase III study of sorafenib after transarterial chemoembolisation in Japanese and Korean patients with unresectable hepatocellular carcinoma. Eur J Cancer 2011;47(14):2117-27.

What are the different staging systems for hepatocellular carcinoma (HCC)?

Key concept

HCC is a unique malignancy with several staging classifications that help determine its stage and prognosis. However, there is no consensus on which is the best staging system to use.[1-3] The most commonly used staging systems include the TNM system, Barcelona Clinic Liver Cancer (BCLC) staging classification (Figure 7-2), Okuda, and Cancer of the Liver Italian Program (CLIP) Score, which includes the cirrhosis severity and Child-Pugh score.[1-3]

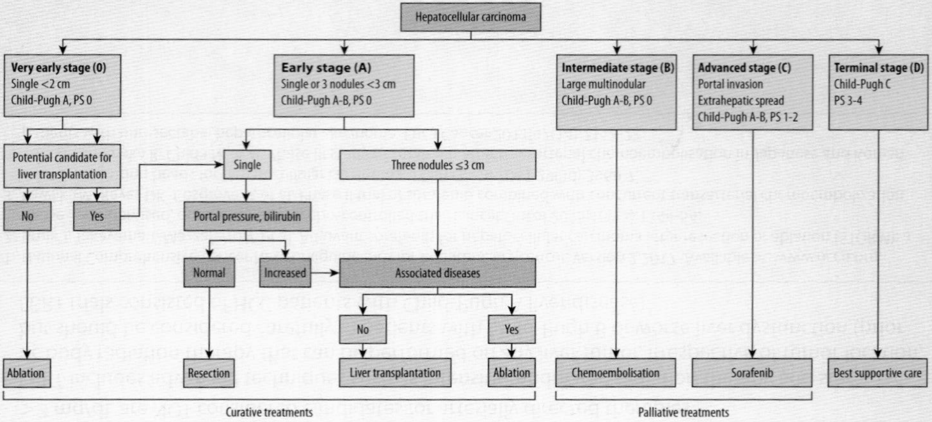

Figure 7-2. Barcelona Clinic Liver Center Staging System. (Reproduced with permission from Springer: Faria SC et al. TNM/Okuda/Barcelona/UNOS/CLIP international multidisciplinary classification of hepatocellular carcinoma: concepts, perspectives, and radiologic implications. Abdom Imaging 2014 39(5):1070-1087. Copyright © 2014.)

Clinical scenario	A 63-year-old obese white man with a history of hepatitis C and diabetes undergoes triple-phase CT and is found to have a 5-cm liver mass and 2 additional masses measuring 2 and 3 cm. There is evidence of portal vein thrombosis. He has no history of encephalopathy, ascites, or GI bleeds. His laboratory results are significant for albumin 3.3, total bilirubin of 1.0, and INR of 1.2. What is his disease stage?
Discussion	• Developed in 1984, **Okuda** staging was the first staging system for HCC; it combines tumor characteristics and hepatic function but does not effectively stratify patients with early disease[2] • **TNM staging** describes the extent of the tumor and vascular invasion and does not include hepatic function[1-3] • The **BCLC** is the *only* staging system that stratifies patients into 5 categories and includes a treatment algorithm with treatment recommendations based on the stage[2,3] • The **CLIP** system consists of 4 variables including tumor characteristics (ie, tumor extent and morphology), alpha-fetoprotein, portal vein thrombosis, and Child-Pugh score[3] • The **Child-Pugh score** was originally developed to estimate outcomes after surgical management of bleeding varices with cirrhosis and portal hypertension. The score includes the following parameters: albumin, prothrombin time, bilirubin, the presence of ascites, and history of encephalopathy[1-3]
Pearl	Due to the heterogeneity of HCC and disease characteristics based on geography, no universal staging system is used.[1-3]
References	1. National Comprehensive Cancer Network guidelines for hepatobiliary cancer. Version 2.2017. Available at: www.nccn.org. 2. Faria SC, Szklaruk J, Kaseb AO, et al. TNM/Okuda/Barcelona/UNOS/CLIP international multidisciplinary classification of hepatocellular carcinoma: concepts, perspectives, and radiologic implications. Abdom Imaging 2014;39(5):1070-87. 3. Maida M, Orlando E, Cammà C, et al. Staging systems of hepatocellular carcinoma: a review of literature. World J Gastroenterol 2014;20(15):4141-50.

What systemic therapy can be used to treat multifocal, advanced hepatocellular carcinoma (HCC)?

Key concept	Sorafenib, an oral multikinase inhibitor of serine–threonine kinases Raf-1 and B-Raf and the receptor tyrosine kinase activity of vascular endothelial growth factor receptors (VEGFRs) 1, 2, and 3 and platelet-derived growth factor receptor β (PDGFR-β), is the mainstay of treatment for patients with Child-Pugh score A or B multifocal, advanced HCC.[1] Sorafenib inhibits tumor-cell proliferation and angiogenesis and induces apoptosis.[1] A recent phase III study evaluated lenvatinib (L) versus sorafenib (S) for first line treatment in multifocal, advanced HCC and demonstrated non-inferiority in overall survival between the two arms. However, the progression-free survival was improved in the lenvatinib arm (L: 7.4 months vs. S: 3.7 months).[2] Multiple second-line treatments have been developed for HCC patients who have failed sorafenib, including other multikinase inhibitors such as regorafenib,[3] which targets similar pathways as sorafenib, and cabozantinib,[4] a MET, VEGFR, and AXL inhibitor. The role of checkpoint inhibitors such as nivolumab and pembrolizumab is being further evaluated based on promising results in early phase 1–2 studies that have shown overall response rates (ORR) around 14%–16%.[5,6]

Clinical scenario

A 62-year-old African-American man with a history of hepatitis C and alcoholic cirrhosis presents with a triple-phase CT of the abdomen demonstrating innumerable liver lesions consistent with HCC. The patient denies any history of encephalopathy, and his ascites is controlled with diuretics. His albumin is 3.0, total bilirubin is 1.5, and international normalized ratio (INR) is 1.7. What systemic treatment options does he have?

Discussion

Two landmark phase III, double-blind, placebo-controlled trials have demonstrated improvements in median overall survival using sorafenib[1,7]:

TRIAL	PATIENT POPULATION	STUDY ENDPOINT	SORAFENIB ARM	PLACEBO ARM
SHARP[1]	602 patients (Europe, North America, South America, Australia)	Median OS	10.7 months	7.9 months
		Median time to radiologic progression	5.5 months	2.8 months
Asia-Pacific[7]	271 patients (China, South Korea, Taiwan)	Median OS	6.5 months	4.2 months
		Median TTP	2.8 months	1.4 months

Abbreviations: OS, overall survival; TTP, time to progression

(continued on following page)

	(continued from previous page) • In patients with Child-Pugh score C, there is limited data on the safety of sorafenib; a CALGB trial evaluated the safety of sorafenib in patients with hepatic or renal dysfunction and found a possible association with elevated bilirubin and hepatoxicity[8] • The RESORCE trial investigated regorafenib vs. placebo in 573 patients who progressed or were previously treated with sorafenib. Results showed an improvement in median OS (regorafenib 10.6 months vs. placebo 7.8 months)[3] • In a phase 1/2 trial of nivolumab in patients who had received prior sorafenib, the ORR was 14.3%, with 2 complete responses and 19 partial response. This trial included patients with chronic viral hepatitis[5] • In a phase 2 trial of pembrolizumab, the ORR was similar, at ~16.3%; responses were observed for hepatitis B or C and uninfected patients with HCC[6]
Pearls	• Sorafenib is the first-line treatment for patients with multifocal, advanced HCC • Regorafenib is the second-line treatment for patients previously treated with or whose disease progressed on sorafenib • Checkpoint inhibitors are being further evaluated in first- and second-line treatment of HCC

References

1. Llovet JM, Ricci S, Mazzaferro V, et al. Sorafenib in advanced hepatocellular carcinoma. N Engl J Med 2008;359(4):378-90.
2. Cheng A-L, Finn RS, Qin S, et al. Phase III trial of lenvatinib (LEN) vs sorafenib (SOR) in first-line treatment of patients (pts) with unresectable hepatocellular carcinoma (uHCC). J Clin Oncol 2017;35 (suppl; abstr 4001).
3. Bruix J, Qin S, Merle P, et al. Regorafenib for patients with hepatocellular carcinoma who progressed on sorafenib treatment (RESORCE): a randomised, double-blind, placebo-controlled, phase 3 trial. Lancet 2017;389(10064):56-66.
4. Abou-Alfa GK, Meyer T, Cheng A-L. Cabozantinib versus placebo in patients with advanced hepatocellular carcinoma who have received prior sorafenib: results from the randomized phase III CELESTIAL trial. J Clin Oncol 2018;36(suppl 4S; abstr 207).
5. El-Khoueiry AB, Sangro B, Yau T, et al. Nivolumab in patients with advanced hepatocellular carcinoma (CheckMate 040): an open-label, non-comparative, phase 1/2 dose escalation and expansion trial. Lancet 2017;389(10088):2492-502.
6. Zhu AX, Knox JJ, Kudo M, et al. KEYNOTE-224: Phase II study of pembrolizumab in patients with previously treated advanced hepatocellular carcinoma. J Clin Oncol 2017;35(4 suppl):TPS504-TPS504.
7. Cheng AL, Kang YK, Chen Z, et al. Efficacy and safety of sorafenib in patients in the Asia-Pacific region with advanced hepatocellular carcinoma: a phase III randomised, double blind, and placebo-controlled trial. Lancet Oncol 2009;10(1):25-34.
8. Miller AA, Murry DJ, Owzar K, et al. Phase I and pharmacokinetic study of sorafenib in patients with hepatic or renal dysfunction: CALGB 60301. J Clin Oncol 2009;27(11):1800-5.

What are the surgical options for colon and rectal cancer?

Key concept	In 2017, ~135,430 new cases of colon and rectal cancers were expected to be diagnosed in the United States.[1] This results in 50,000 cancer-related deaths per year. Five-year survival approaches 90% for patients with localized disease (that has not spread to regional lymph nodes).[2]
Clinical scenario	A 61-year-old African-American woman presents to her primary care physician with complaints of a 15-pound weight loss, new-onset constipation, and occasional bright red blood per rectum. On digital rectal exam, there is no appreciable mass. A colonoscopy demonstrates a circumferential mass 12 cm from the anal verge. CT scan of the chest/abdomen and pelvis demonstrates the mass at the pelvic inlet (rectosigmoid). There is no evidence of metastatic disease. Patient is referred to surgical oncology. What are potential surgical options for the patient?

Discussion	• Surgical treatment options for colon and rectal cancer will vary based on the location of the tumor[2]
	• Treatment for clinically localized (eg, nonmetastatic) colon cancer includes partial colectomy, wide mesenteric resection, and primary anastomosis[3,4]
	• Minimally invasive colon surgery (eg, laparoscopic) is an acceptable option for patients with non-obstructed, non-perforated colon cancer
	  • Several small incisions (5–10 mm) are made in the abdominal wall
	  • A small video camera (5 or 10 mm) is used to assist visualization of the abdominal organs during the procedure
	• The choice of treatment for rectal cancer depends on clinical stage: neoadjuvant chemoradiation is indicated for larger tumors, T3/T4 tumors, or lymph node–positive disease as detected preoperatively by MRI or endorectal ultrasound[5]

	• Surgical options for rectal cancer are more complex and include sphincter-sparing surgeries such as low anterior resection with possible colorectal or coloanal anastomosis versus abdominoperineal resection • The distal margin from the tumor is an important criterion in determining surgical options[5] • Postoperative radiation for rectal cancer should be avoided, if possible, due to significant bowel dysfunction and anastomotic stricture formation[6]
Pearl	Oxaliplatin-based chemotherapy is indicated for stage III disease (ideally started within 8 weeks after surgery).[3,4]
References	1. Siegel RL, Miller KD, Jemal A. Cancer statistics, 2017. CA Cancer J Clin 2017;67(1):7-30. 2. Howlader N, Noone AM, Kraphcho M, et al. SEER cancer statistics review, 1975–2013. National Cancer Institute, Bethesda, MD. Available at: http://seer.cancer.gov/csr/1975_2013/. 3. Andre T, Boni C, Navarro M, et al. Improved survival with oxaliplatin, fluorouracil, and leucovorin as adjuvant treatment in stage II or III colon cancer in the MOSAIC trial. J Clin Oncol 2009;27(19):3109-16. 4. Klein M, Azaquoun N, Jensen BV, et al. Improved survival with early adjuvant chemotherapy after colonic resection for stage III colonic cancer: a nationwide study. J Surg Oncol 2015;112(5):538-43. 5. National Comprehensive Cancer Network guidelines for colon cancer. Version 2.2017. Available at: http://www.nccn.org. 6. Sauer R, Becker H, Hohenberger W, et al. Preoperative versus postoperative chemoradiotherapy for rectal cancer. N Engl J Med 2004;351(17):1731-40.

What are mismatch repair (MMR) genes and microsatellite instability (MSI), and how do we test for them in colorectal cancer (CRC)?

Key concept	Around 15% of CRCs have a defect in MMR pathways.[1] Testing for MMR deficiency and MSI are helpful tools in CRC in determining cases with possible underlying Lynch syndrome due to mutation in MMR genes (*MLH1, MSH2, MSH6, PMS2,* and *EPCAM*) as well as whether adjuvant chemotherapy is appropriate.[2] MSI tumors are usually right sided, well-differentiated, with a mucinous phenotype and intratumoral lymphocytes, and have better prognosis.[1,2] Tumors do not respond well to 5-fluorouracil (5FU) chemotherapy.[2,3]
Clinical scenario	A 55-year-old woman with stage II (pT3 N0) CRC who has undergone right hemicolectomy. Does she need adjuvant chemotherapy, and what tools can be used to help with risk assessment?
Action items	Clinician and patient should discuss benefits and risks of adjuvant chemotherapy[2] Risk assessment should include factors such as number of lymph nodes removed, poor prognostic features (ie, poor differentiation, lymphovascular invasion, perineural invasion, bowel obstruction, perforation, or resection margins)[2] MMR and MSI testing can be done through MMR immunohistochemistry (IHC) or polymerase chain reaction (PCR)[1]

TEST	RESULTS	DEFINITION
MMR protein expression by IHC	Defect in MMR (dMMR)	Absence or loss of protein expression (*MLH1, PMS2, MSH2,* and *MSH6*).
	Intact MMR expression	Presence of protein expression (*MLH1, PMS2, MSH2,* and *MSH6*).

	Microsatellite stable by PCR	MSI—high or unstable	Presence of instability in ≥30% of markers.
		MSI—low	Presence of instability in 10%–29% of markers.
		MSS or stable	NO unstable markers detected.
Discussion	The MMR mechanism identifies and fixes DNA damage from base-pair mismatches. Due to defects in the MMR mechanism, microsatellites, short tandem repeats that make up about 3% of the genome, become hypermutated and are considered "MSI-high." *MLH1/PMS2* and *MSH2/MSH6* are the most common heterodimers involved in CRC pathogenesis.[1-3]		
Pearls	• Tumors with dMMR or that are MSI high are less likely to benefit from 5FU adjuvant chemotherapy[2] • Tumors with sporadic dMMR that demonstrates loss of *MLH1* and *PMS2* should obtain follow-up testing with *MLH-1* promoter hypermethylation and/or *BRAF* V600E mutational analysis to determine whether they are of sporadic or germline etiology: the latter requires further genetic testing to confirm diagnosis but may be performed in a targeted manner using IHC results[1,2]		
References	1. Chen W, Swanson BJ, Frankel WL. Molecular genetics of microsatellite-unstable colorectal cancer for pathologists. Diagn Pathol 2017;12(1):24. 2. National Comprehensive Cancer Network guidelines for colon cancer. Version 2.2017. Available at: www.nccn.org. 3. Armaghany T, Wilson JD, Chu Q, Mills G. Genetic alterations in colorectal cancer. Gastrointest Cancer Res 2012;5(1):19-27.		

What are the common molecular pathways of colorectal cancer (CRC), and what mutations are clinically applicable?

<table>
<tr><td>Key concept</td><td>There are at least 3 pathways (ie, chromosomal instability, microsatellite instability [MSI], and CpG island methylator phenotype) identified in CRC carcinogenesis.[1] Testing of KRAS, NRAS, BRAF, and MSI can be helpful in determining what agents can be used to treat CRC.[2]</td></tr>
<tr><td>Clinical scenario</td><td>A 64-year-old man is diagnosed with metastatic adenocarcinoma of the descending colon with metastatic lesions in the liver and lungs. What are the treatment options, and what tests can you order?</td></tr>
<tr><td>Action items</td><td>
<table>
<tr><th>TEST</th><th>COMMON MUTATIONS</th><th>CLINICAL IMPLICATIONS</th></tr>
<tr><td>KRAS</td><td>Exon 2, codons 12 & 13 (40%)
Exon 3
Exon 4</td><td rowspan="3">Recommend against use of anti–epidermal growth factor (EGFR) agents (ie, cetuximab or panitumumab)</td></tr>
<tr><td>NRAS</td><td>Exon 2, 3, 4</td></tr>
<tr><td>BRAF</td><td>V600E (5%–7%)</td></tr>
<tr><td>MSI by polymerase chain reaction</td><td>MSI—high or unstable</td><td>Less likely to benefit from 5-fluorouracil chemotherapy.</td></tr>
</table>
</td></tr>
</table>

Discussion	The chromosomal instability pathway is also known as the adenoma-carcinoma sequence, which describes the progression of cancer from genomic changes including activation of proto-oncogene *KRAS* and inactivation of tumor suppressor genes (*APC, p53,* and loss of heterozygosity for long arm of chromosome 18, 18 q LOH). Defects in mismatch repair pathways and MSI are seen in >95% of patients with Lynch syndrome, compared to 15%–20% of patients with sporadic CRC. CpG island methylation is an aberrant epigenetic change resulting in genomic instability. This subtype with this phenotype also has *BRAF-V600E* mutations.[2] Downstream effectors of EGFR signaling include *RAS, RAF, MEK, PI3K,* and *PTEN*. Clinical studies have demonstrated a better response to therapy in unmutated CRC.
Pearls	CRC patients with *KRAS, NRAS,* and *BRAF* mutations do not benefit from anti-EGFR agents.[1] However, recent trials demonstrated an improved progression-free survival benefit in patients with *BRAF* V600E treated with irinotecan, cetuximab, and vermurafenib.[2]
References	1. Armaghany T, Wilson JD, Chu Q, Mills G. Genetic alterations in colorectal cancer. Gastrointest Cancer Res 2012;5(1):19-27. 2. National Comprehensive Cancer Network guidelines for colon cancer. Version 2.2017. Available at: www.nccn.org.

Should the elderly receive adjuvant chemotherapy for colon cancer?

Key concept	Adjuvant chemotherapy (single-agent 5-fluorouracil (5FU)/leucovorin versus FOLFOX) in elderly patients with stage III CRC should be carefully evaluated based on patient's performance status, comorbid conditions, and organ function.[1]
Clinical scenario	A 72-year-old woman presents after recent right colon resection and is found to have stage III pT3 N1 Mx adenocarcinoma of the proximal cecum. Two of 15 assessed lymph nodes had cancer involvement. She wants to talk about treatment options. She has a history of hypertension and hypothyroidism. She lives by herself and is able to perform her daily activities. She is able to drive herself to run errands. She walks about 30 minutes a day. She denies any history of peripheral neuropathy. What are possible adjuvant chemotherapy options for this patient?

Discussion	• The benefit of adjuvant chemotherapy with 5FU/leucovorin in both elderly and younger patients has been demonstrated in population studies in stage III colon cancer[1]
	• Studies are not conclusive on the benefit of adding oxaliplatin in stage III elderly patients
	  • An evaluation of >4800 stage III colon cancer patients found a disease-free–survival benefit regardless of age and comorbidities. However, patients ≥70 years old had a more modest benefit and experienced a higher proportion of serious grade 3/4 adverse effects[2]
	  • ACCENT database demonstrated patients ≥70 years old had a reduced benefit with the addition of oxaliplatin[3]

Pearl	A comprehensive geriatric assessment, often performed by a geriatrician, includes a thorough evaluation of overall health including comorbidities, functional status, and nutritional and cognitive function. This is a powerful tool that can predict toxicity from treatment and the presence of geriatric syndromes.[4]

References

1. National Comprehensive Cancer Network guidelines for colon cancer. Version 2.2017. Available at: www.nccn.org.
2. Haller DG, O'Connell MJ, Cartwright TH, et al. Impact of age and medical comorbidity on adjuvant treatment outcomes for stage III colon cancer: a pooled analysis of individual patient data from four randomized controlled trials. Ann Oncol 2015;26(4):715-24.
3. McCleary NJ, Meyerhardt JA, Green E, et al. Impact of age on the efficacy of newer adjuvant therapies in patients with stage II/III colon cancer: findings from the ACCENT database. J Clin Oncol 2013;31(20):2600-6.
4. National Comprehensive Cancer Network guidelines for Older Adult Oncology. Version 2.2017. Available at: www.nccn.org.

What are secondary/lifestyle modifications and survivorship strategies for colorectal cancer (CRC)?

Key concept	Survivorship plans should include disease prevention measures such as screening for secondary cancers, immunizations, monitoring for long-term sequelae from prior treatment (ie, chemotherapy, radiation, or surgery), and management of long-term problems associated with treatment.[1] Evidence supports chemoprevention strategies including healthy lifestyle with diet, exercise, and limited alcohol consumption.[2] The role of aspirin in chemoprevention is controversial, although some studies have demonstrated a benefit. However, there is increased risk of bleeding and stroke. The optimal dose of aspirin has not been determined.[3]	
Clinical scenario	A 58-year-old woman with stage IIIA adenocarcinoma of the transverse colon has completed adjuvant chemotherapy. She asks about strategies to prevent colon cancer. What are the recommendations?	

Action items	**SCREENING SECONDARY CANCERS**
	• The overall cancer rate is higher among cancer survivors
	
	LONG-TERM ADVERSE EFFECTS
	• Peripheral neuropathy
	• Chronic gastrointestinal/urinary or pelvic problems
	• Fatigue, insomnia
	• Cognitive dysfunction
	• Psychosocial distress
	• Sexual dysfunction
		IMMUNIZATIONS
		• Influenza vaccine annually
		• Pneumococcal vaccine
		  • 13-valent pneumococcal conjugate vaccine (PCV13) × 1 dose if never vaccinated
		  • 23-valent pneumococcal polysaccharide (PPSV23) administered at least 8 weeks after PCV13
		  • For those who have received PPV23, PCV13 administered >1 year after PPSV23 administration
		• Tetanus/diphtheria/pertussis (Td/Tdap)
		  • Tdap × 1 dose to adults ≤65 years old who have received it previously or for whom vaccine status is unknown
		  • Td booster yearly
		• Zoster: if ≥60 years old, then administer once

	DIET • Intake of larger amounts of whole grains, fruits, vegetables, poultry, and fish • Decreased intake of red and processed meat	**SOCIAL** • Smoking cessation • Alcohol abstinence
	EXERCISE • Moderate exercise (at least 150 minutes/week)	**CHEMOPREVENTION** • Aspirin
References	1. National Comprehensive Cancer Network guidelines for colon cancer. Version 2.2017. Available at: www.nccn.org. 2. Wu W, Guo F, Ye J, et al. Pre- and post-diagnosis physical activity is associated with survival benefits of colorectal cancer patients: a systematic review and meta-analysis. Oncotarget 2016;7:52095-103. 3. Bains SJ, Mahic M, Myklebust TA, et al. Aspirin as secondary prevention in patients with colorectal cancer: an unselected population-based Study. J Clin Oncol 2016;34(21):2501-8.	

What are the different type of neuroendocrine tumors (NETs)?

Key concept

NETs include carcinoid tumors in the lung and bronchi and entire gastrointestinal tract such as the stomach, small intestine, appendix, colon and rectum, and pancreas.[1-3] The pathological evaluation of neuroendocrine tumors includes differentiation, grade, mitotic rate, and proliferation index of Ki67.[1] Several general neuroendocrine markers are known: chromogranin, synaptophysin, protein cell product 9.5, neural cell adhesion molecule (NCAM/CD56), neuron-specific enolase, and Leu 7.[1-3] Biochemical testing for "functional" tumors of NETs include serum chromogranin A and 24-hour urine 5-HIAA; testing for pancreatic NETs includes chromogranin A, serum pancreatic polypeptide, insulin, pro-insulin, C-peptide, VIP, glucagon, and gastrin.

Clinical scenario

A 48-year-old woman underwent evaluation for early satiety and anorexia. She denies any flushing or diarrhea. She had a laboratory work-up that was remarkable for elevated serum chromogranin A of 50. CT of the abdomen and pelvis with contrast demonstrated a 5-cm mesenteric mass. CT-guided biopsy was done, and pathology demonstrated a neuroendocrine tumor. What additional pathologic evaluation should be performed?

Action items

GASTROENTEROPANCREATIC NETS[1-3]

TUMOR DIFFERENTIATION	TUMOR GRADE	MITOTIC COUNT	KI-67 INDEX
Well-differentiated	Low grade (G1)	<2/10 HPF*	<3%
Well-differentiated	Intermediate grade (G2)	2–20/10 HPF	3%–20%
Poorly differentiated	High grade (G3)	>20/10 HPF	>20%

LUNG AND BRONCHUS CARCINOIDS

Well-differentiated	Low grade (G1)	<2 mitoses/10 HPF AND no necrosis
Well-differentiated	Intermediate grade (G2)	2–10/10 HPF and/or foci of necrosis
Poorly differentiated	High grade (G3)	>10 mitoses/10 HPF

*HPF, high-power field.

References

1. National Comprehensive Cancer Network guidelines for neuroendocrine tumors. Version 3.2017. Available at: www.nccn.org.
2. Kim JY, Hong SM. Recent updates on neuroendocrine tumors from the gastrointestinal and pancreatobiliary tracts. Arch Pathol Lab Med 2016;140(5):437-48.
3. Hirabayashi K, Zamboni G, Nishi T, et al. Histopathology of gastrointestinal neuroendocrine neoplasms. Front Oncol 2013;3:2.

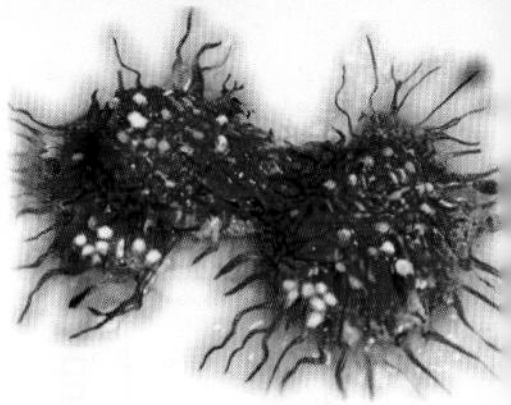

CHAPTER 8
GENITOURINARY CANCERS

What is the first-line systemic treatment for metastatic transitional cell bladder cancer?

Key concept	Cisplatin-based combination chemotherapy is the backbone treatment for metastatic urothelial carcinoma. In patients who are not candidates for cisplatin-based therapy, other options include carboplatin-based regimens, non–platinum-based regimens, and immunotherapy.
Clinical scenario	A 45-year-old woman with a history of bladder cancer treated with neoadjuvant chemotherapy and radical cystectomy presents with weight loss and back pain. CT scan of chest, abdomen, and pelvis reveal diffuse bony lesions for which the biopsy is positive for urothelial carcinoma. The patient has no other medical problems and has good performance status (PS). How should this patient be treated?
Action items	Systemic treatment depends on whether the patient is deemed fit for cisplatin-based chemotherapy. Patients who have any of the following are deemed at higher risk of complications from cisplatin: ECOG PS $\geq$2, estimated glomerular filtration rate $<$60 mL/min, hearing loss, grade $\geq$2 peripheral neuropathy, NY Heart Association congestive heart failure score $\geq$3. For patients with impaired renal function, it is important to correct any reversible etiologies (such as obstruction) before deeming a patient not a candidate for cisplatin.[1,2] **For patients who are candidates for cisplatin-based combination chemotherapy:** • Methotrexate/vinblastine/doxorubicin/cisplatin (MVAC), dose-dense administration preferred • Gemcitabine/cisplatin (GC) • Paclitaxel/gemcitabine/cisplatin (PGC) **For patients who are not candidates for cisplatin-based combination chemotherapy:** • Carboplatin-based regimen (ie, carboplatin and gemcitabine) • Non–platinum-based regimen (ie, paclitaxel and gemcitabine) • PD1/PD-L1 inhibitors (both atezolizumab and pembrolizumab are FDA-approved in this setting)

Discussion

In a randomized multicenter trial, the MVAC regimen proved superior to single-agent cisplatin in term of overall response rate (ORR), progression-free survival (PFS), and overall survival (OS) at the expense of increased toxicity.[3] In another clinical trial, dose-dense (every 2 weeks) administration of MVAC with growth factor support was shown to be associated with greater PFS and complete response, trend toward improved OS, and less myelotoxicity.[4] Another large international study revealed that the GC regimen resulted in equal clinical efficacy compared to standard MVAC but with less serious toxicity in patients with metastatic urothelial carcinoma.[5] In the EORTC30987 trial, the addition of paclitaxel to the GC regimen yielded a higher response rate and a non-significant improvement in OS, at the expense of increased rates of grade 3/4 toxicities.[6]

Although carboplatin-based regimens have not been compared head to head with cisplatin-based regimens, they have proven efficacy in patients unable to receive cisplatin. For example, in the EORTC30896 trial, carboplatin/gemcitabine was equal to methotrexate/carboplatin/vinblastine with fewer adverse effects.[7] The data supporting the use of PD1/PD-L1 inhibitors is discussed in another question.

References

1. Up-to-date. Available at: https://www.uptodate.com.
2. NCCN guidelines for bladder cancer. Available at: https://www.nccn.org.
3. Loehrer PJ Sr, Einhorn LH, Elson PJ, et al. A randomized comparison of cisplatin alone or in combination with methotrexate, vinblastine, and doxorubicin in patients with metastatic urothelial carcinoma: a cooperative group study. J Clin Oncol 1992;10(7):1066-73.
4. Sternberg CN, de Mulder P, Schornagel JH, et al. Seven year update of an EORTC phase III trial of high-dose intensity M-VAC chemotherapy and G-CSF versus classic M-VAC in advanced urothelial tract tumours. Eur J Cancer 2006;42(1):50-4.
5. Von der Maase H, Hansen SW, Roberts JT, et al. Gemcitabine and cisplatin versus methotrexate, vinblastine, doxorubicin, and cisplatin in advanced or metastatic bladder cancer: results of a large, randomized, multinational, multicenter, phase III study. J Clin Oncol 2000;18(17):3068-77.
6. Bellmunt J, von der Maase H, Mead GM, et al. Randomized phase III study comparing paclitaxel/cisplatin/gemcitabine and gemcitabine/cisplatin in patients with locally advanced or metastatic urothelial cancer without prior systemic therapy: EORTC Intergroup Study 30987. J Clin Oncol 2012;30(10):1107-13.
7. De Santis M, Bellmunt J, Mead G, et al. Randomized phase II/III trial assessing gemcitabine/carboplatin and methotrexate/carboplatin/vinblastine in patients with advanced urothelial cancer who are unfit for cisplatin-based chemotherapy: EORTC study 30986. J Clin Oncol 2012;30(2):191-9.

What is the role of immunotherapy in advanced bladder cancer?

Key concept	Cisplatin-based chemotherapy is the backbone of systemic therapy in metastatic urothelial cancer. Although initial response rates are high, median overall survival (OS) remains relatively modest, and not all patients are appropriate candidates for cisplatin-based combination chemotherapy (ie, those with poor renal function, poor performance status, severe congestive heart failure, hearing loss, or peripheral neuropathy). Currently, multiple antibodies targeting the PD1/PD-L1 axis are approved for patients with metastatic urothelial carcinoma who are ineligible for cisplatin-based regimen or whose disease has progressed during or after platinum-based therapy.
Clinical scenario	A 66-year-old man with metastatic urothelial carcinoma of bladder origin received 4 cycles of dose-dense methotrexate/vinblastine/doxorubicin/cisplatin (MVAC) with progressive disease. Patient maintains a good performance status and is interested in immunotherapy. What immunotherapy agent should he be offered?

Action items	• Currently, there are 5 monoclonal antibodies targeting the PD-1/PD-L1 axis that are approved for patients with advanced urothelial carcinoma who have progressed during or following cisplatin-based therapy:
	  • PD1 inhibitors: pembrolizumab, nivolumab
	  • PD-L1 inhibitors: atezolizumab, durvalumab, avelumab
	• Both pembrolizumab and atezolizumab are also indicated in patients with advanced urothelial carcinoma who are deemed ineligible for a cisplatin-based regimen

Discussion	In the Keynote-045 trial, patients with bladder cancer who had recurred or progressed on a platinum-based chemotherapy were randomized to receive either pembrolizumab or investigator-choice chemotherapy (single-agent docetaxel, paclitaxel, or vinflunine). Pembrolizumab was associated with increases in response rate and OS and fewer treatment-related toxicities.[1] Atezolizumab was also approved in the second-line setting. This was based on results of a phase I trial that revealed an overall response rate (ORR) of 15%, with 84% of responses lasting 12 months. Severe immune-related adverse events occurred in 5% of patients.[2] Nivolumab in the second-line setting has shown an ORR of 19.6% and OS of 8.7 months.[3] Both durvalumab and avelumab were approved in the second-line setting on the basis of their efficacy in phase I trial showing ORRs of 17% and 18%, respectively. The median OS with avelumab was 13.7 months.[4,5] *(continued on following page)*

What is the role of immunotherapy in advanced bladder cancer?

	(continued from previous page) Atezolizumab is also indicated in the first-line setting for patients who are not appropriate candidates for cisplatin-based chemotherapy. This was based on the results of a single-arm phase II trial that showed an ORR of 23%, including 9% complete response, unreached median duration of response, and a median OS of 16 months, which is comparable to historical controls using MVAC and gemcitabine/cisplatin chemotherapy.[6] Similarly, the Keynote-052 single-arm study examined the role of pembrolizumab in cisplatin-ineligible patients with advanced urothelial cancer. The ORR was 29%, with 7% being complete responses. The median duration of response was unreached.[7]
Pearls	The PD1 inhibitors (nivolumab and pembrolizumab) and PD-L1 inhibitors (atezolizumab, durvalumab, and avelumab) are indicated for the treatment of advanced urothelial carcinoma that progresses during or after treatment with platinum-based chemotherapy. Additionally, both pembrolizumab and atezolizumab are indicated for use in the first-line setting for patients ineligible for cisplatin-based chemotherapy.

References

1. Bellmunt J, de Wit R, Vaughn DJ, et al. Pembrolizumab as second-line therapy for advanced urothelial carcinoma. N Engl J Med 2017;376:1015-26.
2. Rosenberg GE, Hoffman-Censits J, Powles T, et al. Atezolizumab in patients with locally advanced and metastatic urothelial carcinoma who have progressed following treatment with platinum-based chemotherapy: a single-arm, multicentre, phase 2 trial. Lancet 2016;387(10031):1909-20.
3. Sharma P, Retz M, Siefker-Radtke A, et al. Nivolumab in metastatic urothelial carcinoma after platinum therapy (CheckMate 275): a multicentre, single-arm, phase 2 trial. Lancet Oncol 2017;18(3):312-22.
4. Massard C, Gordon MS, Sharma S, et al. Safety and efficacy of durvalumab (MEDI4736), an anti-programmed cell death ligand-1 immune checkpoint inhibitor, in patients with advanced urothelial bladder cancer. J Clin Oncol 2016;34(26):3119-25.
5. Apolo AB, Infante JR, Balmanoukian A, et al. Avelumab, an anti-programmed death-ligand 1 antibody, in patients with refractory metastatic urothelial carcinoma: results from a multicenter, phase Ib study. J Clin Oncol 2017;35(19):2117-24.
6. Balar AV, Galsky MD, Rosenberg JE, et al. Atezolizumab as first-line treatment in cisplatin-ineligible patients with locally advanced and metastatic urothelial carcinoma: a single-arm, multicentre, phase 2 trial. Lancet 2017;389(10064):67-76.
7. Balar A, Bellmunt J, O'Donnell PH, et al. Pembrolizumab as first-line therapy for advanced/unresectable or metastatic urothelial cancer: preliminary results from the phase 2 KEYNOTE-052 study. Ann Oncol 2016;27(suppl_6):LBA32_PR.

What is the role of neoadjuvant chemotherapy in bladder cancer?

Key concept	Radical cystectomy with bilateral pelvic lymphadenectomy is the backbone treatment of nonmetastatic, muscle-invasive urothelial bladder cancer. Despite improvements in surgical techniques, more than half of these patients will eventually develop metastatic disease. Administration of 3–4 cycles of cisplatin-based chemotherapy prior to radical cystectomy has been shown to improve outcome and survival.
Clinical scenario	A 53-year-old man with a history of smoking presents with hematuria. Cystoscopy reveals a bladder polyp in the posterior wall of the bladder. He underwent transurethral resection of the bladder tumor, which was positive for muscle-invasive urothelial cancer. CT scan of the chest, abdomen, and pelvis was negative for regional and distant metastasis. The patient is amenable to pursue radical cystectomy. How should this patient be treated?

Action items	• This patient will benefit from 3–4 cycles of cisplatin-based chemotherapy prior to radical cystectomy; multiple options are reasonable[1,2]:
	  • Methotrexate/vinblastine/doxorubicin/cisplatin (MVAC) (a dose-dense regimen with growth factor support is preferred)
	  • Gemcitabine/cisplatin (GC)
	  • Methotrexate/vinblastine/cisplatin (CMV)
	• Neoadjuvant chemotherapy is preferred over adjuvant chemotherapy
	• If the patient has been referred following radical cystectomy, adjuvant chemotherapy is advised in the case of pathologic T3, T4, or N+ disease

Discussion	The use of neoadjuvant cisplatin-based chemotherapy in bladder cancer is supported by multiple randomized trials and meta-analyses. In the INT-0080 trial, patients with muscle-invasive bladder cancer were randomized to undergo radical cystectomy alone vs. 3 cycles of standard MVAC therapy followed by surgery. The addition of neoadjuvant chemotherapy was associated with increased rates of pathologic complete response, longer overall survival, and higher toxicity.[3]

	Although randomized trials are lacking about the usage of dose-dense MVAC in the neoadjuvant setting, it has proved effective in single-arm studies and has been shown to be more effective than the standard regimen in the advanced/metastatic setting and thus is preferred over standard MVAC.[2,4] Another randomized trial showed a survival advantage for a CMV regimen given for 3 cycles prior to radical cystectomy.[5] A GC regimen proved to be equally effective and less toxic than MVAC in metastatic bladder cancer. By extrapolation, this regimen is thus a reasonable alternative in the neoadjuvant setting as well.[2] A meta-analysis of 10 randomized trials showed that cisplatin-based chemotherapy preceding radical cystectomy is associated with a 5% absolute overall survival advantage and a 7% absolute disease-free survival at 5 years.[6] In patients ineligible for cisplatin, the role of carboplatin as substitution for cisplatin is not well defined.[2] Although neo-adjuvant chemotherapy remains preferred over adjuvant chemotherapy, based on more evidence, in the instance when chemotherapy was not given prior to surgery, patients with pT3/T4 or pN+ stage disease may benefit from adjuvant chemotherapy. This is supported by a meta-analysis of 6 randomized trials indicating a 25% relative reduction in the risk of death.[1,2,7]
References	1. Up-to-date. Available at: https://www.uptodate.com. 2. NCCN guidelines for bladder cancer. Available at: https://www.nccn.org. 3. Grossman HB, Natale RB, Tangen CM, et al. Neoadjuvant chemotherapy plus cystectomy compared with cystectomy alone for locally advanced bladder cancer. N Engl J Med 2003;349(9):859-66. 4. Choueiri TK, Jacobus S2, Bellmunt J, et al. Neoadjuvant dose-dense methotrexate, vinblastine, doxorubicin, and cisplatin with pegfilgrastim support in muscle-invasive urothelial cancer: pathologic, radiologic, and biomarker correlates. J Clin Oncol 2014;32(18):1889-94. 5. International Collaboration of Trialists, Medical Research Council Advanced Bladder Cancer Working Party (now the National Cancer Research Institute Bladder Cancer Clinical Studies Group), European Organisation for Research and Treatment of Cancer Genito-Urinary Tract Cancer Group, et al. International phase III trial assessing neoadjuvant cisplatin, methotrexate, and vinblastine chemotherapy for muscle-invasive bladder cancer: long-term results of the BA06 30894 trial. J Clin Oncol 2011;29(16):2171-7. 6. Advanced Bladder Cancer Meta-analysis Collaboration. Neoadjuvant chemotherapy in invasive bladder cancer: a systematic review and meta-analysis. Lancet 2003;361(9373):1927-34. 7. Advanced Bladder Cancer Meta-analysis Collaboration. Adjuvant chemotherapy in invasive bladder cancer: a systematic review and meta-analysis of individual patient data. Eur Urol 2005;48:189-99.

What are the initial evaluation and treatment options of localized renal cell carcinoma (RCC)?

Key concept	With the more frequent use of imaging studies such as CT scans and ultrasounds, a kidney mass is sometimes incidentally identified.[1] Evaluation of RCC includes CT of the abdomen (± pelvis) and chest imaging (which can include either chest X-ray or CT chest with contrast). Additional imaging with MRI of the abdomen can be obtained for further evaluation of the vasculature involvement, including the inferior vena cava (IVC). Biopsy of the kidney mass is not considered necessary, as there are characteristic radiographic features of RCC.[1]
Clinical scenario	A 67-year-old woman presents to the emergency room for evaluation of abdominal pain. CT of the abdomen without contrast demonstrates a 4-cm kidney mass. Her labs show adequate kidney function, with creatinine of 0.89, mild anemia with hemoglobin of 11.2, and lactate dehydrogenase and calcium within normal limits. Urology is consulted for discussion of treatment options. What surgical options can be considered for this patient?
Discussion	Surgical options for localized RCC include radical nephrectomy and nephron-sparing surgery; the choice depends on tumor location and involvement or extension into the IVC. Lymph node dissection and adrenalectomy are considered in clinical situations in the case of abnormal radiological findings.[1] Adjuvant therapy for RCC has been controversial. Most recently, a phase 3 S-TRAC trial evaluated the role of adjuvant sunitinib and demonstrated prolonged disease-free survival (DFS) by 1.2 years compared with placebo (6.8 years in sunitinib arm vs. 5.6 years in placebo arm) following nephrectomy for patients with clear-cell RCC. In higher risk patients, the median DFS was 6.2 vs. 4.0 years for sunitinib and placebo, respectively. High-risk RCC included Fuhrman grade ≥ 2 and ECOG score ≥ 1 vs. low-risk (any Fuhrman grade and ECOG score 0 or Fuhrman grade 1 and ECOG score ≥ 1).[2,3]

Pearls	• Nephron-sparing surgery should be considered in special clinical situations including solitary kidney, bilateral synchronous RCC, or patients with hereditary RCC (such as von Hippel–Lindau disease)[1] • Adjuvant sunitinib can be considered in high-risk RCC[2,3]
References	1. National Comprehensive Cancer Network guidelines for kidney cancer. Version 2.2018. Available at: www.nccn.org. 2. Ravaud A, Motzer RJ, Pandha HS, et al. Adjuvant sunitinib in high-risk renal-cell carcinoma after nephrectomy. N Engl J Med 2016;375(23):2246-54. 3. Ravaud A, Motzer RJ, Pandha HS, et al. Phase III trial of sunitinib (SU) vs placebo (PBO) as adjuvant treatment for high-risk renal cell carcinoma (RCC) after nephrectomy (S-TRAC) [abstract]. Presented at: 2016 ESMO Congress. Ann Oncol 2016;27(6):1-36.

What is a prognostic factor model used in metastatic renal cell carcinoma (RCC), and how is it applied in treatment decision-making?

Key concept	Consideration of prognostic factors and prior therapy (ie, cytokines vs. tyrosine kinase inhibitors) is helpful in determining treatment options for patients with metastatic RCC.[1-3] The Memorial Sloan Kettering Cancer Center (MSKCC) prognostic model was derived from 6 clinical trials involving 463 patients with advanced RCC who were given interferon-α as first-line systemic therapy.[1-3]
Clinical scenario	A 67-year-old well-appearing woman without any significant medical issues presents to the emergency room for an evaluation of abdominal pain. CT of the abdomen without contrast demonstrates a 4-cm large kidney mass. Her labs show adequate kidney function, with creatinine of 0.89, mild anemia with hemoglobin of 11.2, and lactate dehydrogenase (LDH) and calcium within normal limits. Further evaluation demonstrates multiple pulmonary nodules, with the largest measuring 1.4 cm. She states that she lives with her husband and volunteers at her church. She exercises 3–4 times per week. What is her prognostic risk group, and what treatment options can be considered based on her prognostic risk group?
Action items	• The MSKCC prognostic model stratifies patients with mRCC into three groups based on the following prognostic factors[1]: • Interval from diagnosis to treatment <1 year • Karnofsky performance status <80% • Serum LDH >1.5 times the upper limit of normal (ULN) • Corrected serum calcium >ULN • Serum hemoglobin <lower limit of normal (LLN)

PROGNOSTIC RISK GROUP	NUMBER OF FACTORS	MEDIAN SURVIVAL TIME (MONTHS)
Low-risk	None	20
Intermediate	1–2	10
Poor	>3	4

- Amato et al. evaluated patients who received prior mTOR therapy and developed a prognostic model and identified 4 risk factors associated with progression-free overall survival: the presence of bony metastasis, LDH >1.5 the upper limit, alkaline phosphatase >120 U/L, and lymphocytes <25 cells/μL[4]

Pearls

- For low- or intermediate-risk patients, sunitinib, pazopanib, or bevacizumab and interferon-α can be considered as first-line treatment[5–7]
- For poor-risk patients, temsirolimus can be considered as first-line treatment[8]

1. National Comprehensive Cancer Network guidelines for kidney cancer. Version 2.2018. Available at: www.nccn.org.
2. Tsui KH, Shvarts O, Smith RB, et al. Prognostic indicators for renal cell carcinoma: a multivariate analysis of 643 patients using the revised 1997 TNM staging criteria. J Urol 2000;163(4):1090-5.
3. Motzer RJ, Mazumdar M, Bacik J, et al. Survival and prognostic stratification of 670 patients with advanced renal cell carcinoma. J Clin Oncol 1999;17(8):2530-40.
4. Amato RJ, Flaherty A, Zhang Y, et al. Clinical prognostic factors associated with outcome in patients with renal cell cancer with prior tyrosine kinase inhibitors or immunotherapy treated with everolimus. Urol Oncol 2014;32(3):345-54.
5. Escudier B, Pluzanska A, Koralewski P, et al. Bevacizumab plus interferon alfa-2a for treatment of metastatic renal cell carcinoma: a randomized, double-blind phase III trial. Lancet 2007;370(9605):2103-11.
6. Motzer RJ, Hutson TE, Cella D, et al. Pazopanib versus sunitinib in metastatic renal-cell carcinoma. N Engl J Med 2013;369(8):722-31.
7. Sternberg CN, Davis ID, Mardiak J, et al. Pazopanib in locally advanced or metastatic renal cell carcinoma: results of a randomized phase III trial. J Clin Oncol 2010;28(6):1061-8.
8. Hudes G, Carducci M, Tomczak P, et al. Temsirolimus, interferon alfa, or both for advanced renal-cell carcinoma. N Engl J Med 2007;356(22):2271-81.

In what patient population do we consider cytoreductive nephrectomy (CN)?

Key concept	CN can be considered in select patients presenting with metastatic renal cell cancer (RCC) with pulmonary metastases only and with good prognostic features and performance status.[1] Additionally, patients presenting with severe gross hematuria or other symptoms from the primary kidney tumor can be offered CN with palliative intent.[1] Surgical treatment in the form of radical nephrectomy also has a role in the care of select patients with metastatic disease. Two prospective randomized trials have demonstrated a survival advantage among those undergoing CN prior to immunotherapy, defining the role of surgery in this setting. Survival advantage among those undergoing CN prior to immunotherapy has been demonstrated in 2 prospective randomized clinical trials.[2-4]
Clinical scenario	A 67-year-old woman presents to the emergency room for evaluation of abdominal pain. CT of the abdomen without contrast demonstrates a 4-cm large kidney mass. Her labs show adequate kidney function with creatinine of 0.89, mild anemia with hemoglobin of 11.2, and lactate dehydrogenase (LDH) and calcium within normal limits. Urology is consulted for a discussion of treatment options. Can CN be considered for this patient?
Discussion	A combined analysis of >300 metastatic RCC patients enrolled in the European Organization for the Research and Treatment of Cancer trial 30947 and Southwest Oncology Group trial 8949 who either underwent nephrectomy followed by interferon (IFN)-α or received IFN-α alone demonstrated that the median overall survival (OS) was longer in patients who underwent nephrectomy compared with patients who received IFN-α alone (13.6 vs. 7.8 months).[2-4]

	Predictors of inferior OS in patients undergoing CN include being clinically symptomatic, LDH >upper limit of normal, albumin <lower limit of normal, liver metastasis, retroperitoneal or supra-diaphragmatic adenopathy, and stage T3 tumors. Surgical patients who had 4 risk factors did not appear to benefit from CN and had an increased risk of death and inferior OS.[5] In the era of molecularly targeted therapies, the applicability of CN is unclear. A recent study by the International Metastatic Database Consortium evaluated 201 patients who underwent CN vs. 113 patients treated non-surgically. There was improved OS (median, 19.8 vs. 9.4 months) in those who underwent CN vs. no CN, respectively. Poor prognostic factors were also identified in those who had $\geq$4 risk factors, including anemia, thrombocytosis, neutrophilia, Karnofsky Performance Status <80%, and <1 year from diagnosis to treatment.[6]
Pearl	CN can be considered in select patients presenting with metastatic RCC as a potential treatment option and in patients presenting with symptoms related to the primary tumor for palliative intent.

References

1. National Comprehensive Cancer Network guidelines for kidney cancer. Version 2.2018. Available at: www.nccn.org.
2. Flanigan RC, Mickisch G, Sylvester R, et al. Cytoreductive nephrectomy in patients with metastatic renal cancer: a combined analysis. J Urol 2004;171:1071-6.
3. Flanigan RC, Salmon SE, Blumenstein BA, et al. Nephrectomy followed by interferon alfa-2b compared with interferon alfa-2b alone for metastatic renal-cell cancer. N Engl J Med 2001;345(23):1655-9.
4. Mickisch GHJ, Garin A, Van Poppel H, et al. Radical nephrectomy plus interferon-alfa-based immunotherapy compared with interferon alfa alone in metastatic renal-cell carcinoma: a randomised trial. Lancet 2001;358(9286):966-70.
5. Culp SH, Tannir NM, Abel EJ, et al. Can we better select patients with metastatic renal cell carcinoma for cytoreductive nephrectomy? Cancer 2010;116(14):3378-88.
6. Choueiri TK, Xie W, Kollmannsberger C, et al. The impact of cytoreductive nephrectomy on survival of patients with metastatic renal cell carcinoma receiving vascular endothelial growth factor targeted therapy. J Urol 2011;185(1):60-6.

What are the systemic treatment options for metastatic clear-cell renal cell carcinoma (RCC)?

Key concept	Interferon (IFN)-α has long been utilized in RCC treatment. However, better understanding of the disease biology has led to drastic changes in RCC treatment over the past decade. Novel agents targeting the vascular endothelial growth factor (VEGF), mTOR, and checkpoint pathways and have changed the landscape of RCC therapy.
Clinical scenario	A 53-year-old woman with history of left nephrectomy 1 year previously undergoes surveillance imaging. CT of chest and abdomen/pelvis with contrast demonstrates pulmonary nodules too numerous to count and a left adrenal mass measuring 2 cm. What are treatment options for this patient?
Action items	• Administer one of the following treatment paradigms: • Immunotherapy: high-dose interleukin-2, nivolumab • VEGF pathway inhibitors: sunitinib, pazopanib, cabozantinib, axitinib, sorafenib, bevacizumab (plus IFN-α), lenvatinib (plus everolimus) • mTOR pathway inhibitors: temsirolimus, everolimus

PATIENT POPULATION	TREATMENT STRATEGY
Previously untreated patients	• High dose IL-2 (in carefully selected patients) • Sunitinib (preferred*) • Pazopanib (preferred*) • Temsirolimus (preferred in poor-risk patients*) • Cabozantinib • Axitinib • Bevacizumab plus IFN-α

Prior high-dose IL-2, no prior tyrosine kinase inhibitors (TKIs)	• Axitinib (preferred*) • Pazopanib • Sorafenib • Sunitinib
Prior TKIs	• Nivolumab (preferred*) • Cabozantinib (preferred*) • Axitinib • Lenvatinib plus everolimus • Everolimus • Sorafenib • Other agents (sunitinib, pazopanib, bevacizumab, high-dose IL-2, temsirolimus)

*Preferred is based on Category 1 evidence as recommended by NCCN.

Discussion

FIRST-LINE TREATMENT:

In low- and intermediate-risk patients, sunitinib was associated with a higher overall response rate (ORR), progression-free survival (PFS), and overall survival (OS) than IFN-α.[1]

In treatment-naïve and cytokine-pretreated patients with metastatic RCC (mainly low and intermediate risk), pazopanib improved ORR and PFS compared with placebo.[2] Pazopanib demonstrated higher ORR, equal PFS and OS, and less toxicity than sunitinib.[3]

Bevacizumab plus IFN-α was associated with prolonged PFS and a trend toward prolonged OS compared with IFN-α in untreated patients with metastatic RCC.[4]

(continued on following page)

(continued from previous page)

In poor-risk patients, temsirolimus was associated with superior OS compared with IFN-α.[5]

Cabozantinib demonstrated a significantly higher ORR and PFS and a trend toward higher OS compared with sunitinib in untreated metastatic RCC (intermediate or high risk).[6]

Axitinib was associated with slightly higher PFS but no difference in OS compared with sorafenib in previously untreated patients with metastatic RCC.[7]

SUBSEQUENT THERAPY:

Prior VEGF:

Cabozantinib was superior to everolimus in terms of ORR, PFS, and OS in metastatic RCC previously treated with anti-VEGF receptor agents.[8]

Nivolumab was superior to everolimus in terms of ORR and OS in metastatic RCC previously treated with anti-VEGF receptor agents.[9]

Lenvatinib plus everolimus was associated with prolonged PFS and a trend toward prolonged OS compared with single-agent everolimus in metastatic RCC previously treated with anti-angiogenic therapy.[10]

Prior cytokine therapy:

- Sorafenib was associated with prolonged PFS compared with placebo in patients with metastatic RCC who progressed on cytokine therapy[11]
- Axitinib was associated with improved ORR and PFS compared with sorafenib in patients previously treated with cytokines or sunitinib[12]

Pearls

In carefully selected patients with excellent performance status and good organ function, high-dose IL-2 may be associated with prolonged disease control in a small percentage. For patients who are not fit or have no access to high-dose IL-2, treatment with anti-angiogenic agents is recommended. Sunitinib and pazopanib are the preferred agents. For patients who fail treatment with VEGF pathway inhibitors, nivolumab, cabozantinib, or combination lenvatinib/everolimus are the preferred agents, and they all result in improved OS compared with single-agent everolimus. Nivolumab has a better safety profile.

References

1. Motzer RJ, Hutson TE, Tomczak P, et al. Overall survival and updated results for sunitinib compared with interferon alfa in patients with metastatic renal cell carcinoma. J Clin Oncol 2009;27(22):3584-90.
2. Sternberg CN, Davis ID, Mardiak J, et al. Pazopanib in locally advanced or metastatic renal cell carcinoma: results of a randomized phase III trial. J Clin Oncol 2010;28(6):1061-8.
3. Motzer RJ, Hutson TE, Cella D, et al. Pazopanib versus sunitinib in metastatic renal-cell carcinoma. N Engl J Med 2013;369(8):722-31.
4. Escudier B, Pluzanska A, Koralewski P, et al. Bevacizumab plus interferon alfa-2a for treatment of metastatic renal cell carcinoma: a randomized, double-blind phase III trial. Lancet 2007;370(9605):2103-11.
5. Hudes G, Carducci M, Tomczak P, et al. Temsirolimus, interferon alfa, or both for advanced renal-cell carcinoma. N Engl J Med 2007; 356(22):2271-81.
6. Choueiri TK, Halabi S, Sanford BL, et al. Cabozantinib versus sunitinib as initial targeted therapy for patients with metastatic renal cell carcinoma of poor or intermediate risk: the Alliance A031203 CABOSUN Trial. J Clin Oncol 2017;35(6):591-7.
7. Hutson TE, Al-Shukri S, Stus VP, et al. Axitinib versus sorafenib in first-line metastatic renal cell carcinoma: overall survival from a randomized phase III trial. Clin Genitourin Cancer 2017;15(1):72-6.
8. Choueiri TK, Escudier B, Powles T, et al. Cabozantinib versus everolimus in advanced renal-cell carcinoma. N Engl J Med 2015;373(19):1814-23.
9. Motzer RJ, Escudier B, McDermott DF, et al. Nivolumab versus everolimus in advanced renal-cell carcinoma. N Engl J Med 2015; 373:1803-13.
10. Motzer RJ, Hutson TE, Glen H, et al. Lenvatinib, everolimus, and the combination in patients with metastatic renal cell carcinoma: a randomised, phase 2, open-label, multicentre trial. Lancet Oncol 2015;16(15):1473-82.
11. Escudier B, Eisen T, Stadler WM, et al. Sorafenib in advanced clear-cell renal-cell carcinoma. N Engl J Med 2007;356(2):125-34.
12. Motzer RJ, Escudier B, Tomczak P, et al. Axitinib versus sorafenib as second-line treatment for advanced renal cell carcinoma: overall survival analysis and updated results from a randomised phase 3 trial. Lancet Oncol 2013;14(6):552-62.

How is prostate cancer initially diagnosed?

Key concept	The initial evaluation of prostate cancer can begin either with a prostate-specific antigen (PSA) test as done for PSA screening or with abnormal digital rectal exam (DRE). A PSA level >3 ng/mL (for men age <75) or >4 ng/mL (for men age ≥75) or very suspicious DRE results should be evaluated with prostate biopsy.[1] Transrectal ultrasound (US)–guided biopsy consists of 12 cores.[2] The Gleason score is the sum of the primary and secondary most prevalent differentiation patterns as delineated as a histologic grade from 1 being the most differentiated to 5 being least differentiated (example Gleason 3 + 4 = Gleason 7).[1] Diagnostic imaging with CT scans, multi-parametric MRI of the prostate, and bone scans can be done if there is concern for more advanced disease, such as higher Gleason score, T stage, and lymph-node involvement.[3,4]
Clinical scenario	A 72-year-old man undergoes evaluation for rising PSA of 4.3 (with a prior PSA of 1.3). Transrectal US-guided biopsy of the prostate shows Gleason score 3 + 4 = 7 in 1 of 6 cores on the left with 30% involvement and Gleason score 3 + 3 = 6 in 2 of 6 cores on the right. DRE reveals a small, smooth prostate. Prostate protocol MRI shows organ-confined disease with no extracapsular extension, seminal vesicle invasion, or lymphadenopathy. What additional evaluation should the patient undergo?
Action items	(see table below)

GLEASON SCORE INTERPRETATION[1]

Gleason X	Cannot be processed
Gleason ≤6	Well differentiated (slight anaplasia)
Gleason 7	Moderately differentiated (moderate anaplasia)
Gleason 8–10	Poorly differentiated (marked anaplasia)

GLEASON GRADE GROUP[5,6]	DEFINITION
1	Gleason score ≤6 Only individual, discrete, well-formed glands
2	Gleason score 3 + 4 = 7 Predominantly well-formed glands with a lesser component of poorly formed/fused/cribriform glands
3	Gleason score 4 + 3 = 7 Predominantly poorly formed/fused/cribriform glands with a lesser component of well-formed glands
4	Gleason score 4 + 4 = 8, 3 + 5 = 8, or 5 + 3 = 8 Only poorly formed/fused/cribriform glands or predominantly well-formed glands with a lesser component lacking glands or predominantly lacking glands and a lesser component of well-formed glands
5	Gleason score 9–10 Lack of gland formation or with necrosis with or without poorly formed/fused/cribriform glands

(continued on following page)

(continued from previous page)

TNM STAGING[1]	
T1a	Tumor incidental histologic finding in 5% or less of tissue resected
T1b	Tumor >5% of tissue resected
T1c	Tumor identified by needle biopsy
T2a	Tumor involves ≤half of one lobe or less
T2b	Tumor involves >half of one lobe but not both lobes
T2c	Tumor involves both lobes
T3a	Extracapsular extension (unilateral or bilateral)
T3b	Tumor invades the seminal vesicle(s)
T4	Tumor is fixed or invades adjacent structures other than seminal vesicles, such as bladder, levator muscles, and/or pelvic wall

References

1. National Comprehensive Cancer Network guidelines for prostate cancer. Version 2.2017. Available at: www.nccn.org.
2. Eichler K, Hempel S, Wilby J, et al. Diagnostic value of systematic biopsy methods in the investigation of prostate cancer: a systematic review. J Urol 2006;175(5):1605-12.
3. Risko R, Merdan S, Womble PR, et al. Clinical predictors and recommendations for staging computed tomography scan among men with prostate cancer. Urology 2014;84(6):1329-34.
4. Merdan S, Womble PR, Miller DC, et al. Toward better use of bone scans among men with early-stage prostate cancer. Urology 2014;84(4):793-8.
5. Epstein JI, Egevad L, Amin MB, et al. The 2014 International Society of Urological Pathology (ISUP) consensus conference on Gleason grading of prostatic carcinoma: definition of grading patterns and proposal for a new grading system. Am J Surg Pathol 2016;40(2):244-52.
6. Epstein JI, Zelefsky MJ, Sjoberg DD, et al. A contemporary prostate cancer grading system: a validated alternative to the Gleason score. Eur Urol 2016;69(3):428-35.

Terminology of recurrent/metastatic prostate cancer

TERM	DEFINITION
Biochemical failure or recurrence[1]	Increase or rise of PSA, but no distant metastasis is identified; scenario includes increase in PSA after radical prostatectomy
Castrate-naïve (castration-sensitive)[1]	Androgen sensitive; these patients are not on ADT; therefore ADT is an effective therapy for this population
Castration-resistant[1]	Progressive metastatic disease despite castrate levels of testosterone (ie, testosterone is undetectable [<50 ng/dL] by laboratory tests)
Flare phenomenon	If LHRH agonists are used alone in patients with metastatic prostate cancer with high-volume disease, due to stimulation of LHRH receptors, there is a surge of testosterone. Serious adverse events such as exacerbation of pain, urinary obstruction, or neurologic compromise can occur.[2] *Pearl*: It is important to administer anti-androgen and LHRH agonists (either simultaneously or anti-androgen given 7 days prior to LHRH agonists) in patients with high-volume disease. The anti-androgen inhibits the stimulatory effect of the testosterone surge at the level of the androgen receptor.[2]

References	1. National Comprehensive Cancer Network guidelines for prostate cancer. Version 2.2017. Available at: www.nccn.org. 2. Thompson IM. Flare associated with LHRH-agonist therapy. Rev Urol 2001;3(Suppl 3):S10.

ADT, androgen deprivation therapy; LHRH, luteinizing hormone-releasing hormone; PSA, prostate-specific antigen.

What radiotherapy treatment options are available for patients with localized prostate cancer?

Key concept	• Localized prostate cancer is classified as low, intermediate, or high risk based on criteria that include prostate-specific antigen (PSA), clinical T stage, and pathology • Localized prostate cancer treatment options include (1) radical prostatectomy (RP) ± pelvic lymph node biopsy/dissection ± adjuvant external beam radiation therapy (EBRT), (2) EBRT ± androgen deprivation (ADT),[1] and (3) brachytherapy ± EBRT ± ADT • Treatment recommendations are largely based on risk category • **NO randomized trial has directly compared brachytherapy, EBRT, and RP,** although numerous prospective series and multiple quality of life (QOL) analyses have been reported
Clinical scenario	A 69-year-old man undergoes evaluation for rising PSA of 4.3 (with prior PSA of 1.3). Transrectal ultrasound-guided biopsy of the prostate shows Gleason score 3 + 4 = 7 in 1 of 6 cores on the left with 30% involvement and Gleason score 3 + 3 = 6 in 2 of 6 cores on the right. Digital rectal exam reveals a small, smooth prostate. Prostate protocol MRI shows organ-confined disease with no extracapsular extension, seminal vesicle invasion, or lymphadenopathy. Patient's IPSS urinary score is 5. Prostate size on volume study is 30 mL. Patient is not interested in surgery. In what risk category is this patient, and what treatment options can be offered?

Action items

PATIENT POPULATION	TREATMENT STRATEGIES
<u>Low risk</u> (PSA ≤10, biopsy Gleason ≤6, T1c or T2a)	• Active surveillance,[2] depending on in-depth discussion with patient, age, co-morbidities, life span • Observation if life span is <10 years • RP • Definitive EBRT • Brachytherapy as monotherapy
<u>Favorable intermediate risk</u> (One factor allowed from: PSA >10–20, or biopsy Gleason 3 + 4 = 7 with ≤3 involved cores and <50% positive cores, or T2b)	• If life span is <10 years, observation considered • RP • EBRT with ADT • Brachytherapy as monotherapy
<u>Unfavorable intermediate risk</u> (% positive biopsy cores >50% involved, >1 intermediate risk factor above, Gleason score 4 + 3 = 7)	• RP ± lymph node evaluation • EBRT + short term ADT • Brachytherapy with EBRT ± ADT
<u>High risk</u> (PSA >20, biopsy Gleason 8–10, biopsy Gleason 7 w/ tertiary grade 5, ≥T2c)	• RP ± lymph node evaluation • EBRT + long-term ADT (2 years) • Brachytherapy with EBRT and ADT

(continued on following page)

(continued from previous page)

Discussion	Patients presenting with localized prostate cancer have multiple options available for definitive therapy. Clinical decisions require consultations with both Urology and Radiation Oncology and thorough discussion of QOL issues.[3] RP side effects include 50% occasional leakage, 10% frequent leakage, 3% no urinary control, 70% with erections not sufficient for intercourse, and impotence in 30%–60% of patients.[4] EBRT side effects can be acute (frequency, urgency, nocturia, hesitancy, retention of urine) as well as late (altered urinary/bowel habits, rectal bleeding in 5%–10% of patients, urinary stricture in 1%, loss of sexual function in 30%–50%, and incontinence in <1%–2%). Brachytherapy contraindications are limited life expectancy, unacceptable operative risks, large transurethral resection of the prostate (TURP) defects, excessively large (>120 mL) or small (<20 mL) prostate gland size, and significant urinary obstructive symptoms with International Prostate Symptom Score (IPSS) >15–20. Brachytherapy side effects include pain, dysuria, hematuria, frequency, and urinary retention in the perioperative setting. Obstructive urinary symptoms can take 6 months to resolve, with impotence in 30%, urethral stricture in 3%, incontinence in 3%, rectal bleeding in <10%, and fistula in <1%.[5]
Pearls	• No randomized trial has directly compared efficacy of brachytherapy to EBRT to RP; **each modality is considered equivocal with regard to outcomes**[6] • Brachytherapy is an established technique for definitive monotherapy of low-risk and favorable intermediate-risk prostate cancer[7] • Brachytherapy can be combined with EBRT ± ADT as definitive treatment for unfavorable intermediate-risk and high-risk prostate cancer[8] • Treatment choice should depend on a thorough discussion by both Urology and Radiation Oncology, including QOL issues after treatment

References

1. Zumsteg ZS, Zelefsky MJ. Short-term androgen deprivation therapy for patients with intermediate-risk prostate cancer undergoing dose-escalated radiotherapy: the standard of care. Lancet Oncol 2012;13(6):e259-69.
2. Wilt TJ, Brawer MK, Jones KM, et al. Radical prostatectomy versus observation for localized prostate cancer. N Engl J Med 2012;367(3):203-13.
3. Donovan JL, Hamdy FC, Lane JA, et al. Patient-reported outcomes after monitoring, surgery, or radiotherapy for prostate cancer. N Engl J Med 2016;375(15):1425-37.
4. Penson DF, McLerran D, Feng Z, et al. 5-year urinary and sexual outcomes after radical prostatectomy: results from the Prostate Cancer Outcomes Study. J Urol 2005;173(5):1701-5.
5. Jawad MS, Dilworth JT, Gustafson GS, et al. Outcomes associated with 3 treatment schedules of high-dose-rate brachytherapy monotherapy for favorable-risk prostate cancer. Int J Radiation Oncol Biol Phys 2016;94(4):657-66.
6. Hamdy FC, Donovan JL, Lane JA, et al. 10-year outcomes after monitoring, surgery, or radiotherapy for localized prostate cancer. N Engl J Med 2016;375(15):1415-24.
7. Hauswald H, Kamrava MR, Fallon JM, et al. High-dose-rate monotherapy for localized prostate cancer: 10-year results. Int J Radiation Oncol Biol Phys 2016;94(4):667-74.
8. Stock RG, Ho A, Cesaretti JA, et al. Changing the patterns of failure for high-risk prostate cancer patients by optimizing local control. Int J Radiation Oncol Biol Phys 2006;66(2):389-94.

What is the management of progressive metastatic prostatic castrate-naïve cancer?

Key concept	Initial therapy with androgen deprivation therapy (ADT) with a luteinizing hormone-releasing hormone (LHRH) agonist/antagonist (ie, medical castration) or through bilateral orchiectomy (surgical castration) is the initial treatment for metastatic castrate-naïve prostate cancer.[1]
Clinical scenario	A 65-year-old man with a history of prostate cancer, status post radical prostatectomy 5 years prior, presents with prostate-specific antigen (PSA) increasing from 3 to 10 ng/mL. He is seen by his medical oncologist, who orders further evaluation with imaging. CT scan of the chest and abdomen, MRI pelvis, and bone scan demonstrates no metastatic lesions. What are the different treatment options?
Action items	Factors including the PSA doubling time, patient's co-morbidities, and anxiety should be considered when starting ADT. In addition, it is important to discuss with the patient about the long-term effects of ADT, which can include osteoporosis, obesity, insulin resistance, hyperlipidemia, chronic kidney disease, and cardiovascular disease.[1,2]
Discussion	Because of the adverse effects of long-term ADT, trials have investigated the role of intermittent versus continuous ADT. There is still no consensus. However, two large phase 3 studies investigated this question in non-metastatic biochemical failure patients and found that intermittent administration was non-inferior to continuous ADT in overall survival.[3] In contrast, intermittent vs. continuous ADT in patients with metastatic disease was inconclusive. Patients who were on intermittent ADT did report improved quality of life, mental health, and better erectile function.[4]

References

1. National Comprehensive Cancer Network guidelines for prostate cancer. Version 2.2017. Available at: www.nccn.org.
2. Ahmadi H, Daneshmand S. Androgen deprivation therapy: evidence-based management of side effects. BJU Int 2013;111(4):543-8.
3. Crook JM, O'Callaghan CJ, Duncan G, et al. Intermittent androgen suppression for rising PSA level after radiotherapy. N Engl J Med. 2012;367:895-903.
4. Hussain M, Tangen CM, Berry DL, et al. Intermittent versus continuous androgen deprivation in prostate cancer. N Engl J Med 2013;368(14):1314-25.

How do I manage metastatic castrate-resistant prostate cancer (mCRPC)?

Key concept	Despite initial response to androgen deprivation therapy (ADT), almost all patients will develop castration-resistant disease. Data have shown that docetaxel[1] is associated with improvement in clinical outcome. Several new agents have been approved recently for mCRPC and have resulted in significant survival benefit, including abiraterone acetate, enzalutamide, cabazitaxel, sipuleucel-T, and radium-223.[2-9]
Clinical scenario	A 70-year-old man with mCRPC currently receiving an LHRH agonist presents with increased bone pain. Laboratory results reveal an increase in prostate-specific antigen (PSA) levels from 10 to 50 ng/mL, and CT and bone scans reveal development of new bony metastases but no visceral metastasis. What are the different treatment options?
Action items	Treatment of mCRPC can be stratified by prior treatment with enzalutamide and docetaxel.[9]

PRIOR ENZALUTAMIDE/PRIOR ABIRATERONE	PRIOR DOCETAXEL
1. Docetaxel with prednisone 2. Abiraterone with prednisone* 3. Enzalutamide* 4. Radium-223# 5. Sipuleucel-T 6. Other secondary hormone therapy: antiandrogen, antiandrogen withdrawal, ketoconazole ± hydrocortisone, corticosteroids, diethylstilbestrol (DES), or other estrogen	1. Enzalutamide 2. Abiraterone with prednisone 3. Radium-223# 4. Cabazitaxel with prednisone 5. Sipuleucel-T 6. Docetaxel re-challenge 7. Mitoxantrone with prednisone 8. Other secondary hormone therapy: antiandrogen, antidrogen withdrawal, ketoconazole ± hydrocortisone, corticosteroids, DES, or other estrogen

Discussion

Landmark trials have change the landscape and sequence in which mCRPC patients receive treatment.[2-9] The first vaccine approved for mCRPC, sipuleucel-T, is an autologous dendritic cell vaccine designed to stimulate the T cell immune response against prostatic acid phosphatase.[2]

Two trials (AFFIRM and PREVAIL) have shown benefit in enzalutamide, a potent second-generation anti-androgen, in docetaxel-naïve patients with mCRPC and those who have received prior docetaxel.[3,4]

Similarly, abiraterone, an androgen biosynthesis inhibitor, demonstrated improvement in overall survival (OS) in the randomized clinical trial COU-AA-301 in mCRPC patients who had received prior docetaxel treatment. Interestingly, the survival benefit was also seen in patients with visceral metastasis.[5] In COU-AA-302, which enrolled docetaxel-naïve, asymptomatic, or minimally symptomatic mCRPC patients with no visceral metastasis, OS with abiraterone was significantly longer.[6]

Of note, other secondary end points such as delays in disease progression and onset of pain and increased quality of life were in favor of abiraterone and enzalutamide.[3-6]

TRIAL	**PATIENT POPULATION**	**MEDIAN OS** Treatment arm vs. placebo (months)
AFFIRM[3]	Prior treatment with docetaxel	Enzalutamide 18.4 vs. placebo 13.6
PREVAIL[4]	Docetaxel-naïve (asymptomatic or minimally symptomatic)	Enzalutamide 32.4 vs. placebo 30.2
COU-AA-301[5]	Prior docetaxel treatment	Abiraterone 15.8 vs. placebo 11.2 months
COU-AA-302[6]	Docetaxel-naïve (asymptomatic or minimally symptomatic)	Abiraterone 34.7 vs. placebo 30.3 months

(continued on following page)

	(continued from previous page) The TROPIC trial randomly assigned CRPC patients whose disease progressed during or after docetaxel-based chemotherapy to receive either cabazitaxel/prednisone or mitoxantrone/prednisone. Cabazitaxel, a second-generation tubulin-binding taxane, was superior to mitoxantrone in terms of OS (15.1 vs. 12.7 months) at the expense of more grade 3/4 toxicities.[7] Radium-223 is an alpha-particle–emitting bone-targeting agent. It has been approved for use in CRPC patients with symptomatic bony metastasis and no visceral metastasis. The approval was based on the ALSYMPCA trial, which showed a superior OS with radium-223 compared with best supportive care (14 vs. 11.3 months). Furthermore, the treatment led to a significant delay in time to first symptomatic skeletal event.[8]
Pearl	The choice of therapy is dictated by different factors, including the disease kinetics and aggressiveness, presence of symptoms, evidence of metastatic disease (M0 = no metastatic disease vs. M1 = presence of metastatic disease) or presence of visceral disease, performance status, history of prior treatment, and patient preferences.
References	1. Tannock IF, de Wit R, Berry WR, et al. Docetaxel plus prednisone or mitoxantrone plus prednisone for advanced prostate cancer. N Engl J Med 2004;351(15):1502-12. 2. Kantoff PW, Higano CS, Shore ND, et al. Sipuleucel-T immunotherapy for castration-resistant prostate cancer. N Engl J Med 2010;363(5):411-22. 3. Scher HI, Fizazi K, Saad F, et al. Increased survival with enzalutamide in prostate cancer after chemotherapy. N Engl J Med 2012;367(13):1187-97. 4. Beer TM, Armstrong AJ, Rathkopf DE, et al. Enzalutamide in metastatic prostate cancer before chemotherapy. N Engl J Med 2014;371(5):424-33. 5. De Bono JS, Logothetis CJ, Molina A, et al. Abiraterone and increased survival in metastatic prostate cancer. N Engl J Med 2011;364(21):1995-2005.

6. Ryan CJ, Smith MR, de Bono JS, et al. Abiraterone in metastatic prostate cancer without previous chemotherapy. N Engl J Med 2013;368(2):138-48.
7. De Bono JS, Oudard S, Ozguroglu M, et al. Prednisone plus cabazitaxel or mitoxantrone for metastatic castration-resistant prostate cancer progressing after docetaxel treatment: a randomised open-label trial. Lancet 2010;376(9747):1147-54.
8. Parker C, Nilsson S, Heinrich D, et al. Alpha emitter radium-223 and survival in metastatic prostate cancer. N Engl J Med 2013;369(3):213-23.
9. National Comprehensive Cancer Network guidelines for prostate cancer. Version 2.2017. Available at: www.nccn.org.

Does chemotherapy have a role in castrate-naïve prostate cancer (CNPC)?

Key concept	Androgen deprivation therapy (ADT) to bring testosterone level to castrate level (<50 ng/dL) remains the backbone of treatment in metastatic castrate-naïve prostate cancer (CNPC). Recent studies have shown that early initiation of chemotherapy improves outcomes in high-volume disease.
Clinical scenario	A 65-year-old man was recently diagnosed with prostate cancer, Gleason 4 + 4 = 8, and prostate-specific antigen of 301. A bone scan revealed widespread skeletal metastases, including the pelvis, both femurs, multiple vertebrae, shoulder plates, ribs, and sternum. His oncologist started him on Lupron and bicalutamide. Is chemotherapy indicated in this setting?
Action items	Docetaxel 75 mg/m^2 every 3 weeks for 6 cycles concurrently with ADT is indicated in patients with castrate-naïve prostate cancer and high disease burden, defined by visceral metastasis or the presence of ≥4 bony metastasis with at least one bony metastasis beyond the pelvis and vertebral bodies.
Discussion	The benefit of chemotherapy when started earlier along with ADT in castrate-naïve metastatic prostate cancer has been proved by 3 large randomized controlled trials. In the CHAARTED trial, 790 patients with CNPC were randomized to receive ADT alone or ADT with 6 cycles of docetaxel. The median overall survival (OS) was 13.6 months longer in the combination group. Subgroup analysis showed that the survival benefit was significant in patients with high volume disease but not in those with low-volume disease.[1] The STAMPEDE trial enrolled patients with high-risk CNPC and revealed the superiority of docetaxel/ADT over ADT alone, with no additional benefit of added zoledronic acid.[2] In the GETUG-AFU 15 trial, there was a marginal benefit with chemotherapy + hormone over ADT alone, yet the OS benefit was not statistically significant. Unlike the previous 2 studies, docetaxel was administered for to up 9 cycles.[3]

Pearls	The addition of 6 cycles of docetaxel added to ADT in CNPC improves OS in patients with high-volume disease.
References	1. Sweeney CJ, Chen YH, Carducci M, et al. Chemohormonal therapy in metastatic hormone-sensitive prostate cancer. N Engl J Med 2015;373(8):737-46. 2. James ND, Sydes MR, Clarke NW, et al. Addition of docetaxel, zoledronic acid, or both to first-line long-term hormone therapy in prostate cancer (STAMPEDE): survival results from an adaptive, multiarm, multistage, platform randomised controlled trial. Lancet 2016;387(10024):1163-77. 3. Gravis G, Fizazi K, Joly F, et al. Androgen-deprivation therapy alone or with docetaxel in non-castrate metastatic prostate cancer (GETUG-AFU 15): a randomised, open-label, phase 3 trial. Lancet Oncol 2013;14(2):149-58.

What is sipuleucel-T, and what is its role in metastatic prostate cancer?

Key concept	Sipuleucel-T is a therapeutic cancer vaccine consisting of an autologous dendritic cell vaccine designed to stimulate the T cell immune response against prostatic acid phosphatase.[1,2]
Clinical scenario	A 65-year-old man was recently diagnosed with prostate cancer, Gleason $4 + 4 = 8$, and prostate-specific antigen of 301. He is overall healthy and has no significant past medical history other than hypertension, with ECOG 0. His bone scan reveals widespread skeletal metastases, including the pelvis, both femurs, multiple vertebrae, shoulder plates, ribs, and sternum. Is he a candidate for sipuleucel-T therapy?
Discussion	The phase 3 randomized, double-blind, placebo-controlled, multicenter IMPACT (Immunotherapy for Prostate Adenocarcinoma Treatment) trial involved 512 patients with metastatic castration-resistant prostate cancer (CRPC). The patients were generally asymptomatic or minimally symptomatic. Patients with ECOG performance status of ≥ 2 or visceral metastases, pathologic long-bone fractures, or spinal cord compression were excluded. There was improvement in median survival of 4.1 months in the sipuleucel-T arm (25.8 months vs. 21.7 months in the placebo group).[1] Two prior phase 3 studies evaluated sipuleucel-T in asymptomatic metastatic CRPC and demonstrated discrepancies with respect to benefit: one trial did not meet its primary end point of time to disease progression (TTP) but did show improvement in overall survival (OS), and the other trial did meet its TTP but showed a trend for prolonged OS that did not meet statistical significance.[2] To receive sipuleucel-T, each patient undergoes leukapheresis to obtain peripheral blood mononuclear cells (PMBCs). The PMBCs are activated ex vivo with a recombinant fusion protein (PA2024), which is composed of the prostate antigen prostatic acid phosphatase, which is fused to granulocyte–macrophage colony-stimulating factor, an immune-cell activator. The ensuing T cell response results in production of antigen-presenting cells, which are isolated from the leukapheresis product and then re-infused back into the patient (Figure 8-1).[1]

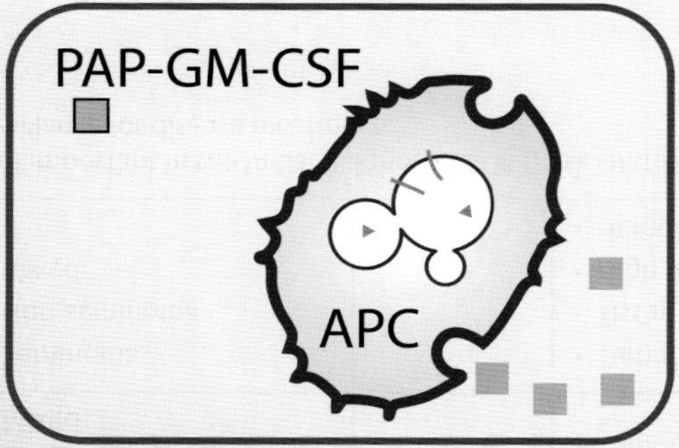

Figure 8-1. Mechanism of action of sipuleucel-T.

Pearls	Sipuleucel-T can be considered for metastatic CRPC patients with good performance status (ECOG 0–1) and who are asymptomatic or minimally symptomatic and with no visceral disease. The vaccine has been shown to prolong OS, although it had no effect on progression-free survival.[1]
References	1. Kantoff PW, Higano CS, Shore ND, et al. Sipuleucel-T immunotherapy for castration-resistant prostate cancer. N Engl J Med 2010;363(5):41122. 2. Cha E, Fong L. Immunotherapy for prostate cancer: biology and therapeutic approaches. J Clin Oncol 2011;29(27):3677-85.

Tumor markers for germ cell tumors (GCT)

TUMOR MARKER[1,2]	HISTOLOGY	HALF-LIFE, DAYS	CAUSE OF FALSE-POSITIVE RESULT	COMMENTS
Beta HCG	• Non-seminoma (typically in choriocarcinoma and embryonal carcinoma) • Seminoma • Mixed	1.5–3	• Hypogonadal state • Tumor lysis • Heterophile antibodies • Marijuana use • Other malignancies	A very elevated BHCG level with normal AFP is classically observed in pure choriocarcinoma
AFP	• Non-seminoma (typical in yolk sac and embryonal carcinoma) • Mixed	5–7	• Liver disease • Hepatocellular carcinoma • Tumor lysis	Normal in pure seminoma
LDH	• Seminoma • Non-seminoma • Mixed		• Tumor lysis • Tissue injury • High tissue turnover • Hemolysis	Not sensitive or specific

Tumor markers are important in the initial diagnosis of GCT, risk stratification, prognosis, monitoring response to therapy, and surveillance for disease recurrence.

References

1. Up-to-date. Serum tumor markers in testicular germ cell tumors. Available at: https://www.uptodate.com/contents/serum-tumor-markers-in-testicular-germ-cell-tumors.
2. Gilligan T, Seidenfeld J, Basch E, et al. American Society of Clinical Oncology practice guideline on uses of serum tumor markers in adult males with germ cell tumors. J Clin Oncol 2010;28(20):3388-404.

AFP, alpha-fetoprotein; BHCG, beta-human chorionic gonadotropin.

How do I treat a patient with testicular seminoma?

Key concept	About 80% of testicular seminomas present as localized disease, whereas 15% of cases presents as stage II disease (extension to retroperitoneal lymph nodes [RPLN]); cases rarely present with stage III (metastatic) disease. Initial treatment consists of radical orchiectomy. Subsequent therapeutic approaches consist of active surveillance, adjuvant radiation, or adjuvant chemotherapy, and the choice of approach depends on the disease staging.
Clinical scenario	A 24-year-old man presented to his primary care physician for a lump on his left testicle. Tumor markers revealed lactate dehydrogenase 3 times normal, alpha fetoprotein normal, and beta-human chorionic gonadotropin 1.5 times normal. Testicular ultrasound showed a hypoechoic left testicular mass. CT scan of the chest, abdomen, and pelvis revealed the presence of a 4-cm RPLN. He underwent sperm cryopreservation and radical left orchiectomy, which was positive for pure seminoma. How he should be treated next?
Action items	Unless a patient presents with rapidly progressing systemic disease requiring urgent administration of chemotherapy, radical orchiectomy is the initial treatment. Sperm cryopreservation prior to orchiectomy is advised in patients wishing to preserve their fertility. Subsequent approaches are as follows[1,2]: • Stage I: active surveillance (preferred), 1–2 cycles of carboplatin, or adjuvant radiation therapy • Stage IIA (RPLN ≤2 cm): adjuvant radiation therapy (preferred) or cisplatin-based chemotherapy (3 cycles of BEP or 4 cycles of EP) • Stage IIB (RPLN >2 and ≤5 cm) or stage IIC (>5 cm): cisplatin-based chemotherapy (3 cycles of BEP or 4 cycles of EP) or radiation therapy (in selected cases)

	• Stage III (extension beyond RPLN): • Favorable risk: cisplatin-based chemotherapy (BEP×3 or EP×4) • Intermediate risk (metastasis to organ other than lungs and lymph nodes): cisplatin-based chemotherapy (BEP×4 or VIP×4) BEP = bleomycin/etoposide/cisplatin; EP = etoposide/cisplatin; VIP = etoposide/ifosfamide/cisplatin
Pearls	Radical orchiectomy is often curative in pure seminoma limited to the testicle. Adjuvant radiation therapy is recommended when metastasis to RPLN is <2 cm in size, whereas cisplatin-based chemotherapy is recommended in the case of more advanced disease.
Discussion	In stage I seminoma, following orchiectomy, active surveillance with periodic scans, clinical evaluation, and serum tumor markers is preferred. For patients who wish to pursue more aggressive therapy, adjuvant carboplatin AUC 7 for 2 cycles is a reasonable option and is preferred over adjuvant low-dose radiation to the para-aortic lymph node. Patients should understand that adjuvant chemotherapy or radiation therapy will not improve overall survival but may prolong the time to recurrence yet be associated with toxicities. In stage IIA disease, adjuvant radiation therapy remains the treatment of choice and has been shown to be associated with 100% overall survival at 5 years (SWENOTECA trial).[3] Adjuvant chemotherapy has been shown to be associated with excellent outcomes in stage IIB and IIC disease.[1-3]
References	1. Up-to-date. Testicular cancer (beyond the basics). Available at: https://www.uptodate.com/contents/testicular-cancer-beyond-the-basics. 2. National Comprehensive Cancer Network. Guidelines for testicular cancer. Available at: https://www.nccn.org. 3. Tandstad T, Smaaland R, Solberg A, et al. Management of seminomatous testicular cancer: a binational prospective population-based study from the Swedish Norwegian testicular cancer study group. J Clin Oncol 2011;29(6):719-25.

How do I treat a patient with metastatic nonseminomatous testicular cancer (NSGCT)?

Key concept	NSGCT is considered to be metastatic whenever it spreads beyond the retroperitoneal lymph nodes. Cisplatin-based chemotherapy is the backbone of therapy. Risk stratification is based on the site of metastasis and tumor markers values following orchiectomy. The number of chemotherapy cycles and regimen are guided by the risk stratification.
Clinical scenario	A 30-year-old man presented with large left testicular mass, and underwent radical left orchiectomy. Pathology was positive for nonseminomatous germ cell tumor. CT scan of the chest, abdomen, and pelvis revealed the presence of bulky retroperitoneal lymphadenopathy as well as of bilateral lung nodules suggestive for metastatic disease. Tumor marker post-orchiectomy are: beta-human chorionic gonadotropin (BHCG) 60,500; alpha-fetoprotein (AFP) 2500, and lactate dehydrogenase (LDH) normal. What chemotherapy should he be offered?

Action items	• Unless the patient presents with rapidly progressing systemic disease requiring urgent administration of chemotherapy, radical orchiectomy is the initial treatment
	• Sperm cryopreservation prior to orchiectomy is advised in patients wishing to preserve their fertility
	• Further chemotherapy is guided by risk stratifications as follows[1,2]:
	  • Favorable risk: 3 cycles of BEP or 4 cycles of EP
	  • Intermediate risk: 4 cycles of BEP or 4 cycles of VIP
	  • Poor risk: 4 cycles of BEP or 4 cycles of VIP
	
	BEP, bleomycin/etoposide/cisplatin; EP, etoposide/cisplatin; VIP, etoposide/ifosfamide/cisplatin

Discussion	The risk stratification depends on the presence or not of metastatic disease beyond the lung and/or lymph nodes, as well as on the value of tumor markers (BHCG, AFP, and LDH) after orchiectomy[1,2]: • Favorable risk if meets all the following criteria:

	• no metastasis beyond the lungs and/or lymph nodes, AND • post-orchiectomy tumor markers are all low (AFP <1000 ng/mL, BHCG <5000 IU/L, and LDH <1.5× the upper limit of normal [ULN]) • Intermediate risk: • testicular or retroperitoneal primary tumors AND • no metastasis beyond the lungs and/or lymph nodes AND • post-orchiectomy tumor markers as follows: • AFP 1000–10,000 ng/mL OR • BHCG 5000–50,000 IU/L OR • LDH 1.5–10× ULN • High risk: • mediastinal primary tumor OR • visceral metastasis other than lungs OR • post-orchiectomy tumor markers as follows: • AFP >10,000 ng/mL OR • BHCG >50,000 IU/L OR • LDH >10× ULN
Pearls	For patients with metastatic NSGCT at favorable risk, chemotherapy consists of 3 cycles of BEP or 4 cycles of EP. In intermediate- and high-risk patients, chemotherapy consists of 4 cycles of BEP or 4 cycles of VIP.
References	1. Up-to-date. Testicular cancer (beyond the basics). Available at: https://www.uptodate.com/contents/testicular-cancer-beyond-the-basics. 2. National Comprehensive Cancer Network. Guidelines for testicular cancer. Available at: https://www.nccn.org.

CHAPTER 9

Gynecolological Malignancies

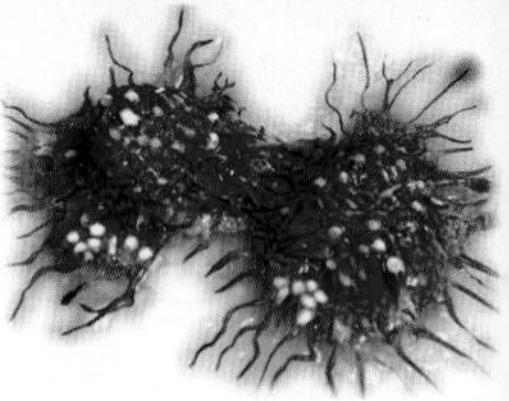

How should I manage patients with locally advanced cervical cancer?

Key concept	Cervical cancer is one of the leading causes of cancer-related death among women in developing countries. It is strongly linked with human papillomavirus (HPV) infection (types 16 and 18). PAP smear is effective for early detection and reduces mortality. In the developed world, women with lower socioeconomic status and those with multiple sexual partners are more likely to develop cervical cancer.[1]
Clinical scenario	A 44-year-old single mother with multiple sexual partners presents with post-coital bleeding. She also reports lower pelvic pain. Local examination reveals a large fungating mass in cervix. Biopsy confirms squamous cell cancer.
Action items	• Pelvic examination should be performed for biopsy and clinical staging • Staging studies such as CT and MRI can be performed • Patients with stage IA1 to IIA1 disease can be treated with surgery • Surgery can be fertility sparing, such as trachelectomy, or radical hysterectomy with bilateral pelvic lymph node dissection
Discussion	Patients are diagnosed at screening, or they may present with symptoms such as post-coital bleeding, vaginal discharge, or pelvic pain. Gynecological examination is needed for diagnosis and clinical staging (International Federation of Gynecology and Obstetrics). Most patients have squamous cell cancer; other types are adenocarcinoma and neuroendocrine histology.

	Patients with stage IB2 to IVA, non-metastatic disease are treated with concurrent chemoradiation.[2] Concurrent chemoradiation reduces risk of death by 30%–50%. Radiation is given by external beam radiation therapy concurrent with weekly cisplatin chemotherapy. Another chemotherapy option includes cisplatin/5-fluorouracil. After concurrent chemoradiation, brachytherapy is considered the standard of care. Patients with metastatic cervical cancer are treated with doublet chemotherapy (cisplatin/paclitaxel or topotecan/paclitaxel) and bevacizumab.
Pearls	HPV vaccines such as Gardasil are very effective against HPV type 16 and 18 infection. They are indicated for female and male patients ages 9–26 years.
References	1. National Comprehensive Cancer Network (NCCN) guidelines for cervical cancer. Version 1.2017. Available at: www.nccn.org. 2. Rose PG, Bundy BN, Watkins EB, et al. Concurrent cisplatin-based radiotherapy and chemotherapy for locally advanced cervical cancer. N Engl J Med 1999;340:1144-53.

How do I treat early stage endometrial cancer?

Key concept	Endometrial cancer is the most common gynecological malignancy in developed countries, including the United States.[1] Risk factors for hormone-sensitive (type 1) endometrial cancer include prolonged unopposed estrogen associated with early age of menarche, nulliparity, late age at menopause, obesity, diabetes, a high-fat diet, Lynch syndrome,* age ≥55 years, unopposed estrogen for control of menopausal symptoms, and tamoxifen use. Smoking and combination oral contraceptives are protective against this type of malignancy.[1,2] Around 70% of endometrial cancers are confined to the uterus at diagnosis and less than 10% present with metastatic disease.[1]
Clinical scenario	A 64-year-old post-menopausal woman presents with vaginal bleeding for the past ~5 days. She undergoes evaluation by a gynecologic oncologist, who performs a transvaginal ultrasound and endometrial biopsy. The pathology demonstrates a grade 2 endometrioid adenocarcinoma. What is the next step in management?
Discussion	Initial work-up and evaluation for suspected endometrial cancer includes a thorough history and physical examination and endometrial assessment with either ultrasound or endometrial biopsy. If endometrial sampling is non-diagnostic, the patient needs to be referred for dilatation and curettage with or without hysteroscopy.[1,3] CA-125 levels can be obtained preoperatively and as a baseline to monitor. CA-125 is frequently elevated in patients with disseminated disease. After a diagnosis of endometrial cancer is made, the treatment of choice is surgical staging, which includes total hysterectomy (minimally invasive or abdominal route is chosen depending on the characteristics of the patient), bilateral salpingo-oophorectomy, pelvic washings, and possibly complete vs. modified lymphadenectomy (sentinel lymph nodes can be considered in appropriate candidates).[2,3]

	After surgical staging is complete, decisions about additional treatment are made based on multiple factors. Radiation of the vaginal cuff (vaginal cuff brachytherapy) or pelvis as well as chemotherapy (carboplatin and paclitaxel) can all be considered, depending on the patient's lymph node status and the characteristics of the cancer in the uterus.[1-3]
Pearls	• Initial treatment of asymptomatic patients presenting with metastatic endometrial cancer of low grade (ie, grade 1 or 2) and that are estrogen and progesterone receptor–positive are hormonal agents with progestational agents such as megestrol acetate • In symptomatic, high-risk patients with metastatic endometrial cancer, cytotoxic therapy with multiple agents including platinum and taxane agents (ie, carboplatin-paclitaxel) can be considered[1]
References	1. National Comprehensive Cancer Network guidelines for uterine neoplasms. Version 1.2018. Available at: www.nccn.org. 2. Burke WM, Orr J, Leitao M, et al. Endometrial cancer: a review and current management strategies: part I. Gynecol Oncol 2014:134(2):385-92. 3. Burke WM, Orr J, Leitao M, et al. Endometrial cancer: a review and current management strategies: part II. Gynecol Oncol 2014:134(2):393-402.

*Endometrial cancers associated with Lynch syndrome make up ~5% of patients. Genetic counseling and testing can be considered in patients <50 years old diagnosed with endometrial cancer.[1]

What is the optimal treatment for non-metastatic ovarian cancer?

Key concept	Ovarian cancer is the leading cause of death from gynecological malignancies. The risk is higher in women with nulliparity and old age at first pregnancy. The presence of BRCA1 and BRCA2 increases the risk of ovarian cancer.[1]
Clinical scenario	A 62-year-old nulliparous woman presents with lower abdominal pain, early satiety, and abdominal fullness. Her appetite is low, and she has lost 20 lb recently. Abdominal ultrasound demonstrates small-volume ascites and a large right ovarian mass. The patient undergoes debulking abdominal surgery. Pathology is consistent with ovarian carcinoma.
Action items	• CA-125 is a reliable tumor marker for ovarian cancer and can be used to monitor the course of disease • Patients should undergo surgical staging and debulking followed by systemic therapy • During surgery, all grossly observable disease should be removed; most patients have hysterectomy with bilateral salpingo-oophorectomy, omentectomy, and lymphadenectomy • Some patients may benefit from neoadjuvant chemotherapy prior to surgery for bulky disease
Discussion	Most women are >50 years old, and nearly two-thirds present with advanced disease at the time of diagnosis. Patients can have vague symptoms that include abdominal pain, a sense of fullness, early satiety, and urinary symptoms. Most patients will need adjuvant chemotherapy after debulking surgery. Intravenous (IV)/intraperitoneal (IP) chemotherapy is the standard of care for patients undergoing optimal debulking (<1 cm residual disease) surgery. IP chemotherapy is associated with catheter complications, nausea, vomiting, dehydration, and abdominal pain.[2]

	Patients who are unable to undergo IP chemotherapy should be given adjuvant IV chemotherapy. Bevacizumab may be considered in select patients with high-risk features.
Pearls	• There is no approved screening test for ovarian cancer • If disease recurs, platinum-based combination chemotherapy can be considered if prior treatment with platinum agent was >6 months previously • If the disease is platinum-resistant (ie, prior platinum treatment <6 months previously), then consider treatment with docetaxel, gemcitabine, or etoposide
References	1. National Comprehensive Cancer Network (NCCN) guidelines for ovarian cancer. Version 1.2017. Available at: www.nccn.org. 2. Armstrong D, Bundy B, Wenzel L, et al. Intraperitoneal cisplatin and paclitaxel in ovarian cancer. N Engl J Med 2006;354:34-43.

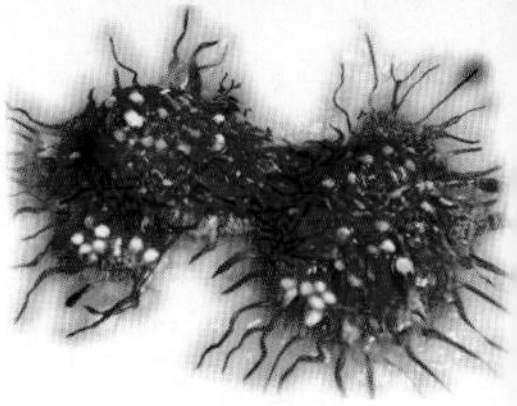

CHAPTER 10

Thoracic Cancers

How do I treat patients presenting with limited-stage small cell lung cancer (LS-SCLC)?

Key concept	Chemotherapy is an integral component of the treatment of patients with LS-SCLC, because of the high likelihood of early dissemination. Radiation therapy is also important, because treatment with chemotherapy alone in LS-SCLC can be associated with a high risk of local progression. Surgery plays a role only in T1-2N0M0 disease.
Clinical scenario	A 52-year-old man with a history of heavy smoking presents for worsening shortness of breath. CT of the chest revealed large mediastinal and right hilar lymph nodes. Endobronchial ultrasound is positive for small-cell lung cancer. An MRI of the brain is normal, and PET/CT scan shows a fluorodeoxyglucose (FDG)-avid, large mediastinal mass and bilateral hilar lymph nodes but no distant metastasis. What will be the next step in the management of this patient?
Action items	• The backbone of LS-SCLC treatment consists of concurrent chemotherapy and radiation therapy followed by prophylactic cranial irradiation if the patient has a good response • Patients with T1-2N0M0 disease might benefit from surgery followed by adjuvant treatment (chemotherapy with or without radiation for nodal disease) • Thoracic radiation therapy must be administered with the first or second cycle of chemotherapy • Standard dose of radiation therapy is 45 Gy (1.5 Gy twice daily for 3 weeks) • Alternative radiation therapy dose is 60–70 Gy (2 Gy daily for 6 weeks) • Chemotherapy consists of 4–6 cycles of platinum doublet (ie, cisplatin and etoposide or cisplatin and irinotecan). Cisplatin is the preferred platinum agent to be used during radiation therapy

Discussion

A meta-analysis has shown that chest radiation therapy, when added to chemotherapy, improves the survival in LS-SCLC, with a 3-year overall survival (OS) rate of 14.3% for the bimodality approach vs. 8.9% for chemotherapy only.[1] Another important randomized controlled study has proved that concurrent chemoradiation is superior to sequential chemotherapy–radiation therapy in LS-SCLC, with a median average survival of 27.2 months for concurrent therapy vs. 19.7 months for sequential therapy.[2] Another meta-analysis showed that early initiation of radiation therapy correlated with better OS than late initiation of radiation therapy.[3] A hyperfractionated accelerated radiation therapy regimen (45 Gy/1.5 Gy twice daily over 3 weeks) proved superior to standard fractionation of 50 Gy (2 Gy daily over 5 weeks).[4] Whether this regimen is superior to 60 Gy (2 Gy daily over 6 weeks) is being assessed in an ongoing trial. Finally, the addition of prophylactic cranial irradiation (PCI) following chemoradiation has been shown to decrease the incidence of brain metastasis and improve OS in LS-SCLC.[5]

Pearls

For patients with LS-SCLC, treatment consists primarily of concurrent chemotherapy (cisplatin-based regimen) and radiation therapy. Radiotherapy preferably should be initiated before cycle 2 of chemotherapy. Patients with a good response to treatment should be offered PCI. In the rare scenario of LS-SCLC with low tumor burden and absence of nodal disease, surgery may be considered instead, followed by adjuvant chemotherapy with or without radiation therapy.

References

1. Pignon JP, Arriagada R, Ihde DC, et al. A meta-analysis of thoracic radiotherapy for small-cell lung cancer. N Engl J Med 1992;327:1618-24.
2. Takada M, Fukuoka M, Kawahara M, et al. Phase III study of concurrent vs. sequential thoracic radiotherapy in combination with cisplatin and etoposide for LS-SCLC: results of the JCOGS 9104. J Clin Oncol 2002;20(14):3054-60.
3. Fried DB, Morris DE, Poole C, et al. Systematic review evaluating the timing of thoracic radiation in combined modality therapy for LS-SCLC. J Clin Oncol 2004;22(23):4837-45.
4. Turrisi AT III, Kim K, Blum R, et al. Twice-daily compared with once-daily thoracic radiotherapy in LS-SCLC treated concurrently with cisplatin and etoposide. N Engl J Med 1999;340(4):265-71.
5. Auperin A, Arriagada R, Pignon JP, et al. PCI for patients with SCLC in complete remission. Prophylactic cranial irradiation overview collaborative group. N Engl J Med 1999;341(7):476-84.

How do I treat patients presenting with extensive-stage small cell lung cancer (ES-SCLC)?

Key concept	SCLC is highly responsive to chemotherapy and radiotherapy initially. However, it is associated with poor prognosis owing to eventual disease relapse, usually within few months, and becoming refractory to further treatment. Chemotherapy is the backbone of treatment and is associated with disease control and improvement in survival. Palliative radiation therapy and prophylactic cranial irradiation (PCI) can be considered in specific settings.
Clinical scenario	A 58-year-old man with a history of heavy smoking presents with worsening facial edema and headaches. CT scan of the chest reveals a bulky mediastinal mass compressing the superior vena cava (SVC). MRI of the brain is negative. CT of the abdomen and pelvis reveal multiple hepatic lesions. Biopsy of one of the hepatic lesions is positive for small cell carcinoma of lung origin. What treatment do you offer him?
Action items	• Systemic therapy consists of 4–6 cycles of platinum-doublet chemotherapy (ie, platinum and etoposide) • Carboplatin can be substituted for cisplatin • Regimens substituting irinotecan, topotecan, or epirubicin for etoposide are acceptable alternatives • In cases of symptomatic brain metastasis or spinal cord compression, palliative radiation therapy should be considered prior to initiation of systemic therapy • In cases of SVC syndrome, lobar obstruction, or asymptomatic brain metastasis, systemic treatment can be initiated first • Consolidation thoracic radiation therapy should be offered for patients with a good response to chemotherapy • PCI may be considered following completion of treatment in cases of good response • The choice of second-line chemotherapy depends on the timing of recurrence: for relapse occurring after >6 months, reinduction with same chemotherapy regimen is recommended; otherwise, different antineoplastic agents can be considered (eg, topotecan, docetaxel, CPT-11, gemcitabine, temozolomide, and nivolumab with or without ipilimumab)

Discussion	Chemotherapy prolongs survival compared with best supportive care only.[1] However, median overall survival (OS) remains <12 months despite chemotherapy. Meta-analysis of 5 clinical trials showed no difference in OS between cisplatin-based and carboplatin-based chemotherapy[2]; thus, these can be used interchangeably in metastatic disease. Consolidative chest radiotherapy may be beneficial for selected patients who respond to chemotherapy and have no extrathoracic disease after chemotherapy.[3] The impact of PCI on OS in ES-SCLC is debatable. Whereas an EORTC trial showed a survival advantage with PCI, a second trial conducted in Japan demonstrated a trend toward reduced OS with PCI.[4,5] PCI with hippocampus-sparing techniques to reduce neurotoxicity and improve outcome are currently being investigated. Maintenance treatment, dose-dense chemotherapy, and multidrug combination regimens (≥3) have not been shown to offer substantial benefits.
Pearls	4–6 cycles of platinum-based (carboplatin or cisplatin) chemotherapy is the backbone of treatment for metastatic SCLC. Thoracic radiotherapy with or without PCI should be considered following completion of chemotherapy in the instance of a good disease response. There is no proven role for maintenance chemotherapy.
References	1. Agra Y, Pelayo M, Sacristan M, et al. Chemotherapy vs. best supportive care for extensive SCLC. Cochrane Database Syst Rev 2003;(4):CD001990. 2. Rossi A, Di Maio M, Chiodini P, et al. Carboplatin or cisplatin-based chemotherapy in first-line treatment of SCLC: the COCIS meta-analysis of individual patient data. J Clin Oncol 2012;30(14):1692-8. 3. Slotman BJ, van Tinteren H, Praag JO, et al. Use of thoracic radiotherapy for ES-SCLC: a phase 3 randomized controlled trial. Lancet 2015;385(9962):36-42. 4. Slotman B, Faivre-Finn C, Kramer G, et al. Prophylactic cranial irradiation in ES-SCLC. N Engl J Med 2007;357(7):664-72. 5. Seto T, Takahashi T, Yamanaka T, et al. Prophylactic cranial irradiation (PCI) has detrimental effect on the overall survival of patients with ES-SCLC: results of a Japanese randomized phase III trial (abstract 7503). 2014 ASCO meeting. J Clin Oncol 2014;32(15_suppl):7503.

Is there a role for radiation therapy following palliative chemotherapy in ES-SCLC?

Key concept	Systemic chemotherapy remains the backbone of treatment for ES-SCLC. Few studies have demonstrated that consolidation thoracic radiation therapy or prophylactic cranial radiation (PCI) may play a therapeutic role in ES-SCLC patients with a favorable response to chemotherapy.
Clinical scenario	A 52-year-old man diagnosed with ES-SCLC completed 6 cycles of carboplatin and etoposide. Repeat imaging showed an excellent response with residual disease in the chest. Should he be referred to radiation oncology?
Action items	• For patients with ES-SCLC achieving a good response to chemotherapy with residual disease in the chest, consolidation with thoracic radiation therapy is recommended • PCI in ES-SCLC following a good response to chemotherapy is suggested in patients with good performance status, since it can reduce the incidence of symptomatic brain metastasis, although its impact on overall survival (OS) is debatable; patients should be encouraged to participate in clinical trials investigating the role of hippocampus-sparing PCI in this context
Discussion	In the Dutch CREST trial, patients with ES-SCLC achieving good response following 4–6 cycles of platinum-based chemotherapy were randomized to receive PCI or PCI plus consolidative chest radiation. At 2 years, OS was higher in the arm receiving chest radiation therapy. Subgroup analysis showed that the survival advantage was limited to patients with residual disease to the chest and not to those with a complete response in the chest.[1] Although an EORTC trial showed an OS advantage associated with PCI in patients with ES-SCLC who had a favorable response to chemotherapy, a recent Japanese randomized trial revealed that although the incidence of brain metastasis was reduced with PCI, OS was shorter, but the difference was not statistically significant.[2,3]

	When used, the dose of PCI is 25 Gy total in 10 daily fractions. A higher dose of 36 Gy was associated with increased mortality and neurotoxicity.[4]
Pearls	Thoracic radiation therapy is recommended following a good response to systemic chemotherapy and residual disease to the chest in ES-SCLC. PCI is suggested in patients with an excellent response to chemotherapy if they have good performance status and no impairment from neurocognitive disorder. Patients should be encouraged to enroll in clinical trials examining the role of hippocampus-sparing PCI in SCLC. If PCI is not an option, patients should be offered close observation with brain MRI.
References	1. Slotman BJ, van Tinteren H, Praag JO, et al. Use of thoracic radiotherapy for extensive stage small-cell lung cancer: a phase 3 randomised controlled trial. Lancet 2015;385(9962):36-42. 2. Slotman B, Faivre-Finn C, Kramer G, et al. Prophylactic cranial irradiation in extensive small-cell lung cancer. N Engl J Med 2007;357(7):664-72. 3. Takahashi T, Yamanaka T, Seto T, et al. Prophylactic cranial irradiation versus observation in patients with extensive-disease small-cell lung cancer: a multicentre, randomised, open-label, phase 3 trial. Lancet Oncol 2017;18(5):663-71. 4. Le Péchoux C, Dunant A, Senan S, et al. Standard-dose versus higher-dose prophylactic cranial irradiation (PCI) in patients with limited-stage small-cell lung cancer in complete remission after chemotherapy and thoracic radiotherapy (PCI 99-01, EORTC 22003-08004, RTOG 0212, and IFCT 99-01): a randomised clinical trial. Lancet Oncol 2009;10(5):467-74.

What molecular tests should I order in a patient diagnosed with non–small cell lung cancer (NSCLC)?

Key concept	Predictive biomarkers identified through molecular testing aid the selection of targeted and personalized therapy for patients with advanced NSCLC. Use of targeted drugs in patients with specific activating "driver mutations" results in a response rate better than that of chemotherapy.[1]
Clinical scenario	A 48-year-old woman never smoker reports an increasing dry cough for the past 4 months. Patient undergoes chest imaging, which shows a large mediastinal mass and bilateral metastatic lung lesions. Biopsy is consistent with lung adenocarcinoma. The medical oncologist orders molecular testing for identifying biomarkers.

Action items	• Lung adenocarcinoma or those with component of adenocarcinoma
	  • epidermal growth factor receptor (EGFR) testing through polymerase chain reaction (PCR)
	  • Anaplastic lymphoma kinase (ALK) testing through fluorescence in-situ hybridization (FISH)
	  • ROS1 testing through FISH
	  • Immunohistochemistry (IHC) for EGFR is not recommended
	• All NSCLC patients irrespective of histology
	• Programmed death ligand-1 (PDL-1) testing through IHC

Discussion	Nearly half of newly diagnosed NSCLC cancer patients present with metastatic disease at the time of diagnosis. Biopsy of a primary or metastatic site is needed to establish the diagnosis. Biopsy should be performed at the most accessible site. Biopsy can be performed through bronchoscopy, including endobronchial ultrasound, interventional radiology, or thoracotomy with preference for the least invasive procedure.

	Histological and IHC analysis of the biopsy specimen is needed to differentiate between various subtypes of NSCLC, such as adenocarcinoma, squamous cell carcinoma, or large cell carcinoma. Additional molecular testing is needed on lung adenocarcinomas to identify specific mutations that help identify personalized or targeted therapy for individual patients. Predictive biomarkers for lung adenocarcinoma include EGFR, ALK translocation, ROS1, and the recently added PD-L1. Detection of an activating driver mutation is a key in selection of therapy for advanced NSCLC patients. If an activating mutation is found, targeted therapy is preferred over chemotherapy. Clinicians should work closely with pathologists to ensure that these tests are performed on all newly diagnosed NSCLC patients.
Pearls	10%–15% of newly diagnosed patients with lung cancer will test positive for activating mutations. Presence of activating mutations is more likely in women, nonsmokers, and those of Asian descent.
References	1. Leighl NB, Rekhtman N, Biermann WA, et al. Molecular testing for selection of patients with lung cancer for epidermal growth factor receptor and anaplastic lymphoma kinase tyrosine kinase inhibitors: American Society of Clinical Oncology endorsement of the College of American Pathologists/International Association for the Study of Lung Cancer/Association for Molecular Pathology Guidelines. J Clin Oncol 2014;32(32):3673-9.

What is the stage of my lung cancer patient's disease?

Key concept	Patients with lung cancer are staged based on anatomic extent of the tumor. For lung cancer, TNM staging is used where T = local tumor spread, N = regional lymph node involvement, and M = distant hematogenous seeding or metastases.[1] Staging determines treatment choice and prognosis for lung cancer patients.
Clinical scenario	A 63-year-old man presents with cough, shortness of breath, and hemoptysis. Physical examination shows decreased breath sounds on the right side. Initial X-ray shows complete whiteout on the right side. Patient undergoes a CT scan that shows complete collapse of right lung with a large right hilar mass and pleural effusion.
Action items	• Obtain CT scan of the chest and abdomen with contrast (if no contraindication to contrast) • Obtain MRI of the brain • Obtain PET scan when clinically indicated • Obtain cytology to look for presence of malignant pleural/pericardial effusion when clinically indicated • Obtain mediastinoscopy for surgical staging of mediastinum when clinically indicated
Discussion	Patients who are newly diagnosed with lung cancer need further investigation to establish tumor stage. For all patients, initial staging is done clinically using physical examination and radiological tests. Patients who undergo surgery will also have pathological staging, which is more accurate than clinical staging. Stages I–IV separate patients into different prognostic groups. The presence of malignant pleural or pericardial effusion automatically upstages patient to stage IV.

Pearls	Patients with small cell lung cancer are generally staged using Veterans Administration Lung Study Group (VALG)[2] staging system into: • Limited stage disease (covered by a single radiation therapy portal) • Extensive stage disease (outside a single radiation therapy portal)
References	1. Goldstraw P. *IASLC Staging Handbook in Thoracic Oncology.* 1st ed. Orange Park, FL: EditorialRx Press; 2009. 2. Zelen M. Keynote address on biostatistics and data retrieval. Cancer Chemother Rep 1973;4:31-42.

Can my patient tolerate lung resection surgery?

Key concept	Surgery offers the chance of cure for patients with early-stage lung cancer. Unlike surgery for breast, prostate, or colon cancer, lung surgery involves removing part of an organ that is vital for optimal physiological functioning. Assessing lung function prior to surgery will increase perioperative morbidity and mortality. Poor lung function alone can make a patient ineligible for surgery in up to one-third of patients with newly diagnosed lung cancer.[1] Optimal surgery for lung cancer is lobectomy or pneumonectomy.
Clinical scenario	A 52-year-old man is recently found to have a left hilar mass. Lesion is PET positive and is consistent on biopsy with squamous cell lung cancer. Patient is referred to thoracic surgery for consideration of surgery. The surgeon is concerned that the patient may require left pneumonectomy.
Action items	• Obtain pulmonary function tests (PFTs), including forced expiratory volume in 1 second (FEV1) and diffusing capacity of lung for carbon monoxide (DLCO) • Ventilation/perfusion scintigraphy when clinically indicated • Cardiopulmonary exercise testing for maximum oxygen consumption (VO_2) max when clinically indicated. • Calculate predictive post-operative (PPO) FEV1
Discussion	For patients whose early-stage lung cancer is anatomically resectable, assessing lung function in addition to general risk of surgery is important. Patients are referred to a pulmonary specialist in order to assess the ability of a patient's lungs to withstand lung resection surgery. • Preoperative FEV1 of 1.5 L for lobectomy and 2 L for pneumonectomy is generally considered safe for lung resection surgery. • A predicted FEV1 of ≥80% and DLCO of ≥60% is also considered safe for lung resection surgery.

	• PPO FEV1 is calculated by the estimating the number of bronchopulmonary segments to be removed during surgery out of a total of 19 segments in both lungs (eg, for a right-upper-lobe lobectomy, 3 segments will be removed). If pre-operative FEV1 is 1.8 L, PPO after right upper lobe lobectomy will be 1.8 × 16/19 = 1.5 L. PPO >40% is considered safe for surgery. • Exercise pulmonary testing showing a VO_2 max >15 mL/kg/min is considered safe for lung resection surgery.
Pearls	• Patients requiring pneumonectomy (as opposed to lobectomy) after neoadjuvant chemoradiotherapy have a high mortality; thus, pneumonectomy is discouraged in these patients.[2] • Patients unable to undergo lung resection surgery can be treated with stereotactic ablative radiotherapy (SABR) for peripheral lesions of <3 cm.[3]
References	1. Mazzone P. Preoperative evaluation of the lung cancer resection candidate. Cleve Clin J Med 2012;79(Electronic Suppl 1): eS17-22. 2. Albain KS. Radiotherapy plus chemotherapy with or without surgical resection for stage III non-small cell lung cancer: a phase III randomized controlled trial. Lancet 2009;374(9687):379-89. 3. Verstegan NE. Stage I-II non-small cell lung cancer treated using either stereotactic ablative radiotherapy (SABR) or lobectomy by a video-assisted thoracoscopic surgery (VATS): outcomes of a propensity-matched analysis. Ann Oncol 2013;24(6):1543-8.

Does my patient need adjuvant chemotherapy after lung cancer surgery?

Key concept	Patients with localized lung cancer can have micro-metastatic disease, which can result in development of distant metastasis after curative lung cancer surgery. Adjuvant chemotherapy can reduce the chance of distant metastasis and prolong survival in early stage lung cancer patients after surgery.
Clinical scenario	A 56-year-old man with a 40 packs/year history of smoking undergoes routine lung cancer screening. CT scan shows a 3-cm right lower lobe with enlarged right hilar lymph nodes. The patient is referred to a thoracic surgeon for evaluation for lung resection surgery.

Action items	Adjuvant chemotherapy is indicated in the following patients[1]:
	• Stage IB (T ≥4 cm)
	• Stage II and III
	• Consider adjuvant chemotherapy in patients with other high-risk features:
	  • Poorly differentiated cancer
	  • Vascular invasion
	  • Visceral pleural involvement
	  • Wedge resection
	  • Unknown lymph node involvement
	  • Micro-papillary and solid predominant histological subtype adenocracinoma[2]
	• Patients with indication for adjuvant chemotherapy should be offered chemotherapy for 4 cycles
	• Platinum doublets, including cisplatin/vinorelbine and carboplatin/etoposide, are reasonable choices
	• Patients should be assessed for adequate performance status and organ function
	• An IV catheter is placed for delivery of adjuvant chemotherapy

Discussion	Patients should be evaluated peri-operatively to assess the need for adjuvant chemotherapy after curative lung resection surgery. Peri-operative radiology images, operative notes, and pathology reports should be reviewed to assess the need for adjuvant chemotherapy. Multiple randomized clinical trials and meta-analysis[3] have shown that adjuvant chemotherapy given to patients after lung resection surgery leads to improvement in disease-free survival and overall survival by 5%. An exception to this is that patients with stage IA disease and those with tumors <4 cm have not been shown to have improved outcome after adjuvant chemotherapy.
Pearls	Patients with positive mediastinal (N2) nodes also benefit from adjuvant radiation.[4]
References	1. National Comprehensive Cancer Network guidelines for lung cancer screening. Available at: www.nccn.org. 2. Travis WD, Brambilla E, Noguchi M, et al. International Association for the Study of Lung Cancer/American Thoracic Society/European Respiratory Society international multidisciplinary classification of lung adenocarcinoma. J Thorac Oncol 2011; 6:244-85. 3. Pignon JP. Lung adjuvant cisplatin evaluation: a pooled analysis by the LACE collaborative Group. J Clin Oncol 2008;26(21): 3552-9. 4. Robinson CG. Postoperative radiotherapy for pathological N2 non-small cell lung cancer treated with adjuvant chemotherapy: a review of the National Cancer Database. J Clin Oncol 2015;33(8):870-6.

When does my patient need adjuvant radiation therapy after lung cancer surgery?

Key concept	Locoregional recurrence after surgery can lead to bad outcomes in resected non–small cell lung cancer (NSCLC). In carefully selected patients, evidence has shown that the addition of adjuvant radiation may reduce the rate of locoregional recurrence and improve overall survival (OS).
Clinical scenario	A 63-year-old woman with a 30 packs/year history of smoking undergoes a right upper lobe lobectomy for a 3-cm right lung lesion. The final pathology is consistent with T2N2 lung adenocarcinoma.

Action items	• Adjuvant radiation therapy is indicated if
	  • Suspected or pN2 disease found postoperatively
	  • Positive surgical margins (R1 or R2 resection)
	• Consider administering concurrently with chemotherapy in case of R2 resection (gross residual disease) in stage II or IIIA NSCLC

Discussion	The National Cancer Database study showed that adjuvant radiation for positive surgical margins in stage II and III NSCLC patients who had undergone lobectomy or pneumonectomy significantly improves OS (median OS 33.5 vs. 23.7 months without radiation, 5-year OS 32.4 vs. 23.7%).[1] Subgroup analysis conducted from a SEER database study that included patients with stage II or III NSCLC who underwent lobectomy or pneumonectomy followed by adjuvant radiation showed that for patients with N2 disease, radiation therapy was associated with improved survival. By contrast, for patients with N0 or N1 disease, adjuvant radiation therapy was associated with reduced survival.[2]

Pearls	Postoperative radiation therapy is indicated in patients with positive surgical margin when additional resection is not possible or in mediastinal lymph node disease. In the case of stage II or IIIA NSCLC with gross residual disease, administration of chemotherapy concurrently with radiation therapy should be considered.
References	1. Wang EH, Corso CD, Rutter CE, et al. Postoperative radiation therapy is associated with improved overall survival in incompletely resected stage II and III non-small-cell lung cancer. J Clin Oncol 2015;33(25):2727-34. 2. Lally BE, Zelterman D, Colasanto JM, et al. Postoperative radiotherapy for stage II or III non-small-cell lung cancer using surveillance, epidemiology and end results database. J Clin Oncol 2006;24(19):2998-3006.

Which systemic treatment should I chose for newly diagnosed patients with advanced or relapsing non–small cell lung cancer (NSCLC)?

Key concept	Patients presenting with metastatic/relapsed NSCLC are treated with systemic therapy with the goal of prolonging survival and improving quality of life. The choice of treatment depends on histology, presence of biomarkers, and comorbidities that personalize therapy for patients with advanced NSCLC.
Clinical scenario	A 73-year-old man presents to his primary care physician for increasing right hip pain. Initial work-up, including MRI of the right hip, shows pathological fracture of right femur. The patient undergoes CT-guided biopsy, which is consistent with metastatic lung adenocarcinoma. The patient is seen in clinic for management of stage IV lung adenocarcinoma.
Action items	• Determine histological subtype of lung cancer • Order predictive biomarker analysis (ie, presence of EGFR, ALK, ROS1, and PDL-1 expression) • Determine performance status • Determine comorbidities (eg, peripheral neuropathy, which limits choice of chemotherapy) • Determine organ function through complete blood count (CBC) and comprehensive metabolic panel (CMP) (eg, pemetrexed not given in patients with glomerular filtration rate <45) • Refer for IV catheter placement in those being considered for chemotherapy
Discussion	Newly diagnosed patients with metastatic NSCLC and those with relapse of disease are carefully evaluated in the clinic to determine choice of systemic therapy. Key determinations of choice of treatment are: • Stage of disease • Histology • Presence of predictive biomarkers • Performance status • Comorbidities

<table>
<tr><td></td><td>Treatment choices include:
• Systemic chemotherapy (platinum doublet chemotherapy, eg, carboplatin-paclitaxel with or without bevacizumab)
• Pemetrexed is not used in patients with squamous histology
• Targeted therapy (small molecule inhibitors for those patients with presence of activating driver mutations, eg, EGFR, ALK, and ROS1)
• Immunotherapy (eg, pembrolizumab in those with ≥50% PDL-1 expression on the surface of tumors)
• Clinical trial

Patients with metastatic NSCLC live for an average of 1 year after receiving systemic therapy.[1] Those with activating mutations who are treated with targeted agents tend to have longer overall survival (2–3 years).[2] Up to 30% of metastatic lung cancer patients are unable to receive any systemic therapy due to poor performance status or comorbidities.[3] Patients who progress on first-line therapy are offered second-line treatment or a clinical trial.[4]</td></tr>
<tr><td>Pearls</td><td>Early use of palliative care in advanced NSCLC patients results in improved quality of life and overall survival.[5]</td></tr>
<tr><td>References</td><td>1. Sandler A, Gray R, Perty M, et al. Paclitaxel-carboplatin alone or with bevacizumab for non-small cell lung cancer. N Engl J Med 2006;355:2542-50.
2. Makoto M, Akira I, Kunihiko K, et al. Gefitinib or chemotherapy for non-small cell lung cancer with mutated EGFR. N Engl J Med 2010;362:2380-8.
3. Keith D, Ravi G, Stephen A, et al. Real-world treatment patterns and costs in a US Medicare population with metastatic squamous non-small cell lung cancer. Lung Cancer 2015;87:176-85.
4. Edward G, Tudor EC, Oscar A, et al. Ramucirumab plus docetaxel versus placebo docetaxel for second-line treatment of stage IV non-small-cell lung cancer after disease progression on platinum-based therapy (REVEL): a multicenter, double blind, randomised phase 3 trial. Lancet 2014;384(9944):665-73.
5. Jennifer ST, Josepht AG, Alna M, et al. Early palliative care for patients with metastatic non-small cell lung cancer. N Engl J Med 2010;363(8):733-42.</td></tr>
</table>

What is the current role of stereotactic radiation therapy (SBRT) in medically inoperable lung cancer?

Key concept	Lung cancer is the leading cause of cancer-related death. However, recent phase 3 data have established decreasing overall mortality associated with lung cancer, as a result of screening of high-risk patients.[1] In addition to screening, increased utilization of diagnostic CT scanning in elderly populations has resulted in an increased number of incidentally detected pulmonary nodules.[2] Prompt, safe treatment with curative intent directed at this patient population is of utmost priority. Stereotactic body radiotherapy (SBRT) offers an attractive treatment option for such patients.
Clinical scenario	A 59-year-old man with a history of ischemic cardiomyopathy, congestive heart failure on left ventricular assist device support, coronary artery disease, and smoking history presents to the hospital for management of *Aspergillus* pneumonia. CT scan of the chest reveals a 1.5-cm, speculated, progressive retrosternal pulmonary nodule. Biopsy is not deemed possible due to anticoagulation requirement and retrosternal tumor location. The tumor doubling time is estimated at approximately 6 months using prior CT studies as a reference. The patient is clinically staged with T1a lung cancer. Treatment options (continued observation, resection, biopsy, radiofrequency ablation, and SBRT) are discussed in multidisciplinary fashion and with the patient and family. The patient opts to receive SBRT empirically. Patient requires relocation of his pacemaker to allow for radiation therapy. Simulation and treatment planning are performed. The patient then receives 50 Gy to the lung nodule and margin using a highly conformal SBRT technique over 4 treatment sessions given every other day (Figure 10-1).

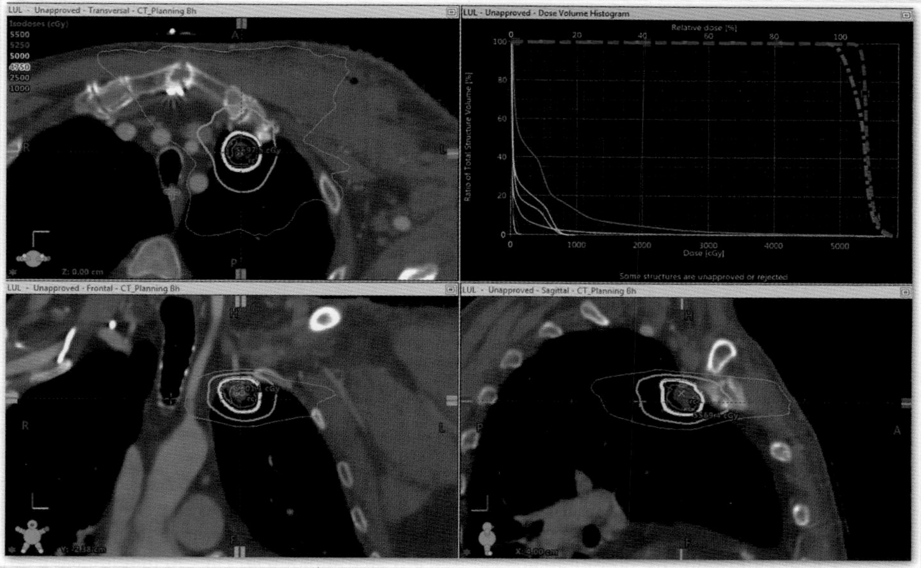

Figure 10-1. Radiation oncology treatment plan of lung cancer with 50 Gy to the lung nodule and margin using a highly conformal SBRT technique over 4 treatment sessions given every other day.

(continued on following page)

What is the current role of SBRT in medically inoperable lung cancer?

(continued from previous page)

Action items	• In medically inoperable lung cancer, treatment options should be discussed in detail in multidisciplinary fashion (interventional radiology, pulmonary, cardiology, and radiation oncology)
Discussion	The development of SBRT technology over the past decade represents an important medical advance that has enabled treatment of small (ideally <4 cm) primary or secondary tumors in the lungs or liver with excellent accuracy and tolerance.[2,3] Ideally, patients should have a histological diagnosis to avoid potential mistreatment, although clinically this is not always possible. Published phase 2 series[3] have demonstrated 3-year tumor control rates of >90% for stage I lung cancer with minimal toxicity and patient exclusion criteria. The adoption of SBRT has been shown to improve overall survival in the elderly lung cancer population.[4]

References

1. Aberle DR, Adams AM, Berg CD, et al. Reduced lung-cancer mortality with low-dose computed tomographic screening. N Engl J Med 2011;365(5):395-409.
2. National Comprehensive Cancer Network guidelines for lung cancer screening. Available at: https://www.nccn.org.
3. Timmerman R, Paulus R, Galvin J, et al. Stereotactic body radiation therapy for inoperable early stage lung cancer. JAMA 2010;303(11):1070-6.
4. Palma D, Visser O, Lagerwaard FJ, et al. Impact of introducing stereotactic lung radiotherapy for elderly patients with stage I non–small-cell lung cancer: a population-based time-trend analysis. J Clin Oncol 2010;28:5153-9.

What are the different strategies of maintenance chemotherapy in advanced NSCLC, and when is it associated with better outcome?

Key concept	For patients with stage IV non-squamous NSCLC without a driver mutation who show no disease progression following induction chemotherapy may benefit from maintenance chemotherapy. This has been shown to improve progression-free survival (PFS) and, in certain settings, overall survival (OS). Close observation may be considered in patients who are at not high risk for rapid disease progression and those with squamous histology.
Clinical scenario	A 54-year-old man with stage IV EGFR/ALK/ROS1 negative, NSCLC completed 6 cycles of carboplatin and pemetrexed with a good response on restaging CT scan. Would he benefit from receiving more chemotherapy?
Action items	There are multiple options for maintenance therapy following no progression on induction chemotherapy[1]: **Non-squamous NSCLC** • Continuation maintenance: bevacizumab (category 1), pemetrexed (category 1), bevacizumab + pemetrexed (category 2A), gemcitabine (category 2B) • Switch maintenance (category 2B): pemetrexed • Close observation (category 2A)

	Squamous NSCLC • Continuation maintenance (category 2B): gemcitabine • Switch maintenance (category 2B): docetaxel • Close observation (category 2A)
Discussion	In a large phase 3 clinical trial, patients with stage IV NSCLC who experienced no disease progression following treatment with platinum doublet chemotherapy (cisplatin or carboplatin plus docetaxel, paclitaxel, or gemcitabine) were randomized to receive either pemetrexed or placebo. Maintenance therapy with pemetrexed was associated with improved PFS and OS. Subgroup analysis showed that the OS benefit was limited to patients with non-squamous histology.[2] In the PARAMOUNT study, patients with stage IV lung adenocarcinoma who had no disease progression following 4 cycles of cisplatin and pemetrexed were randomized to receive continuation therapy with pemetrexed or placebo. Pemetrexed was also associated with significant prolongation of PFS and OS.[3] In the E4599 trial, patients with stage IV non-squamous NSCLC were randomized to receive induction chemotherapy with carboplatin plus paclitaxel or carboplatin, paclitaxel, and bevacizumab. After 6 cycles, bevacizumab was continued for patients on the second treatment arm. Bevacizumab was associated with improved PFS and OS at the expense of increased treatment-related deaths.[4] *(continued on following page)*

(continued from previous page)

In the AVAPERL study, patients were initially treated with cisplatin, pemetrexed, and bevacizumab for 4 cycles, then randomized to receive maintenance bevacizumab or bevacizumab with pemetrexed. Bevacizumab/pemetrexed maintenance was associated with better PFS and a trend toward improved OS.[5]

Maintenance therapy with gemcitabine or docetaxel has also been shown to result in improved PFS and trend toward improved OS.[6,7]

Pearls

Maintenance chemotherapy is associated with improved outcome in stage IV non-squamous NSCLC with no driver mutation. Pemetrexed, when used as continuation or switch maintenance therapy, has resulted in better PFS and OS in non-squamous tumors compared with surveillance. Bevacizumab maintenance following induction chemotherapy with carboplatin/paclitaxel and bevacizumab is also associated with improved PFS and OS compared with induction chemotherapy with carboplatin and paclitaxel followed by observation. The use of erlotinib in maintenance setting is not recommended if no epithelial growth factor receptor mutation is found. Close observation may be considered in patients with squamous histology and can be considered in patients who are not at high risk for rapid disease progression. The role of immunotherapy in this setting is under clinical investigation.

References

1. NCCN guidelines for head and neck cancers. Available at: https://www.nccn.org/.
2. Ciuleanu T, Brodowicz T, Zielinski C, et al. Maintenance pemetrexed plus best supportive care versus placebo plus best supportive care for non-small-cell lung cancer: a randomised, double-blind, phase 3 study. Lancet 2009;374(9699):1432-40.
3. Paz-Ares LG, de Marinis F, Dediu M, et al. PARAMOUNT: Final overall survival results of the phase III study of maintenance pemetrexed versus placebo immediately after induction treatment with pemetrexed plus cisplatin for advanced nonsquamous non-small-cell lung cancer. J Clin Oncol 2013;31(23):2895-902.
4. Sandler A, Gray R, Perry MC, et al. Paclitaxel-carboplatin alone or with bevacizumab for non-small-cell lung cancer. N Engl J Med 2006;355(24):2542-50.

5. Barlesi F, Scherpereel A, Rittmeyer A, et al. Randomized phase III trial of maintenance bevacizumab with or without pemetrexed after first-line induction with bevacizumab, cisplatin, and pemetrexed in advanced nonsquamous non-small-cell lung cancer: AVAPERL (MO22089). J Clin Oncol 2013;31(24):3004-11.
6. Fidias PM, Dakhil SR, Lyss AP, et al. Phase III study of immediate compared with delayed docetaxel after front-line therapy with gemcitabine plus carboplatin in advanced non-small-cell lung cancer. J Clin Oncol 2009;27(4):591-8.
7. Pérol M, Chouaid C, Pérol D, et al. Randomized, phase III study of gemcitabine or erlotinib maintenance therapy versus observation, with predefined second-line treatment, after cisplatin-gemcitabine induction chemotherapy in advanced non-small-cell lung cancer. J Clin Oncol 2012 Oct;30(28):3516-24.

CHAPTER 11

Rare Cancers

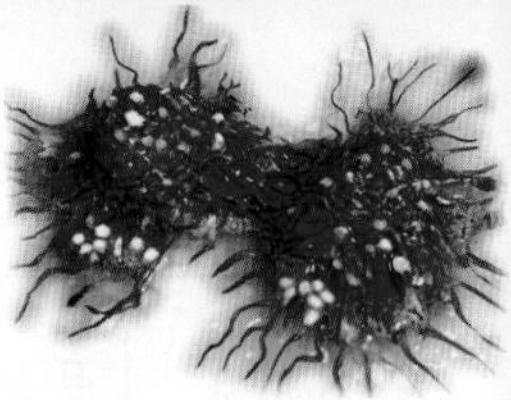

Which targeted drugs are approved for use in thyroid cancer?

Key concept	Systemic therapy with oral kinase inhibitors can be used to treat patients with metastatic thyroid cancer that is not amenable to surgical resection or radiation therapy or is refractory to radioactive iodine (RAI).[1]
Clinical scenario	A 65-year-old man was diagnosed with follicular thyroid cancer 8 years ago. He underwent thyroidectomy followed by RAI. His thyroglobulin has been rising and is unresponsive to RAI. The patient undergoes CT scan which demonstrates multiple bilateral lung nodules that are slowly progressive. He reports mild cough and shortness of breath on exertion.
Action items	• Lenvatinib and sorafenib are recommended for treatment of patients with radioiodine-refractory differentiated thyroid carcinoma[2,3] • Vandetanib and cabozantinib are recommended for the treatment of medullary carcinoma[4,5]
Discussion	The main histological subtypes of thyroid carcinoma are: • Differentiated (papillary, follicular, Hurthle cell) • Medullary • Anaplastic Age is the most important prognostic factor. Patients <45 years old with differentiated thyroid cancer are considered to have stage II disease even in the presence of metastasis. Thyroid-stimulating hormone suppression by giving levothyroxine is used to control differentiated thyroid cancers.

	Patients with slowly progressive asymptomatic metastatic disease may be observed. Oral tyrosine kinase inhibitors (TKIs) have been shown to improve progression-free survival without an overall survival advantage compared to placebo. Patients can have significant toxicity from oral TKIs, including hypertension, fatigue, rash, diarrhea, and cytopenias.
Pearls	• Anaplastic thyroid cancer is a rare, very aggressive tumor seen in older individuals • Patients with unresectable or metastatic disease can be treated with cytotoxic chemotherapy such as doxorubicin alone or in combination
References	1. NCCN guidelines for thyroid cancer. Available at: https://www.nccn.org. 2. Schlumberger M, Tahara M, Wirth L, et al. Lenvatinib versus placebo in radioiodine-refractory thyroid cancer. N Engl J Med 2015;372:621-30. 3. Brose M, Nutting C, Jarzab B, et al. Sorafenib in locally advanced or metastatic, radioactive iodine-refractory, differentiated thyroid cancer: a randomized, double-blind, phase 3 trial. Lancet 2014;384:319-28. 4. Wells SA, Robinson BG, Gagel RF, et al. Vandetanib in patients with locally advanced or metastatic medullary thyroid cancer: a randomized, double-blind phase III trial. J Clin Oncol 2012;30 (2):134-41. 5. Elisei R, Schlumberger M, Muller S, et al. Cabozantinib in progressive medullary thyroid cancer. J Clin Oncol 2013;29:3639-46.

How do I treat a patient with metastatic cutaneous melanoma?

Key concept	Cytotoxic chemotherapy is associated with modest activity in metastatic melanoma. A better understanding of the disease biology has led to the emergence of targeted therapy (BRAF and MEK inhibitors) and immunotherapy (anti-PD1 alone or with anti-CTLA4) that have proved their clinical superiority to chemotherapy.
Clinical scenario	A 50-year-old white woman with a history of stage IA melanoma 3 years previously, treated with wide local excision, presents with increased shortness of breath. Her chest CT reveals numerous bilateral lung nodules, the largest one 4 cm in size. Biopsy of one lung nodule is positive for BRAF V600E mutant metastatic melanoma. The rest of the imaging shows no evidence of disease outside the chest. What are her treatment options?
Action items	**Absence of BRAF V600 mutation** • Anti-PD1 alone (pembrolizumab or nivolumab) • Anti-PD1 in combination with anti-CTLA4 (nivolumab with ipilimumab) **Presence of BRAF V600 mutation** • Anti-PD1 ± anti-CTLA4 (as above) • BRAF and MEK inhibitors (dabrafenib/trametinib or vemurafenib/cobimetinib)—preferred if achieving a quick response is needed, such as symptomatic or high disease burden **Oligometastatic disease** • Addition of local treatment such as metastasectomy or radiosurgery should be considered in addition to systemic treatment

	Failure to immunotherapy and targeted therapy • Chemotherapy (eg, dacarbazine, temozolomide, carboplatin/paclitaxel, or albumin-bound paclitaxel), high-dose interleukin-2 (in very selected cases), or clinical trial can be considered **Presence of KIT mutation** • Consider imatinib
Discussion	BRAF mutations are present in ~40%–60% of advanced melanoma cases. Patients with BRAF mutant advanced melanoma have the option of BRAF and MEK inhibitors in combination or with checkpoint inhibitors. The optimal sequence of therapy is not defined and is currently being tested in clinical trials. Because transient disease worsening may be seen initially with immunotherapy, targeted therapy may need to be considered first in patients with symptomatic disease if they have the BRAF mutation.[1,2] Vemurafenib was the first FDA-approved BRAF inhibitor in BRAF V600 mutant metastatic melanoma after demonstrating superior progression-free survival (PFS) and overall survival (OS) over dacarbazine.[3] Dabrafenib is another FDA-approved BRAF inhibitor. It has shown superior PFS and a trend toward improved OS compared with dacarbazine.[4] Recent studies have demonstrated that the combination of BRAF and MEK inhibitors resulted in higher observed response rates and longer PFS and OS compared with treatment with a single-agent BRAF inhibitor.[5,6] To date, two combinations are approved for BRAF mutant metastatic melanoma: dabrafenib plus trametinib and vemurafenib plus cobimetinib. Pembrolizumab has shown OS superiority to chemotherapy in ipilimumab-refractory advanced melanoma (KEYNOTE-002)[7] and OS superiority to ipilimumab in patients with no prior immunotherapy (KEYNOTE-006).[8] However, in the CheckMate-066 trial, nivolumab was associated with prolonged OS relatively to dacarbazine in previously untreated patients with BRAF wild type disease.[9] *(continued on following page)*

	(continued from previous page) In the Checkmate 067 trial, patients with treatment-naïve advanced melanoma were randomized to receive ipilimumab, nivolumab, or the two agents combined. Nivolumab alone or in combination with ipilimumab corresponded to better PFS and OS compared with ipilimumab alone. The difference in OS between nivolumab alone vs. nivolumab/ipilimumab was not statistically significant. The rate of grade 3–4 immune-related toxicity was significantly higher in patients receiving the combination treatment.[10]
Pearls	First-line treatment for metastatic melanoma consists of immunotherapy (pembrolizumab alone or nivolumab ± ipilimumab) regardless of BRAF status or targeted therapy (vemurafenib/cobimetinib or dabrafenib/trametinib) only in patients with BRAF mutant disease. Local therapy should be considered in patients with oligometastatic disease.

References

1. National Comprehensive Cancer Network guidelines for melanoma. Available at: www.nccn.org.
2. Uptodate. Melanoma treatment: advanced or metastatic melanoma. Available at: www.uptodate.com.
3. Chapman PB, Hauschild A, Robert C, et al. Improved survival with vemurafenib in melanoma with BRAF V600E mutation. N Engl J Med 2011;364(26):2507-16.
4. Hauschild A, Grob JJ, Demidov LV, et al. Dabrafenib in BRAF-mutated metastatic melanoma: a multicentre, open-label, phase 3 randomised controlled trial. Lancet 2012;380(9839):358-65.
5. Long GV, Flaherty KT, Stroyakovskiy D, et al. Dabrafenib plus trametinib versus dabrafenib monotherapy in patients with metastatic BRAF V600E/K-mutant melanoma: long-term survival and safety analysis of a phase 3 study. Ann Oncol 2017;28(7):1631-9.
6. Ascierto PA, McArthur GA, Dréno B, et al. Cobimetinib combined with vemurafenib in advanced BRAF(V600)-mutant melanoma (coBRIM): updated efficacy results from a randomised, double-blind, phase 3 trial. Lancet Oncol 2016;17(9):1248-60.
7. Ribas A, Puzanov I, Dummer R, et al. Pembrolizumab versus investigator-choice chemotherapy for ipilimumab-refractory melanoma (KEYNOTE-002): a randomised, controlled, phase 2 trial. Lancet Oncol 2015;16(8):908-18.

8. Robert C, Schachter J, Long GV, et al. Pembrolizumab versus ipilimumab in advanced melanoma. N Engl J Med 2015;372(26):2521-32.
9. Robert C, Long GV, Brady B, et al. Nivolumab in previously untreated melanoma without BRAF mutation. N Engl J Med 2015;372(4):320-30.
10. Wolchok JD, Chiarion-Sileni V, Gonzalez R, et al. Overall survival with combined nivolumab and ipilimumab in advanced melanoma. N Engl J Med 2017;377(14):1345-56.

How do I manage patients with soft-tissue sarcoma (STS)?

Key concept	Sarcomas account for <1% of all malignancies. Most of them arise from soft tissues, and the remaining ones rise from bones (osteosarcoma). STS is a heterogeneous tumor type that includes many histological subtypes such as liposarcoma, leiomyosarcoma, undifferentiated pleomorphic sarcoma, and synovial sarcoma.[1] Gastrointestinal stromal tumors are discussed under the GI section.
Clinical scenario	A 44-year-old Asian woman presents to her primary care clinic with an increasing right thigh mass. The mass is otherwise asymptomatic. She denies any limitation in movement. Her appetite and weight are stable. Biopsy of the primary mass reveals a pleomorphic STS.
Action items	Patients suspected of having STS should undergo: • Core needle biopsy • Staging studies, including CT scan and MRI, and PET/CT scan • Multidisciplinary evaluation with a surgeon, radiation oncologist, and medical oncologist to determine the treatment plan
Discussion	The anatomical location of STS is an important factor in clinical management. STS can arise in the extremities (43%), trunk (10%), viscera (19%), retroperitoneum (15%), or head and neck (9%). Tumor size and histological grade are also important to management and prognosis. Large tumors with high grade upstage the disease. Any regional lymph node disease, although these are rarely involved, is considered stage IV disease. Lungs are a common site of metastatic spread. **Extremity STS:** Management includes limb-sparing surgery with neoadjuvant or adjuvant radiation depending on the size and grade of the lesion. Some patients benefit from neoadjuvant chemotherapy prior to surgery.

	Retroperitoneal STS: Management involves surgery with or without radiation. **Chemotherapy agents:** Many chemotherapy agents such as doxorubicin, ifosfamide, methotrexate, docetaxel, and gemcitabine are considered active against STS. Olaratumab is a platelet-derived growth factor receptor alpha blocking antibody that is active in STS.
Pearls	Patients with lung-only metastatic disease should be considered for metastasectomy or ablative procedures for local control.
References	1. NCCN guidelines for soft-tissue sarcoma. Available at: https://www.nccn.org.

How should I approach a patient with carcinoma of unknown primary (CUP)?

Key concept	Some 2%–5% of cancer patients have metastatic disease from an unknown primary site. Even after extensive work-up, a primary is found in only 30% of these patients. Patients often require empiric treatment without knowing the definitive primary site, but, overall, they have a poor prognosis.[1]
Clinical scenario	A 62-year-old woman is admitted to the hospital with fatigue, weight loss, and right upper quadrant pain. CT scan shows multiple liver and lung metastases. Biopsy confirms poorly differentiated adenocarcinoma. Work-up for primary—including tumor markers, mammogram, and endoscopies—does not show a primary site of malignancy.
Action items	Patients require extensive diagnostic work-up to rule out a primary site: • Imaging: CT scan, MRI, PET/CT scan • Immunohistochemistry and gene expression profiling (GEP) • Mammogram/breast MRI for women with adenocarcinoma in axilla • β-hCG and α-fetoprotein for mediastinal lymph node involvement • CA-125 for suspected ovarian primary (peritoneal metastasis) • Prostate-specific antigen testing for suspected prostate primary (bone metastasis) • Otorhinolaryngology examination for squamous cell carcinoma (SCC) involving neck lymph nodes (LN) • Upper and lower gastrointestinal (GI) endoscopy for liver metastasis
Discussion	Patients presenting with CUP can often be categorized into one of the following groups: • Well or moderately differentiated adenocarcinoma (60%) • Poorly differentiated or undifferentiated carcinoma (29%) • SCC (5%)

	• Poorly differentiated malignant neoplasm (5%) • Neuroendocrine tumors of unknown primary site (1%) Patients can present with a variety of symptoms and clinical and radiological findings, depending on the location of the tumor. It is important to differentiate carcinoma from other histological subtypes such as lymphoma, sarcoma, and melanoma. Some patients with CUP have a favorable prognosis, including those with poorly differentiated carcinoma in the midline distribution, adenocarcinoma of the peritoneal cavity, adenocarcinoma of the axillary LN only, or SCC of neck or groin only.[2] Others, with poor performance status, visceral involvement, or elevated white blood cell count, have a poor prognosis. Depending on the suspected primary site, treatment can be tailored accordingly (eg, SCC of neck LN is treated like head and neck cancer and adenocarcinoma of axillary lymph nodes like breast cancer). No specific regimen has been shown to be superior then others for CUP. Carboplatin with paclitaxel is a reasonable choice for adenocarcinoma or poorly differentiated carcinoma. Cisplatin and 5-fluororacil–based therapy is used for SCC. Regimens for small cell lung cancer can be used for cancers that have neuroendocrine differentiation. Regimens tailored for suspected GI or ovarian cancer can be used when clinically suspected. Where indicated, radiation may be used.
Pearls	GEP can help with diagnosis, but no clinical benefit in terms of outcome has been demonstrated by using GEP.
References	1. NCCN guidelines for occult primary. Available at: https://www.nccn.org. 2. Petrakis D, Pentheroudakis G, Voulgaris E, et al. Prognostication in cancer of unknown primary (CUP): development of a prognostic algorithm in 311 cases and review of literature. Cancer Treatment Rev 2013;39:701-8.

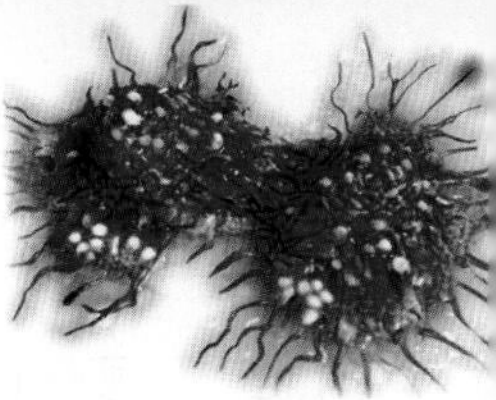

CHAPTER 12

Basics of Bone Marrow Transplantation

What are the indications for a stem cell transplantation (SCT)?

Key concept	The most common indication for an SCT—specifically, autologous SCT—in the United States remains multiple myeloma. Acute myeloid leukemia (AML), by contrast, is the most common indication for allogeneic SCT.[1] The indications for SCTs have continuously been refined by incorporating the cytogenetic composite and biology of tumors, and these are continuously compared against novel therapeutics to determine the safest and most effective approaches.
Clinical scenario	A 47-year-old man is diagnosed with Philadelphia chromosome–negative acute lymphoblastic leukemia (ALL). Cytogenetic analysis reveals a mixed-lineage leukemia translocation. He is treated with modified hyper-CVAD chemotherapy, achieving a complete remission. He relapses 2 months later while on therapy. He receives re-induction therapy with blinatumomab, achieving a second complete remission followed by an allogeneic SCT from a sibling donor who is a 9/10 HLA match.
Action items	The discussion of an SCT should be held with patients and transplant hematologists early during the course of treatment, as soon as it becomes a consideration. The pre-transplant evaluation, and, in allogeneic SCTs, the donor search, can be a lengthy process, and an early referral can prove valuable.
Discussion	***Allogeneic SCT*** AML • Relapsed/refractory disease • Poor-risk disease based on cytogenetics • AML with FLT3-ITD mutation[2] • Treatment-related AML (t-AML) unless good risk cytogenetics • Secondary AML (eg, secondary to myelodysplastic syndrome or myeloproliferative disorders)

ALL

- Poor-risk ALL based on cytogenetics
- Minimal residual disease positivity by flow cytometry at the end of induction[3]
- Consider if presenting with white blood cell counts >30,000/μL in B-ALL, >100,000/μL in T-ALL, age >30–35, or failure to achieve a complete remission in 4 weeks

Myeloproliferative disorders

- Blast-phase chronic myeloid leukemia
- Myelofibrosis: Dynamic international prognostic scoring system-plus intermediate-2 score or high risk, and in high-risk molecular features[4]

Myelodysplastic syndrome

- International Prognostic Scoring System intermediate-2 score or high risk[5]

Bone marrow failure syndromes

- Aplastic anemia
- Congenital marrow failure syndromes

Autologous SCT

- Multiple myeloma
- Relapsed/refractory diffuse large B cell lymphoma
- Mantle cell lymphoma in first complete remission[6]
- Peripheral T cell lymphoma in first complete remission[7]
- Relapsed/refractory Hodgkin lymphoma
- Relapsed follicular lymphoma
- Relapsed acute promyelocytic leukemia (APL) if molecular remission is achieved

(continued on following page)

Pearls

(continued from previous page)

- With the exception of APL, acute leukemias require the graft-versus-tumor effect of an allogeneic SCT in cases when an allogeneic SCT is indicated
- With the exception of ALL, autologous transplantation is used in lymphoid malignancies
- Owing to the defective stem cells in patients with bone marrow failure syndromes, treatment is with an allogeneic SCT when indicated
- Autologous SCT can be a non-curative modality to achieve a prolonged progression-free and treatment-free survival
- The role and sequencing of autologous SCT for multiple myeloma had been and remains a constant topic of discussion among experts, more recently owing to the approval of several anti-myeloma therapeutics
- Allogeneic SCT can be curative in conditions traditionally treated with autologous SCTs or non-transplant approaches; however, its risks outweigh its benefits
- Institutions vary in their morbidity and mortality outcomes of SCTs, and the decision to transplant or not requires a continuous evaluation of patients' comorbidities and social support and should be weighed against the institution's outcomes

References

1. Data from the Center for International Blood and Marrow Transplant Research (CIBMTR). 2014. Available at: https://www.cibmtr.org.
2. DeZern A, Sung A, Kim S, et al. Role of allogeneic transplantation for FLT3/ITD acute myeloid leukemia: outcomes from 133 consecutive newly diagnosed patients from a single institution. Biol Blood Marrow Transplant 2011;17:1404-9.
3. Dhédin N, Huynh A, Maury S, et al. Role of allogeneic stem cell transplantation in adult patients with Ph-negative acute lymphoblastic leukemia. Blood 2015;125(16):2486-96.
4. Tefferi A. Primary myelofibrosis: 2014 update on diagnosis, risk-stratification, and management. Am J Hematol 2014;89(9):915-25.

5. Robin M, Porcher R, Adès L, et al. HLA-matched allogeneic stem cell transplantation improves outcome of higher risk myelodysplastic syndrome. A prospective study on behalf of SFGM-TC and GFM. Leukemia 2015;29(7):1496-501.
6. Campo E, Rule S. Mantle cell lymphoma: evolving management strategies. Blood 2015;125(1):48-55.
7. d'Amore F, Relander T, Lauritzsen GF, et al. Up-front autologous stem-cell transplantation in peripheral T-cell lymphoma: NLG-T-01. J Clin Oncol 2012;30(25):3093-9.

What are the potential complications of a stem cell transplantation (SCT)?

Key concept	It is imperative to perform a thorough evaluation of comorbidities, anticipated benefits of the transplant, social support, and ability to maintain long-term follow-up care in selecting patients appropriate for SCT, to achieve optimal outcomes. Transplant-related morbidity and mortality outcomes vary significantly between allogeneic and autologous SCTs: the former has higher rates, mainly owing to the additional graft-related complications.
Clinical scenario	A 40-year-old man with adverse-risk acute myeloid leukemia achieves a complete remission after induction chemotherapy. Allogeneic SCT consolidation is performed with a 9/10 HLA-matched unrelated donor. On day 15 post-transplantation, he develops a diffuse erythematous maculopapular rash involving >50% of his body surface area and diarrhea passing >1.5 L/day. Active cytomegalovirus infection is ruled out with serum testing. A skin biopsy reveals acute graft-versus-host disease (GVHD).
Action items	• The majority of SCT complications can be attributed to either the pre-transplant conditioning process or to the graft • In an autologous SCT, the graft contains the patient's own cells; therefore, graft-related complications are limited
Discussion	<u>Definitions:</u> • Conditioning: delivering chemotherapy with or without radiation therapy to eliminate residual malignant cells and, in case of an allogeneic transplant, to suppress the host immune response, allowing for successful engraftment; conditioning regimens can be myeloablative, non-myeloablative, or reduced-intensity

- Engraftment: the acceptance of the graft by the host with evidence of graft function (ie, absolute neutrophil count >500/μL for 3 consecutive days)
- HLA-antigen matching: comparing HLA antigen typing (HLA-A, HLA-B, HLA-C, HLA-DR, and HLA-DQ) between the donor and recipient of stem cells

<u>Complications related to the conditioning regimen:</u>

- Myelosuppression: average time to engraftment 7–14 days in an autologous SCT, 14–28 days in an allogeneic SCT; prolonged time to engraftment in umbilical cord allogeneic SCT
- Infections: proportionate with the degree and duration of immunosuppression
- Skin toxicity: secondary to total body irradiation (TBI)
- GI toxicity: nausea, vomiting, mucositis, diarrhea
- Hepatic veno-occlusive disease (VOD): potentially fatal, treated with defibrotide[1]
- Idiopathic pulmonary syndrome: diffuse alveolar injury, associated with the use of carmustine and TBI[2]
- Diffuse alveolar hemorrhage: seen within the first 4 weeks of transplantation, fatal in most cases[3]
- Transplant-associated thrombotic microangiopathy: secondary to calcineurin inhibitors in allogeneic SCTs

(continued on following page)

What are the potential complications of a stem cell transplantation (SCT)?

<table>
<tr><td></td><td>(continued from previous page)
<u>Complications related to the graft</u>
• Graft failure: secondary to immune rejection, infections, drugs, inadequate dose of graft
• GVHD: a donor T cell–mediated reaction to host antigens; treated with immunosuppression
  • Acute GVHD: skin rash, transaminitis, diarrhea, interstitial pneumonitis
  • Chronic GVHD: resembles autoimmune conditions; skin thickening, xerophthalmia, esophageal strictures, bronchiolitis obliterans, myasthenia gravis</td></tr>
<tr><td>Pearls</td><td>• Transplant-related infections vary by the phase of transplant; prophylactic antimicrobials should be chosen accordingly
• The most common cause of death within 100 days post-transplantation is related to the underlying disease; therefore, optimal disease control should be achieved prior to transplantation[4]
• In adults, donor stem cells in the majority of cases are collected for an allogeneic SCT from peripheral blood via apheresis or from the bone marrow, which is preferred in SCTs for bone marrow failure syndromes
• Matched, unrelated donor graft allogeneic SCT poses a greater risk of GVHD than matched, related donor graft counterpart, given the higher degree of minor HLA antigen mismatching
• The National Marrow Donor Program provides clinicians and patients access to a large and diverse stem cell registry
• For patients with no available HLA-matched related or unrelated graft, a haploidentical (50% match) graft can be obtained from a parent or child; however, additional measures may be deployed to prevent GVHD or graft failure[5]</td></tr>
</table>

References

1. Dignan FL, Wynn RF, Hadzic N, et al. BCSH/BSBMT guideline: diagnosis and management of veno-occlusive disease (sinusoidal obstruction syndrome) following haematopoietic stem cell transplantation. Br J Haematol 2013;163(4):444-57.
2. Fukuda T, Hackman RC, Guthrie KA, et al. Risks and outcomes of idiopathic pneumonia syndrome after nonmyeloablative and conventional conditioning regimens for allogeneic hematopoietic stem cell transplantation. Blood 2003;102(8):2777-85.
3. Majhail NS, Parks K, Defor TE, et al. Diffuse alveolar hemorrhage and infection-associated alveolar hemorrhage following hematopoietic stem cell transplantation: related and high-risk clinical syndromes. Biol Blood Marrow Transplant 2006;12:1038-46.
4. Center for International Blood and Marrow Transplant Research. Available at: https://www.cibmtr.org.
5. Ciurea SO, Zhang MJ, Bacigalupo AA, et al. Haploidentical transplant with posttransplant cyclophosphamide vs matched unrelated donor transplant for acute myeloid leukemia. Blood 2015;126:1033-40.

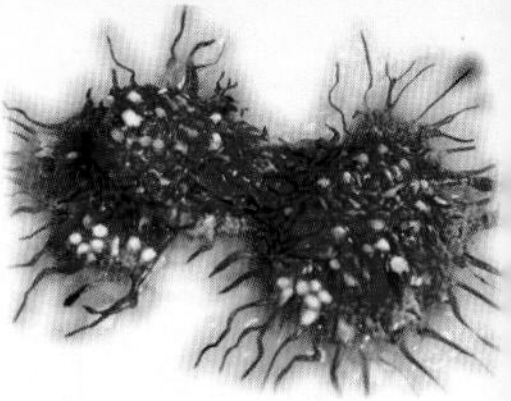

CHAPTER 13
Leukemia

How should I treat my patient with leukostasis?

Key concept	Leukostasis is a major cause of early mortality in patients with acute leukemias. Signs of leukostasis include altered sensorium, ischemic heart signs, respiratory distress, and priapism and are a function of the size, number, and type of leukemic cells.[1] Of these, immediate reduction of the number of leukemic cells can restore organ function and allow for subsequent anti-leukemia therapy.
Clinical scenario	A 64-year-old man in acute respiratory distress is found to have a white blood cell (WBC) count of 153×10^9/L with 71% blasts. Labs reveal an elevated troponin level, and chest radiography demonstrates scattered bilateral opacifications. Peripheral smear review shows large immature cells with Auer rods. Peripheral blood flow cytometry was requested. Rapid leukocyte reduction was achieved with oral hydroxyurea.
Action items	Both pharmacological and mechanical methods of cytoreduction have been deployed in treating patients with hyperleukocytosis and signs of leukostasis. <u>Pharmacological cytoreduction</u> **Diagnosis confirmed:** • Induction chemotherapy in suitable patients **Diagnosis confirmation pending:** • Hydroxyurea is effective in myeloid hyperleukocytosis; patients should be capable of enteral intake • Systemic steroids can be effective against malignant lymphoid hyperleukocytosis and can be given orally or parenterally • Vincristine is effective against malignant lymphoid cells and is given intravenously • Cytarabine is effective in both myeloid and lymphoid hyperleukocytosis • Anthracyclines are used in protocols in acute promyelocytic leukemia (APL) <u>Mechanical cytoreduction</u> • Leukapheresis is effective in both myeloid and lymphoid hyperleukocytosis[2] • Leukapheresis is contraindicated in APL due to risks of disseminated intravascular coagulation (DIC)[2]

Discussion	Hyperleukocytosis is arbitrarily defined as circulating WBC or blast count $>100 \times 10^9$/L. Leukostasis is a complication of hyperleukocytosis and results in end-organ ischemia and/or hemorrhage. Myeloid cells are larger and more rigid than lymphoid cells and produce cytokines, resulting in inflammatory endothelial changes; therefore, myeloid leukemias result in leukostasis at lower counts than their lymphoid counterparts. Pros and cons of different leukoreduction methods: <u>Pharmacological methods</u> • **Pros:** No invasive procedures required, rapid administration, safer method in APL • **Cons:** Off-target toxicities of pharmacological agents and higher rates of post-therapy respiratory distress in monocytic leukemias <u>Mechanical methods</u> • **Pros:** *Rapid cytoreduction and possible role in asymptomatic hyperleukocytosis (prophylactic)*[3] • **Cons:** *Requires central catheter placement and invasive procedures, requires special equipment and technical expertise, may trigger bleeding complications in APL, and does not obviate the need for chemotherapy*
Pearls	• Aggressive supportive care is equally important in the acute management of hyperleukocytosis and leukostasis and improves early mortality outcomes • It is common practice to administer cytoreduction methods with cross-reactivity against both myeloid and lymphoid cells empirically until the diagnosis is established • The number of treatment occurrences depends on the patient's response; repeated treatment is often warranted • Continue to monitor for signs of tumor lysis syndrome while treating hyperleukocytosis
References	1. Röllig C, Ehninger G. How I treat hyperleukocytosis in acute myeloid leukemia. Blood 2015;125(21):3246-52. 2. Schwartz J, Padmanabhan A, Aqui N, et al. Guidelines on the use of therapeutic apheresis in clinical practice—evidence-based approach from the Writing Committee of the American Society for Apheresis: The seventh special issue. J Clin Apher 2016;31:149-62. 3. Ventura GJ, Hester JP, Smith TL, et al. Acute myeloblastic leukemia with hyperleukocytosis: risk factors for early mortality in induction. Am J Hematol 1988;27:34-7.

Why is it important to consider the diagnosis of acute promyelocytic leukemia (APL) in any patient presenting with an acute leukemia?

Key concept	APL, also classified as acute myeloid leukemia (AML)–M3, is a subtype of AML with a distinct biology and cytogenetic signature.[1] Patients with APL have the propensity for life-threatening complications on presentation; therefore, prompt recognition and empiric treatment are vital and can mitigate early disease-related mortality.
Clinical scenario	A 53-year-old man presents to the emergency room with gingival bleeding and oral "blood blisters." A complete blood count shows a white blood cell count of 0.4×10^9/L, hemoglobin of 10.2 g/dL, and platelets of 11/μL. Peripheral blood smear review shows a few blasts with numerous granules, some with bi-lobed nuclei. A coagulation profile and fibrinogen are within normal limits.
Action items	• Empiric administration of all-*trans*-retinoic acid (ATRA) in patients with APL can reverse or prevent the coagulopathy often associated with this form of acute leukemia[2] • APL blasts are exquisitely sensitive to and undergo differentiation when exposed to ATRA[3] • Patients should be closely monitored for the development of differentiation syndrome, manifested as respiratory distress, pulmonary infiltrates, weight gain, and effusions • Prompt administration of dexamethasone 10 mg intravenously twice daily, with or without interruption of ATRA therapy, is indicated with the earliest manifestations of differentiation syndrome
Discussion	APL accounts for 5%–15% of all adult AML cases and is considered its most curable form. It occurs with a higher incidence in young adults and in Hispanics, and patients generally have a higher mean body mass index (BMI) than patients with other AML subtypes.[4] In the vast majority of cases, the leukemic blasts carry a reciprocal translocation between the promyelocytic leukemia gene (PML) and the retinoic acid receptor-α gene (RARα), resulting in the PML-RARα fusion gene, which arrests normal differentiation at the level of the promyelocyte. Leukemic promyelocytes interact with the

coagulation system, which can result in catastrophic bleeding complications. Early institution of ATRA can reverse this coagulopathy, yet there remains an early mortality rate of ~10%, mainly due to these hemorrhagic complications. APL blasts have a characteristic immunophenotype,[5] and confirmation of the diagnosis requires the demonstration of the PML-RARα fusion gene. Once the diagnosis of APL is confirmed, induction-phase therapy using cytotoxic chemotherapy or non-chemotherapy approaches can be delivered. Outcomes of either approach have been highly favorable, with complete remission rates between 95% and 100%.[6]

Pearls

- APL cytogenetic variants other than t(15;17)/PML-RARα exist and are resistant to ATRA
- Await confirmation of the presence of the PML-RARα fusion gene before initiating induction therapy, as highly effective non-chemotherapeutic regimens can be used for this subtype, potentially sparing patients the toxicities of chemotherapy
- Granulocyte colony-stimulating factor preferentially stimulates the growth of APL leukemic cells, therefore increasing the number of circulating promyelocytes and potentiating coagulopathy; use is contraindicated in APL except in the presence of life-threatening infections in patients with neutropenia
- ATRA is teratogenic, therefore, in women of child-bearing age diagnosed with APL, abstinence or 2 simultaneous methods of contraception are recommended
- Non-chemotherapeutic regimens in APL combine ATRA and arsenic trioxide and are very well tolerated compared to chemotherapy

References

1. Ablain J, de The H. Revisiting the differentiation paradigm in acute promyelocytic leukemia. Blood 2011;117:5795-802.
2. Avvisati G. Coagulopathy in APL: a step forward? Blood 2012;120:4-6.
3. Miyauchi J. All-*trans* retinoic acid and hematopoietic growth factors regulating the growth and differentiation of blast progenitors in acute promyelocytic leukemia. Leuk Lymphoma 1999;33:267-80.
4. Smith BD, Stein E. Acute myeloid leukemia. *American Society of Hematology Self-Assessment Program.* 6th ed.; 2017:521-9.
5. San Miguel JF, Gonzalez M Cañizo MC, et al. Surface marker analysis in acute myeloid leukaemia and correlation with FAB classification. Br J Haematol 1986;64(3):547-60.
6. Lo-Coco F, Avvisati G, Vignetti M, et al. Retinoic acid and arsenic trioxide for acute promyelocytic leukemia. N Engl J Med 2013;369:111-21.

How do I prepare my patient for induction chemotherapy?

Key concept	Timely administration of effective therapy in the induction phase of acute leukemia is critical; however, attempts to mitigate early treatment and disease-related mortality rates should be made by performing a proper evaluation of the patients' characteristics and organ functions prior to choosing the induction regimen and initiation of treatment.
Clinical scenario	A 33-year-old man with precursor T acute lymphoblastic leukemia presents with leukocytosis with circulating blasts, hepatosplenomegaly, and an elevated total bilirubin of 4.5 mg/dL with direct hyperbilirubinemia. A 2D echocardiogram shows no evidence of systolic or diastolic dysfunction or valvular abnormalities. His renal function is preserved. He has no pre-existing neuropathy. He is treated with a modified hyper-CVAD regimen by administration of 25% of the dose of doxorubicin, and vincristine is omitted due to the underlying hyperbilirubinemia. If hyperbilirubinemia proves to be secondary to leukemic liver infiltration and improves with therapy, reassessment of dosing will be made.
Action items	• Chemotherapy dosing should follow published guidelines and be adjusted for organ dysfunction • When dosage adjustment guidelines are not available for certain therapeutics, best clinical judgment should be used
Discussion	Although there are high early mortality rates associated with acute leukemias, proper steps to optimize reversible comorbidities prior to initiation of therapy must be taken when possible. Patients should be assessed for organ dysfunction, active infections, fluid balances, and performance status. A central catheter should be in place to provide a stable access for potential resuscitative measures and due to the vesicant and irritant nature of certain chemotherapeutic agents.

	A study that set out to determine the effects of delaying induction therapy in select acute myeloid leukemia (AML) patients with a white blood cell count of $\leq 50 \times 10^9$/L reported unfavorable overall survival and complete remission rates in patients ≤ 60 years old when induction therapy was delayed for ≥ 5 days and no difference in patients >60 years old.[1] Once a full assessment is performed, an appropriate regimen is chosen with potential alterations in dosing, sequencing, and duration of infusions as needed.
Pearls	• Elderly AML patients may benefit from delaying therapy until cytogenetic data become available for guidance • Rituximab and other anti-CD20 monoclonal antibodies should be avoided in HIV patients with CD4 counts $<50/mm^3$ due to higher rates of infectious deaths[2] • It is common to deliver one or two agents from the induction regimen prior to the full initiation of the induction phase to serve as an attempt to control the disease while patients are being managed for acute inter-current illnesses
References	1. Sekeres MA, Elson P, Kalaycio ME, et al. Time from diagnosis to treatment initiation predicts survival in younger, but not older, acute myeloid leukemia patients. Blood 2009;113(1):28-36. 2. Kaplan L, Lee J, Ambinder RF, et al. Rituximab does not improve clinical outcome in a randomized phase 3 trial of CHOP with or without rituximab in patients with HIV-associated non-Hodgkin lymphoma: AIDS-Malignancies Consortium Trial 010. Blood 2005;106(5):1538-43.

Do I need to evaluate cytogenetic and molecular data in my patient with acute leukemia?

Key concept	Historically, acute myeloid leukemia (AML) and acute lymphoblastic leukemia (ALL) subtypes were classified according to their morphological features into AML M0-M7 and ALL L1-L3, respectively. However, the adoption of cytogenetic and molecular data in classifying acute leukemias led to a better understanding of individual subtypes and advances in guiding therapy and prognostication.
Clinical scenario	A 24-year-old woman presents with headaches and fatigue. A complete blood count shows a white blood cell count of 64×10^9/L with 30% circulating blasts. A bone marrow biopsy shows 90% cellularity with diffuse involvement by myeloblasts. Cytogenetic analysis using fluorescent in-situ hybridization of marrow leukemic blasts shows the presence of t(8;21).
Action items	• Chromosomal and molecular cytogenetic analysis techniques are best performed on bone marrow cells of patients with acute leukemia • In conditions when a bone marrow biopsy is not readily feasible, cytogenetic data may also be obtained from peripheral blood specimens, although the routine practice of peripheral blood cytogenetic testing should be discouraged given its lower yield • In the majority of cases, initiation of induction chemotherapy occurs prior to the availability of cytogenetic data
Discussion	<u>Cytogenetic profile and prognostication</u> **AML**[1] *Favorable:* t(15;17), t(8;21), and Inversion 16/t(16;16) *Intermediate:* Normal karyotype and -Y *Adverse:* inversion 3/t(3;3), -5, -7, and complex karyotype *Other mutations:* NPM1, bi-allelic CEBPA (favorable), FLT3-ITD, and Kit (adverse)

	ALL[2] *Favorable:* High hyperdiploid *Adverse:* Hypodiploid <44, t(9;22)/BCR-ABL1, t(v;11)/MLL-rearrangement Cytogenetic profile and therapy **AML** *FLT3 mutation:* add a FLT3 inhibitor, consider allogeneic stem cell transplantation (SCT) in first remission[3] *IDH2 mutation:* add an IDH2 inhibitor[4] *Kit:* consider an allogeneic SCT in first remission **ALL**[2] *t(9;22):* add a BCR-ABL1 tyrosine kinase inhibitor, consider an allogeneic SCT after first remission *t(4;11):* consider an allogeneic SCT after first remission
Pearls	• Diagnosis of AML does not require >20% blasts in the presence of the following genetic alterations: t(15;17), t(8;21), or inversion 16/t(16;16) • Several cytogenetic risk classifications exist across institutions and collaborative groups • Induction chemotherapy should not be delayed in the absence of cytogenetic data, with the exception of acute promyelocytic leukemia • Combinations of chromosomal and molecular cytogenetic abnormalities may exist in an individual patient
References	1. Marcucci G, Haferlach T, Döhner H. Molecular genetics of adult acute myeloid leukemia: prognostic and therapeutic implications. J Clin Oncol 2011;29(5)475-86. 2. Litzow M, Heyman M. Acute lymphoblastic leukemia and lymphoblastic lymphoma. *American Society of Hematology Self-Assessment Program*. 6th ed.; 2017:531-46. 3. Stone R, Mandrekar S, Sanford BL, et al. Midostaurin plus chemotherapy for acute myeloid leukemia with a FLT3 mutation. N Engl J Med 2017;377:454-64. 4. Stein E, DiNardo C, Pollyea D, et al. Enasidenib in mutant-IDH2 relapsed or refractory acute myeloid leukemia. Blood 2017;130(6):722-31.

What are the supportive care measures in patients being treated for acute leukemia?

Key concept	Patients with acute leukemia, by nature of their disease and by its treatment, invariably suffer acute toxicities, such as profound and prolonged myelosuppression, hyperuricemia, electrolyte imbalance, and fluid overload. Improvements in supportive care measures allow more patients to emerge from these toxicities and achieve improved outcomes of treatments, leading to improvements in overall survival rates.
Clinical scenario	A 41-year-old man is undergoing induction chemotherapy with hyper-CVAD for his newly diagnosed pre–B acute lymphoblastic leukemia. He is started on allopurinol prior to initiation of chemotherapy and requires rasburicase for hyperuricemia and acute kidney injury. Infection prophylaxis is with a fluoroquinolone, an azole antifungal agent, and an antiviral. Granulocyte colony-stimulating factor (G-CSF) is given daily after chemotherapy. He develops bacteremia with an alpha streptococcus and septic shock requiring resuscitative measures and intensive care unit (ICU) care. After several days in the ICU, he recovers and is transferred to the regular medical floor. A day-28 marrow shows a complete remission.
Action item	• Prophylactic antimicrobials, anti-hyperuricemia agents, hematopoietic growth factors, electrolyte replacement therapies, and readily available subspecialty services are all necessary for the safe administration of anti-leukemia therapy and have a significant impact on outcomes

Discussion

Neutropenic infections

Historically, the majority of patients with acute leukemia died of their disease as a direct result of infections, which contributed to 70% of deaths.[1] In 1966, Bodey et al. described the inverse relationship between the number of circulating neutrophils and severe infections. Based on this observation, antimicrobial agents were incorporated into the supportive management of acute leukemia, leading to a significant reduction in severe infections and mortality. Leading infectious complications remain respiratory tract infections followed by gastrointestinal infections and bacteremia, and while gram-negative bacteria were the cause of the majority of neutropenic infections in these patients in the past, the addition of prophylactic fluoroquinolones has halved these rates. The prompt institution of broad-spectrum antimicrobials and escalation of acuity of care can be lifesaving in patients with early signs of neutropenic infections, and ongoing diligence during their period of neutropenia is vital to their survival.

Hematopoietic growth factors

Hematopoietic growth factors (ie, G-CSF) are used for the primary prevention of neutropenic fevers in patients undergoing chemotherapy for acute leukemia.[2] Institutional practices vary as to their use in acute myeloid leukemia.

Blood product transfusion

Patients with acute leukemia inevitably have myelosuppression owing to the clonal expansion of marrow leukemic blasts impairing marrow function and later to chemotherapy-induced marrow hypoplasia. Therefore, blood-product transfusion support through the period of myelosuppression and until bone marrow recovery is part of the supportive care measures that have a positive impact on outcomes. The AABB (formerly American Association of Blood Banks) recommends prophylactic platelet transfusions with a single apheresis unit or equivalent in the following scenarios[3]:

- A platelet count of $\leq 10 \times 10^9$/L to prevent spontaneous bleeding (*strong recommendation*)
- A platelet count of $\leq 20 \times 10^9$/L for patients having central venous catheter placement (*weak recommendation*)

(continued on following page)

(continued from previous page)

	• A platelet count of $\leq 50 \times 10^9$/L for patients having an elective lumbar puncture (*weak recommendation*) The transfusion threshold for a hemoglobin level of 7 g/dL was associated with fewer units of packed red blood cell units needed and had comparable outcomes to higher thresholds.[4] Anti-emetics[5] Intensive chemotherapy for acute leukemias results in a moderate to high emetogenic risk, with a frequency of chemotherapy-induced nausea and vomiting of 30%–90%. To prevent the acute and delayed emesis of chemotherapy, patients are given a 5HT3 receptor antagonist and dexamethasone with the addition of a neurokinin1 receptor antagonist in highly emetogenic regimens, both before initiating chemotherapy and with subsequent dosing. Combinations and dosing of antiemetics differ according to the chosen chemotherapeutic regimen. Tumor lysis syndrome Tumor lysis syndrome is a well-recognized complication of the rapid cell turnover of acute leukemias, whether occurring spontaneously or due to the cytotoxicity of chemotherapy. Preventive measures include initiation of allopurinol at the time of diagnosis along with initial aggressive hydration at signs of renal insufficiency. The acute management of hyperuricemia involves the use of rasburicase.
Pearls	• Prophylaxis against *Pneumocystis jiroveci* pneumonia may also be included • Fluoroquinolone- and β-lactam–resistant gram-negative organisms are increasing in frequency • G-CSF is not recommended in the treatment of an established neutropenic fever, as it has not proven to improve survival rates • Monitor fluid intake and output closely in patients undergoing chemotherapy for acute leukemia and treat volume overload with diuretics

References

1. Hersh E, Bodey G, Nies BA, et al. Causes of death in acute leukemia: a ten-year study of 414 patients from 1954-1963. JAMA 1965;193(2):105-9.
2. Smith TJ, Bohlke K, Lyman GH, et al. Recommendations for the use of WBC growth factors: American Society of Clinical Oncology Clinical Practice Guideline Update. J Clin Oncol 2015;33(28):3199-212.
3. Kaufman R, Djulbegovic B, Gernsheimer T, et al. Platelet transfusion: a clinical practice guideline from the AABB. Intern Med 2015;162:205-13.
4. DeZern A, Williams K, Zahurak M, et al. Red blood cell transfusion triggers in acute leukemia: a randomized pilot study. Transfusion 2016;56(7):1750-7.
5. National Comprehensive Cancer Network guidelines for supportive care. Version 2.2017. Available at: www.nccn.org.

How do I know whether my patient with acute leukemia has achieved a complete remission (CR)?

Key concept	Patients with acute leukemia often present with signs of bone marrow failure. The goal of induction chemotherapy is to eradicate bone marrow leukemic blasts and restore marrow function, evidenced by normalization, or near-normalization, of peripheral blood counts.
Clinical scenario	A 54-year-old man presents to the emergency room with profound fatigue, gingival hyperplasia, and bleeding. His white blood cell count is found to be 180×10^9 with 84% blasts. A bone marrow biopsy reveals sheets of blasts involving 90%–95% of the marrow. Immunophenotyping is consistent with the diagnosis of acute myelomonocytic leukemia.
Action items	• The induction phase of acute leukemia management aims to induce a bone marrow remission and allow for post-remission therapy[1,2] • During this phase, patients are supported with blood products, antimicrobials, and clinical diligence through the toxicities of the induction regimen, most notably myelosuppression • Upon bone marrow recovery, the peripheral blood and bone marrow are evaluated for the presence of leukemic blasts • Patients who are found to be in a complete remission (CR) can proceed to post-remission therapy; however, patients who have not achieved a CR will require a second induction phase
Discussion	A CR is the outcome of a successful induction phase, defined as clearance of peripheral blood blasts and the presence of <5% blasts on a marrow sample obtained after demonstration of an absolute neutrophil count $>1000 \times 10^3/\mu L$ and a platelet count $>100/\mu L$ for 2 consecutive days, independent of transfusions, on peripheral blood evaluation.[3,4] This is based on a morphological evaluation of the bone marrow specimen and is termed "morphological CR." Minimal residual disease (MRD) refers to the amount of disease detected by advanced techniques after achieving a CR and has a significant impact on the prognosis and risk of relapse. An MRD-negative CR is the ultimate goal of treatment in acute leukemias.[1,2]

Pearls	• A CR with incomplete platelet recovery, or CRi, refers to the above definition of CR but without full recovery of platelets counts at the time of evaluation • Different techniques of MRD detection with higher sensitivity than morphological evaluation have been deployed, including flow cytometry and real-time polymerase chain reaction • The administration of granulocyte colony-stimulating factor can alter the evaluation of the bone marrow morphology by affecting the number of blasts
References	1. Smith BD, Stein E. Acute myeloid leukemia. *American Society of Hematology Self-Assessment Program*. 6th ed.; 2017:521-9. 2. Litzow M, Heyman M. Acute lymphoblastic leukemia and lymphoblastic lymphoma. *American Society of Hematology Self-Assessment Program*. 6th ed.; 2017:531-46 3. National Comprehensive Cancer Network guidelines for acute myeloid leukemia. Version 3.2017. Available at: www.nccn.org. 4. National Comprehensive Cancer Network guidelines for acute lymphoblastic leukemia. Version 3.2017. Available at: www.nccn.org.

Should my patient receive intrathecal (IT) chemotherapy?

Key concept	Systemic chemotherapy at traditional doses is excluded from the central nervous system (CNS) by the blood-brain barrier (BBB), creating a sanctuary site for leukemic cells. IT chemotherapy administered into the subarachnoid space can be delivered via a lumbar puncture (LP) or into an Ommaya reservoir. Prophylactic or therapeutic IT chemotherapy is given to patients with leukemias with a high propensity of CNS involvement.
Clinical scenario	A 59-year-old woman presents with fatigue and fevers. A complete blood count shows a white blood cell count (WBC) of 217.8×10^9/L with 43% blasts. Peripheral blood smear microscopy shows these blasts to be variable in size, and no Auer rods are seen. Immunophenotyping of leukemic blasts is consistent with the diagnosis of pre-B acute lymphoblastic leukemia (ALL). A bone marrow evaluation confirms the diagnosis.
Action items	• Cytarabine, methotrexate, and hydrocortisone, as single agents or in combination, are administered intrathecally to eradicate CNS disease or for prophylaxis in patients with leukemias of high risk of CNS relapse • Alternatively, high-dose systemic chemotherapy can overcome the BBB but may result in significant systemic toxicities
Discussion	<u>Leukemia-specific indications for IT chemotherapy</u> **Acute myeloid leukemia[1]:** • In the presence of CNS symptoms, cerebrospinal fluid (CSF) is also sent for cytological evaluation and/or flow cytometry testing[1] • *Suggested* in high-risk scenarios at the time of bone marrow remission: monocytic leukemias, presenting WBC $>100 \times 10^9$/L, relapsed APL, or certain immunophenotypic and cytogenetic features[1-3]

	ALL: • All patients starting in induction phase; incidence of CNS relapse is nearly 80%[4] **Chronic myeloid and lymphoid leukemias:** • In the presence of CNS symptoms, CSF is also sent for cytological evaluation and/or flow cytometry
Pearls	• In the event of CNS involvement with leukemia (or lymphoma), IT chemotherapy is administered 2–3 times weekly until clearance, followed by administration at increased intervals for up to 1 year • In patients with hyperleukocytosis on presentation, initial cytoreduction is recommended prior to performing a lumbar puncture due to the theoretical risk of introducing leukemic blasts into the thecal space during an LP • Our understanding of the biology and treatment effectiveness, including CNS-directed therapy, in ALL is largely extrapolated from childhood ALL literature • IT chemotherapy is incorporated into the standard protocols for Burkitt leukemia/lymphoma and in certain aggressive lymphomas with high-risk features
References	1. Alakel N, Stölzel F, Mohr B, et al. Symptomatic central nervous system involvement in adult patients with acute myeloid leukemia. Cancer Manag Res 2017;9:97-102. 2. Holmes R, Keating MJ, Cork A, et al. A unique pattern of central nervous system leukemia in acute myelomonocytic leukemia associated with inv(16)(p13q22). Blood 1985;65:1071-8. 3. Shihadeh F, Reed V, Faderl S, et al. Cytogenetic profile of patients with acute myeloid leukemia and central nervous system disease. Cancer 2012;118:112-7. 4. Evans AE, Gilbert ES, Zandstra R. The increasing incidence of central nervous system leukemia in children. (Children's Cancer Study Group A). Cancer 1970;26:404-9.

How do I manage an elderly patient or patients with comorbidities diagnosed with acute leukemia?

Key concept	Optimal remission-induction therapy for acute leukemia requires intensive, combinatorial cytotoxic chemotherapy. Elderly patients and patients with comorbidities suffer higher rates of treatment-related mortality; therefore, "abbreviated" or low-intensity therapies should be used, despite the less favorable disease outcomes.
Clinical scenario	A 71-year-old woman presents to the emergency department due to profound fatigue. A complete blood count shows pancytopenia with 7% circulating blasts. A bone marrow biopsy shows hypercellularity approaching 100% and 25%–30% blasts. Underlying myelodysplasia is noted morphologically. Cytogenetic analysis shows unfavorable features.
Action item	• A clear and comprehensive discussion of risks and benefits of anti-leukemia therapy in elderly patients and patients with comorbidities should be held prior to initiating or withholding therapy, with an emphasis on the higher rates of early mortality compared to younger healthy patients
Discussion	The management of elderly patients with acute leukemias has posed a significant challenge over the years and continues to produce dismal outcomes and median survival durations of 8–12 months at best. Patients treated with aggressive chemotherapeutic regimens historically had a significantly higher rate of treatment-related deaths. By contrast, patients treated with low-intensity approaches had survival times limited by disease progression.[1] Leukemic blasts in the elderly tend to possess unfavorable cytogenetic features compared with those in younger patients, inferring higher disease resistance and rates of relapse. Additionally, elderly patients often have underlying chronic comorbidities that prohibit aggressive therapies. Secondary leukemias, described as those emerging in the background of a preceding hematological disorder (ie, myelodysplastic syndrome or myeloproliferative disorder) or secondary to prior therapy (ie, alkylating agents or topoisomerase inhibitors) are also more common in elderly patients and carry similar poor outcomes. Assessment of physiologic,

	rather than chronologic, age should guide therapeutic decisions. In "unfit" patients, abbreviated versions of standard therapies or targeted therapies added to a backbone of low-intensity agents have been used with variable success. This field has attracted the attention of clinicians and industry leaders alike over the past decade, and referral for clinical trials should be encouraged.
Pearls	• Acute myeloid leukemia (AML) is a disease of the elderly, with a median age at diagnosis of 67 years[2] • Hypomethylating agents in AML can achieve disease stability and transfusion independence and induce remissions in 10%–20% of patients[1] • In elderly patients with acute lymphoblastic leukemia (ALL), ongoing clinical trials with abbreviated standard induction regimens plus targeted agents show promise[3] • In the presence of actionable mutations in an "unfit" patient, maintenance therapy strategies have been devised • In "fit" patients with secondary AML, an allogeneic stem cell transplantation in first remission can be considered • BCR-ABL1 is more common in older adults with ALL and is a poor prognostic feature[4]
References	1. Smith BD, Stein E. Acute myeloid leukemia. *American Society of Hematology Self-Assessment Program.* 6th ed.; 2017:521-9. 2. Röllig C, Bornhäuser M, Thiede C, et al. Long-term prognosis of acute myeloid leukemia according to the new genetic risk classification of the European LeukemiaNet recommendations: evaluation of the proposed reporting system. J Clin Oncol 2011;29:2758-65. 3. Jabbour E, O'Brien S, Thomas DA, et al. Inotuzumab ozogamicin in combination with low-intensity chemotherapy (mini-hyper-CVD) as frontline therapy for older patients (≥60 years) with acute lymphoblastic leukemia (ALL). Blood 2014;124:794. 4. Pui C, Relling M, Downing JR. Acute lymphoblastic leukemia. N Engl J Med 2004;350:1535-48.

How do I monitor my patient in a sustained complete remission for disease relapse and late toxicities after completion of chemotherapy?

Key concept	With the advances in supportive care and the advent of novel agents in the upfront management of acute leukemias over the past few decades, more patients have emerged from treatment phases with ongoing remissions and begun their post-remission surveillance. Additionally, having undergone prolonged therapies, patients are periodically evaluated for late toxicities.
Clinical scenario	A 49-year-old man with B acute lymphoblastic leukemia who completed the induction and consolidation/intensification phases of the modified hyper-CVAD regimen and 8 doses of intrathecal chemotherapy followed by 2 years of maintenance chemotherapy is currently on active surveillance after sustaining a complete remission. He was evaluated with a history, physical examination, and laboratory testing on his first surveillance visit 1 month previously that revealed no evidence of disease relapse. He had a 10% decrease in his left ventricular ejection fraction, and a DEXA scan showed osteopenia in the lumbar spine. Subsequent monthly visits were uneventful. On his sixth surveillance visit, he reports headaches and nuchal rigidity; cerebrospinal fluid analysis reveals central nervous system relapse.
Action items	• Recommendations from collaborative groups provide guidance on rational surveillance and long-term care of cancer survivors • Physical and mental well-being should be evaluated periodically and appropriate diagnostics and referrals instituted guided by signs and symptoms

Discussion	Post-remission surveillance after completion of anti-leukemia therapies requires periodic assessments for disease relapse, bone marrow function, and a focused history and physical examination. Targeted investigations should be performed to evaluate new symptoms or abnormal findings. Patients with acute leukemia are commonly exposed to multi-agent chemotherapies, including anthracyclines, steroids, and alkylating agents, which can result in late toxicities including cardiomyopathy, secondary malignancies, loss of bone density, renal impairment, and gonadal dysfunction. Routine bone marrow biopsies for surveillance are an uncommon practice and marrow evaluations are reserved for patients with abnormal laboratory findings.[1–4] Patients are encouraged to maintain a relationship with their primary care providers for routine health issues.
References	1. National Comprehensive Cancer Network guidelines for acute myeloid leukemia. Version 3.2017. Available at: www.nccn.org. 2. National Comprehensive Cancer Network guidelines for acute lymphoblastic leukemia. Version 3.2017. Available at: www.nccn.org. 3. National Comprehensive Cancer Network guidelines for adolescent and young adult oncology. Version 1.2018. Available at: www.nccn.org. 4. Children's Oncology Group. Long-term follow-up guidelines for survivors of childhood, adolescent, and young adult cancer. Version 4.0. Available at: https://childrensoncologygroup.org/index.php/survivorshipguidelines.

How do I treat relapsed and refractory acute leukemia?

Key concept	Relapsed and refractory acute leukemia represents an area of great challenge due to its dismal survival outcomes and higher rates of failed remission (re)induction. Referral for investigational trials is encouraged.
Clinical scenario	A 29-year-old woman diagnosed with CD20-positive B acute lymphoblastic leukemia (ALL) with complex cytogenetics undergoes induction chemotherapy with hyper-CVAD plus rituximab, achieving a minimal residual disease (MRD)–negative complete remission (CR). She receives consolidation chemotherapy but relapses 2 months later with evidence of circulating lymphoblasts, confirmed by a bone marrow evaluation showing a leukemic relapse. She is referred for a clinical trial and treated with inotuzumab ozogamicin plus hyper-CVAD re-induction and achieves a second CR. She is being considered for a consolidative allogeneic stem cell transplantation.
Action items	• Investigative clinical trials remain the best option for patients with relapsed and refractory leukemias • If a second CR is achieved, patients are usually considered for a consolidative allogeneic stem cell transplantation
Discussion	The induction phase of acute leukemia management aims to deliver chemotherapy to eradicate leukemic blasts and restore marrow function. Once a patient is deemed to be in a CR after induction chemotherapy, the consolidation phase begins, which in turn aims to eradicate disease below the level of detection, also known as MRD, in order to prevent leukemic relapse. The last phase of treatment deployed in certain leukemias is the maintenance (continuation) phase, during which slow-growing leukemic clones not affected by induction or consolidation chemotherapy are exposed to anti-neoplastic agents over a prolonged period of time.[1] Relapse is defined as the re-emergence of leukemic blasts after attaining an initial CR, whereas refractory disease results

	from the failure to attain an initial CR with induction therapy. Both disease states are more commonly encountered in leukemias with poor-risk cytogenetics at diagnosis and secondary leukemias; therefore, these patients should be regarded as candidates for investigational trials upfront.[2] MRD positivity is regarded as a marker for a higher risk of relapse in acute leukemias after initial CR and is incorporated into the risk-adapted management of ALL.[3] The management of relapsed/refractory leukemias follows the same paradigm as newly diagnosed acute leukemia, with the choice of re-induction regimens tailored to cytogenetics, host characteristics, and duration of remission in relapsed patients. Consolidation after a second remission is by allogeneic stem cell transplantation, although alternative investigational therapies are under way.
Pearls	• Early relapses are associated with low rates of CR after re-induction therapy • The majority of patients with acute myeloid leukemia experience disease relapse despite reaching an initial CR • Relapses can occur in extramedullary sites
References	1. Smith BD, Stein E. Acute myeloid leukemia. *American Society of Hematology Self-Assessment Program*. 6th ed.; 2017:521-9. 2. Breems DA, Van Putten WL, Huijgens PC, et al. Prognostic index for adult patients with acute myeloid leukemia in first relapse. J Clin Oncol 2005;23(9):1969-78. 3. Beldjord K, Chevret S, Asnafi V, et al. Oncogenetics and minimal residual disease are independent outcome predictors in adult patients with acute lymphoblastic leukemia. Blood 2014;123:3739-49.

What is leukemia cutis (LC)?

Key concept	Although acute leukemia is a disease of the bone marrow that manifests primarily in the peripheral blood, it can also present in extramedullary tissues. LC is the infiltration of the epidermis, dermis, or subcutis by leukemia cells in the form of cutaneous lesions.
Clinical scenario	A 68-year-old man with a history of chronic myeloid leukemia (CML) presents to the emergency room of a local hospital in blast crisis. A diagnosis of acute leukemia secondary to a CML in blast crisis is made. During the physical examination, multiple nodules in both lower extremities are noted. The nodules are raised, painless, and of a violaceous color. A skin biopsy reveals an infiltrate of the skin by leukemic cells.
Action item	• Always biopsy suspicious skin lesions in patients presenting with a diagnosis of acute leukemia
Discussion	Leukemia cutis has been mostly described in acute myeloid leukemia (AML). It occurs in ~3% of patients with AML and less frequently in CML and myelodysplastic syndrome. A biopsy is always necessary, as CL can be confused with similar lesions of different etiology, including inflammatory and infectious etiology. The most frequent sites of involvement are the legs, arms, skin of the back, anterior part of the thorax, and face. CL lesions have predilection for sites of acute or chronic skin inflammation and in children produce what is known as "blueberry muffin" appearance." "Aleukemic LC" is the occurrence of a generalized papulo-nodular presentation prior to the initiation of systemic leukemia. The infiltrates of LC are mostly of mononuclear cells in a diffuse and infiltrative pattern. Scattered macrophages and neutrophils may be present. Immunohistochemistry may help to establish the diagnosis of leukemia. The treatment of the LC is based on the systemic treatment of the leukemia.[1]

Pearls	• The immunohistochemical profile may be discordant with the immunophenotype of the leukemic blasts • LC is most commonly associated with myelomonocytic and monocytic leukemia • LC is rarely described in acute lymphoblastic leukemia
References	1. Bakst RL, Tallman MS, Douer D, et al. How I treat extramedullary acute myeloid leukemia. Blood 2011;118:3785-93.

Do all acute lymphoblastic leukemia (ALL) patients require a bone marrow evaluation?

Key concept	ALL is a cancer of the lymphoid line of blood cells, characterized by the rapid growth of abnormal cells in the bone marrow. From there the cells can be found in the peripheral blood and invade other organs. Because the bone marrow is the site of origin of the disease, a bone marrow evaluation is necessary and required in every case of ALL.[1]
Clinical scenario	A 25-year-old woman develops anemia, fatigue, and tiredness with easy bruisability and bleeding of the gums. She goes to an emergency room and, as part of her evaluation, an examination of the peripheral blood reveals >20% blasts in the peripheral circulation. During the observation period, reports of a flow cytometry evaluation of the peripheral blood confirm a diagnosis of ALL as per WHO criteria: ≥20% lymphoid lineage blasts in the peripheral blood or bone marrow. Because the diagnosis of ALL has been confirmed in the peripheral blood, should you schedule a bone marrow aspiration and biopsy?

Action items	• Schedule a bone marrow aspiration and biopsy
	• This should include a core biopsy and aspiration material
	  • The core biopsy is used for touch preparations and immunohistochemistry
	  • The aspiration material is used to prepare a clot and aspirate smears; portions are submitted for flow cytometry, cytogenetics, molecular diagnostics, and tumor markers

Discussion	The diagnosis of ALL starts with a combination of clinical and a peripheral blood smear findings. Flow cytometry can confirm the diagnosis in the peripheral blood. However, a bone marrow aspiration and biopsy is always required to establish a disease baseline and evaluate therapeutic responses. In >95% of cases, flow cytometry can assign lineage. Mixed-phenotype acute leukemia is rare. ALL blasts are negative for myeloperoxidase (MPO). Low-level + MPO (<5%) can occur with myeloid markers. Terminal deoxynucleotidyl transferase (TdT) separates ALL from reactive processes.[1] ALL has three immunophenotypic groups: precursor B cell, mature B cell, and T cell ALL (T-ALL). Precursor B cell ALL (B-ALL) stains positive for TdT, HLA-DR, CD19, CD22, and CD79a. Expression of CD10 (common ALL antigen [CALLA]) distinguishes common ALL (early pre–B-ALL). Mature B-ALL (Burkitt leukemia) is TdT-negative/CD20+. BCR-ABL translocation is expressed in 20%–30% of ALL cases. A Philadelphia chromosome–like signature lacking expression of the BCR-ABL1 fusion protein is seen in 10% of children and as many as 25%–30% of young adults.[2]
Pearls	Surface CD3 is positive in mature T-ALL, with positivity for either CD4 or CD8, but not both. Only thymic T-ALL has good outcome with chemotherapy alone.
References	1. Kantarjian HM. *The MD Anderson Manual of Medical Oncology*. 3rd ed. Columbus, OH: McGraw-Hill Education/Medical; 2016. 2. Boer JM, den Boer ML. BCR-ABL1-like acute lymphoblastic leukemia: from bench to bedside. Eur J Cancer 2017;82:203-18.

What are the targeted therapies for acute lymphoblastic leukemia (ALL)?

Key concept	Targeted cancer therapies are drugs or other substances that interfere with molecular targets involved in the growth of tumor cells. By contrast, standard chemotherapies act on all rapidly dividing normal and cancerous cells. Targeted therapies are often cytostatic, whereas standard chemotherapy agents are *cytotoxic*. Molecular targets have been identified in ALL, and specific drugs targeting such molecules have been characterized, adding to the effect of standard chemotherapy in the treatment of ALL.[1]
Clinical scenario	A 56-year-old man was found in a routine CBC to have a significantly elevated white blood cell count, with >50% blasts in the peripheral blood. A bone marrow biopsy and aspiration confirmed the diagnosis of ALL, positive for aBCR-ABL fusion protein by fluorescence in-situ hybridization (FISH). He started treatment with hyperCVAD and a BCR-ABL1 tyrosine kinase inhibitor (TKI), which continued after completion of induction and maintenance therapy. He has remained in complete remission (CR) for 6 years after his diagnosis.
Action items	• All new patients diagnosed with ALL must be tested for BCR-ABL1 fusion protein • If BCR-ABL1 negative, consider testing for other fusions associated with Philadelphia chromosome positive–like ALL
Discussion	The response of ALL to therapy is 80%–91% in adults, but only 25%–45% remain in remission after 5 years. This has made the need for development of new and complementary therapies an important problem in ALL. The addition of targeted therapy in some instances has increased the proportion of patients who achieve and maintain CR and has also been the key element in ensuring a response during relapse and a bridge to transplantation. Monoclonal antibodies and specific molecular agents such as BCR-ABL TKIs are the major examples of targeted therapy in ALL.

	In the case of BCR-ABL1 fusion–positive patients, second-generation TKIs have shown improvements in complete molecular responses and 5-year survival rates of 50%. These rates at 3 years have now been improved even further with ponatinib, a third-generation TKI. In ALL-relapsed patients, salvage chemotherapy CR rates can range from 20% to 45%, with median survival durations of 3–9 months. Achieving a CR is a first and necessary step in order to realize the curative potential of hematopoietic stem cell transplantation. The bispecific T cell antibody blinatumomab directs lysis of CD19-positive B cells by CD3-positive cytotoxic T cells. Blinatumomab can achieve a CR or CR with partial hematological recovery (CRh) rate of 43% within the first 2 treatment cycles. Other promising targeted therapies of ALL in development include chimeric antigen receptor therapies, agents targeting NOTCH, FLT3, and the proteasome. Studies are in development to find their safe and effective combinations.[2,3]
Pearls	To avoid a cytokine release syndrome associated to the administration of blinatumomab, consider pretreatment with 25 mg meperidine and 20 mg SIVP + dexamethasone IV prior to the first dose of each cycle and prior to each intra-cycle dose increase (eg, as occurs on cycle 1 day 8). If the infusion is interrupted for >4 hours, administer another dose of meperidine and dexamethasone.
References	1. Portell CA, Advani AS. Novel targeted therapies in acute lymphoblastic leukemia. Leuk Lymphoma 2014;55:737-48. 2. Maude S, Frey N, Shaw PA, et al. Chimeric antigen receptor T cells for sustained remissions in leukemia. N Engl J Med 2014;37:1507-17. 3. Jabbour E, Kantarjian H, Ravandi F, et al. Combination of hyper-CVAD with ponatinib as first-line therapy for patients with Philadelphia chromosome-positive acute lymphoblastic leukemia: a single-centre, phase 2 study. Lancet Oncol 2015;16(15):1547-55.

What are the differences in acute lymphoblastic leukemia (ALL) treatment by patient age?

Key concept	Age is the most important factor in predicting tolerance to ALL treatment.
Clinical scenario	A 55-year-old man presents to an emergency department complaining of severe headache. He becomes comatose, and a CT scan reveals left acute subdural hematoma. A complete blood cell count and peripheral smear show a white blood cell count of 55,400/dL, with 50% blasts in the peripheral circulation. Due to significant midline shift, he undergoes a successful evacuation of the hematoma. The question is raised about the best treatment for his ALL.
Discussion	In elderly patients with ALL (patients >55 years old), intensive chemotherapy results in a complete remission (CR) rate of 80%, albeit with a high rate of toxicities. One-third of patients achieving CR may die of myelosuppression-associated complications during consolidation-maintenance therapy. The long-term cure rate among such patients is 15%–20%. Median survival is 10 months. Based on these statistics, the goal with modern regimens focuses on maintaining efficacy with a reduced toxicity. An example of this approach is the use of dose reductions in chemotherapy and the use of targeted therapy to maintain therapeutic efficacy. In this scenario, the regular hyper-CVAD is converted to a mini-hyper-CVD in which no anthracycline is used, 50% dose reduction of steroid and cyclophosphamide, 75% dose reduction of methotrexate, and 83% dose reduction of cytarabine + inotuzumab ozogamicin, a CD22 monoclonal antibody that is covalently linked to calicheamicin, a potent cytotoxic agent that causes a break between double-stranded DNA. When compared the hyper-CVAD regimen, the combination of low-intensity chemotherapy with inotuzumab improves the outcome of these patients population. Recently, 4 cycles of blinatumomab were added to this regimen to further improve efficacy.[1]

Pearl	• Always asses end organ reserve, particularly kidney function and liver function, and make appropriate pharmacokinetic dose adjustments
References	1. National Comprehensive Cancer Network guidelines for older adult oncology. Version 2.2017. Available at: www.nccn.org.

What is the rationale for multi-agent chemotherapy in acute lymphoblastic leukemia (ALL)?

Key concept	ALL is treated in adults with the same pattern of combination chemotherapy developed for the treatment of ALL in children. In children, there is a direct correlation between the number of agents used and the cure rate; hence the use of combination chemotherapy in adults.[1]
Clinical scenario	A patient is to be started on combination chemotherapy for ALL. He expresses a desire that the treatment not be "too complicated" and limited to one drug. The physician argues for combination chemotherapy, and the patient accepts.
Action items	• Always confirm that the use of agents is done with documented evidence of lack of added toxicity and potential therapeutic benefit • Do not start empirical combinations of agents based on assumed efficacy or benefit
Discussion	The rationale for combination chemotherapy in ALL is based on the well-known tumor cell heterogeneity and its implication for drug resistance, and of course the success of combination chemotherapy in the clinic. It has been shown that curative chemotherapy in a variety of human and animal tumors involves combinations of 2 and usually ≥ 3 agents. In some cases, there is clear evidence for synergy or an additive effect between chemotherapeutic agents and agents representing other classes. For example, the addition of the complement-fixing monoclonal antibody rituximab to ALL regimens in patients expressing CD20 increases response without increased toxicity. Another established combination highly potent for ALL is the combination of vincristine and prednisone. Whereas tumors are clonal in origin, they are characterized by DNA instability, which leads to increased variation of daughter cells (clonal evolution) and thus tumor cell heterogeneity. This biological fact is associated with an increase in the number and diversity of potential target sites and the need for combining therapeutic agents.

Pearls	The augmented Berlin-Frankfurt-Munster (BFM) and hyper-CVAD regimens for treatment of adolescents and young adults with ALL have similar efficacy outcomes with different toxicity profiles. Asparaginase-related toxicity (hepatotoxicity, pancreatitis, and thrombosis) is associated with augmented BFM and myelosuppression with hyper-CVAD.[2]
References	1. Lister TA, Whitehouse JMA, Beard MEJ, et al. Combination chemotherapy for acute lymphoblastic leukemia in adults. BMJ 1978;1:199-203. 2. Rytting M, Jabbour EJ, Jorgensen JL, et al. Final results of a single institution experience with a pediatric-based regimen, the augmented Berlin-Frankfurt-Münster, in adolescents and young adults with acute lymphoblastic leukemia, and comparison to the hyper-CVAD regimen. Am J Hematol 2016;91(8):819-23.

Do all acute lymphoblastic leukemia (ALL) patients receive intrathecal chemotherapy?

Key concept	Despite the intense administration of systemic chemotherapy in ALL, there are leukemic cells that can persist within sites and cannot reach the central nervous system (CNS) because of the blood-brain barrier.
Clinical scenario	A 23-year-old woman developed anemia, fatigue, and tiredness with easy bruisability and bleeding of the gums. She is confirmed to have ALL and started on hyper-CVAD. When started on treatment, she is told she will need to receive intrathecal (IT) chemotherapy. The patient asks why and how many times.
Action item	• As soon as the patient is initiated on systemic chemotherapy, schedule the administration of IT chemotherapy with the neuro-radiology department
Discussion	The CNS constitutes a sanctuary site where cells of ALL can persist despite systemic chemotherapy. At our institution we extensively use hyper-CVAD in the treatment of adult patients with ALL (hyperfractionated cyclophosphamide, vincristine, doxorubicin, and dexamethasone alternating with high-dose methotrexate and cytarabine for a total of 8 alternating cycles every ~3–4 weeks). They then receive 2 years of POMP maintenance therapy, interspersed with intensification courses during months 6, 7, 18, and 19. All patients are scheduled for 2 IT injections per course with 8 ITs for nonmature B-ALL and 16 ITs for mature B-ALL due to their higher risk of CNS relapse.[1]

Pearl	• Cerebrospinal fluid can always be sent in addition to regular cytology for flow cytometry, particularly in patients at high risk of CNS relapse
References	1. Pui CH. Central nervous system disease in acute lymphoblastic leukemia: prophylaxis and treatment. Hematology Am Soc Hematol Educ Program 2006:142-6.

Is it common to use asparaginase compounds in all acute lymphoblastic leukemia (ALL) patients?

Key concept	Lymphoblastic leukemia cells are unable to synthesize L-asparagine (Asn or N). Asparagine is necessary for DNA, RNA, and protein synthesis. Its depletion ultimately leads to the death of the leukemic cell.[1]
Clinical scenario	A 40-year-old woman develops anemia, fatigue, and tiredness with easy bruisability and bleeding of the gums. She is confirmed to have ALL. She has read that asparaginase "is a good drug for ALL." Her liver functions are abnormal. She asks her doctor whether she should receive asparaginase.
Discussion	There are three available asparaginase preparations: asparaginase from *Escherichia coli*, a pegylated form (PEG-asparaginase), and an *Dickeya dadantii* asparaginase. Asparaginases are used in treatment of pediatric ALL for remission induction and intensification with proven improvements in clinical outcome. However, in young adolescents and adults its use is infrequent because of increased toxicity in this population, including hypersensitivity reactions, pancreatitis, and thrombosis. Clinical hypersensitivity reactions and silent inactivation due to inactivation of *E. coli* asparaginase is seen in up to 60% of cases. PEG-asparaginase is used in first-line treatment of ALL.[2] A recent analysis showed that there is equivalent therapeutic efficacy between hyper-CVAD and the BMF regimen (an asparaginase-containing regimen) in the treatment of ALL, with the difference mostly due to the different toxicities attributable to asparaginase.[2]
Pearl	• An asparaginase activity level of 0.1 IU/mL is the target necessary to ensure adequate Asn depletion[3]

References

1. Ho DH, Whitecar JP Jr, Luce JK, et al. L-Asparagine requirement and the effect of L-asparaginase on the normal and leukemic human bone marrow. Cancer Res 1970;30:466-72.
2. Rytting ME, Jabbour EJ, Jorgensen JL, et al. Final results of a single institution experience with a pediatric-based regimen, the augmented Berlin-Frankfurt-Münster, in adolescents and young adults with acute lymphoblastic leukemia, and comparison to the hyper-CVAD regimen. Am J Hematol 2016;91:819-23.
3. Riccardi R, Holcenberg JS, Glaubiger DL, et al. L-Asparaginase pharmacokinetics and asparagine levels in cerebrospinal fluid of rhesus monkeys and humans. Cancer Res 1981;41(11 Pt 1):4554-8.

Why is consolidation therapy given after induction if patients achieve remission?

Key concept	Induction, intensified consolidation, maintenance, and central nervous system (CNS) prophylaxis are the phases of treatment for acute lymphoblastic leukemia (ALL).[1] Consolidation or intensified consolidation involves the use of anti-leukemic agents on specific schedules of administration with the objective of restoring normal hematopoiesis and eradicating resistant sub-clones, protecting sanctuary sites (CNS, testicles) with CNS prophylaxis.
Clinical scenario	A 44-year-old man with a diagnosis of ALL completed his first course of hyper-CVAD. A bone marrow is done and he is advised that he is in complete remission. He asks what comes next.
Action item	• Bone marrow aspiration and biopsy should be done as soon as there is hematological recovery in the peripheral blood after the first induction treatment
Discussion	It is known from animal models of leukemia and from clinical empirical experience that the achievement of complete remission with one course of chemotherapy is not enough to eliminate all leukemic cells that give rise to the clinical presentation of ALL.[2] The post-remission phase can be considered as a form of therapeutic intensification. Because the achievement of a complete response is the goal of treatment, the same drugs used during induction are usually used during the consolidation phase.
Pearl	• In contrast to acute leukemia of myeloid lineage, the use of granulocyte colony-stimulating factor is customary during induction and consolidation of acute leukemia of lymphoid lineage

References	1. Faderl S, O'Brien S, Pui C-H, et al. Adult acute lymphoblastic leukemia: concepts and strategies. Cancer 2010;116(5):1165-76. 2. Momparler RL. A model for the chemotherapy of acute leukemia with 1-β-D-arabinofuranosylcytosine. Cancer Res 1974; 34:1775-87.

What are the key differences between allogeneic and autologous stem cell transplantation (SCT)?

Key concept	SCTs differ in the source of stem cells (SCs),[1] indications, mechanism of action, and potential complications. The strategies deployed to eradicate malignancies with SCTs differ according to the underlying malignancy as well as host factors.[2] If a graft-versus-tumor (GVT) effect is the desired strategy to eradicate tumor cells, an allogeneic SCT is performed in suitable patients, whereas when the goal is eradicating tumor cells using high doses of chemotherapy, an autologous SCT is performed.
Clinical scenario	A 37-year-old man with newly diagnosed acute myeloid leukemia (AML) with poor-risk cytogenetic features was treated with induction chemotherapy without attaining a complete remission (CR). A second induction was delivered, resulting in a CR. Post-remission allogeneic stem cell transplant from an HLA-matched unrelated donor is planned.
Action items	Patients with conditions warranting an SCT undergo an extensive pretransplant work-up to evaluate their candidacy, including evaluation of performance status, organ function, and comorbidity index.[2] If a patient is a candidate, they will undergo the following procedures in order of occurrence: • Donor search for allogeneic SCTs or SC collection for autologous SCTs • Maximization of underlying disease control • Conditioning: therapies given to eradicate residual tumor cells and, in the case of allogeneic SCTs, also suppress the host immune response to allow engraftment of the donor graft • Transplant (day 0): infusion of collected SCs • Engraftment: signs of bone marrow recovery; duration varies according to the type of SCT and source of SCs • Long-term post-transplant care

Discussion	Allogeneic and autologous SCTs are conceptually different means of therapy; in an allogeneic SCT, the SCs—or graft—are procured from a healthy donor and given to the patient. The T lymphocytes transferred with the graft from the donor exert an anti-tumor effect also known as the GVT effect, thereby eradicating residual disease. In an autologous SCT, the SCs are procured from the patient; this is followed by delivering high doses of chemotherapy (conditioning regimen) to eradicate the disease. SCs are then re-infused in order to "rescue" the marrow, which was also eradicated in the process by the high-dose chemotherapy. Autologous SCs do not exert a GVT effect.
Pearls	• The role and timing of stem cell transplantation is continuously evaluated as novel therapies become available • Allogeneic SCTs are most commonly used in leukemias and bone marrow failure syndromes[3]; autologous SCTs are most commonly used in plasma cell dyscrasias and lymphomas • The intent behind a transplant can be curative (eg, allogeneic SCT for AML, acute lymphoblastic leukemia, and aplastic anemia) or to achieve a deeper response (non-curative, eg, autologous SCT for multiple myeloma)[4]
References	1. Ballen KK, Koreth J, Chen YB, et al. Selection of optimal alternative graft source: mismatched unrelated donor, umbilical cord blood, or haploidentical transplant. Blood 2012;119:1972-80. 2. Sorror M, Maris MB, Storb R, et al. Hematopoietic cell transplantation (HCT)-specific comorbidity index: a new tool for risk assessment before allogeneic HCT. Blood 2005;106:2912-9. 3. Scheinberg P, Young NS. How I treat acquired aplastic anemia. Blood 2012;120(6):1185-96. 4. Palumbo A, Cavallo F, Gay F, et al. Autologous transplantation and maintenance therapy in multiple myeloma. N Engl J Med 2014;371:895-905.

Which acute lymphoblastic leukemia (ALL) patients are recommended an allogeneic stem cell transplant (AHSCT)?

Key concept	High-risk features can segregate patients with ALL who are candidates for AHSCT in first complete remission (CR). Given that standard-risk disease patients can also benefit significantly from AHSCT, for this latter group the guidance for decision is provided by whether they achieve minimal residual disease (MRD) as evaluated by flow cytometry (FCM) or RT-PCR.[1]
Clinical scenario	A 24-year-old patient has a peripheral blood smear compatible with the diagnosis of acute leukemia. A bone marrow aspiration and diagnosis confirm the diagnosis of ALL. On the first month of maintenance therapy, a surveillance bone marrow aspiration and biopsy reveal the presence of MRD by FCM. The patient is referred to a tertiary center for evaluation of an AHSCT.
Action item	• Always request follow-up surveillance bone marrow evaluations for MRD
Discussion	AHSCT has traditionally been reserved for patients with high-risk ALL features, such as B-lineage with WBC $\geq 30 \times 10^9$/L, T-lineage with WBC $\geq 100 \times 10^9$/L, hypodiploid, Philadelphia chromosome–positive, or mixed-lineage leukemia translocation ALL [eg, t(4;11)]. For patients with standard-risk disease, failure to achieve MRD is a powerful indicator of future relapse. In some centers, this is an indication for AHSCT. By contrast, patients who achieve MRD-negative status have a significantly improved 5-year overall survival (75% vs. 33%; P = .001).
Pearl	• A post-induction MRD level $\geq 10^{-4}$ and unfavorable genetic characteristics (ie, MLL gene rearrangement or focal IKZF1 gene deletion in B-cell precursor ALL and no NOTCH1/FBXW7 mutation and/or N/K-RAS mutation and/or PTEN gene alteration in T-ALL) are independently associated with worse outcome[2]

References

1. Goldstone AH, Richards SM, Lazarus HM, et al. In adults with standard-risk acute lymphoblastic leukemia, the greatest benefit is achieved from a matched sibling allogeneic transplantation in first complete remission, and an autologous transplantation is less effective than conventional consolidation. Blood 2008;111(4):1827-33.
2. Campana D. Minimal residual disease in acute lymphoblastic leukemia. Hematology Am Soc Hematol Educ Program 2010;2010:7-12.

Are steroids effective in acute lymphoblastic leukemia (ALL)?

Key concept	Glucocorticoids, generically referred to as steroids, were one of the first agents with demonstrable activity against ALL, first in children and then in adults. They remain an essential component of the therapy of ALL in both children and adults.[1]
Clinical scenario	A 55-year-old hypertensive, diabetic man is diagnosed with ALL. His diabetes and arterial hypertension are poorly controlled. Because of this, his oncologist initially omits steroids from the induction regimen. Realizing that it is more important to control the leukemia, the physician opts for better control of the patient's diabetes and blood pressure and proceeds to incorporate the steroids in the therapy of the patient's ALL.

Action items	• Using steroids for the treatment of ALL requires the following measures:
	  • Control of arterial blood pressure
	  • Monitoring of glucose intolerance
	  • Promoting exercise to avoid significant osteoporosis and steroid-associated myopathy
	  • Use of prophylactic antibiotics, because the immunosuppression of steroids is additive with the use of the chemotherapy
	  • Monitoring for emotional and mental changes (steroid psychosis)

Discussion	Steroids are one of the most effective agents against ALL. Part of the reason for this effectiveness is that steroids have a cytotoxic effect on the malignant cells. This effect appears to be mediated by the binding of these agents to glucocorticoid receptors in the cytoplasm, from which they can homodimerize, translocate to the nucleus, and interact with glucocorticoid response elements. In addition, when monomeric, they can repress the activity of transcription factors (activating protein-1 of the nuclear factor–κB). This results in overall inhibition of cytokine production, alteration of the expression of oncogenes, and induction of cell cycle arrest and apoptosis.

Pearl	• Dexamethasone is superior to prednisone in preventing central nervous system relapse in ALL when used at a prednisone:dexamethasone ratio of 6:7
References	1. Hiroto I, Ching-Hon P. Glucocorticoid use in acute lymphoblastic leukemia: comparison of prednisone and dexamethasone. Lancet Oncol 2010;11:1096-106.

What is chronic myelogenous leukemia (CML), and why is it classified separately from other myeloproliferative neoplasms?

Key concept	CML is the only myeloproliferative neoplasm with an associated identifiable genetic cause: reciprocal translocation t(9:22), also known as the Philadelphia chromosome.
Clinical scenario	A 72-year-old man presents to the emergency room with complaints of fever, fatigue, and cough. A chest X-ray shows a left lung infiltrate, and complete blood count shows a white blood cell count of 400,000 and hemoglobin of 7.7. He is started on allopurinol, fluids, and hydroxyurea. A bone marrow biopsy confirms the presence of a Philadelphia chromosome. He is treated for his pneumonia, given a blood transfusion for his anemia, and discharged on imatinib (Gleevec, a BCR-ABL1 tyrosine kinase inhibitor). He is given a diagnosis of CML.
Action items	• Order a bone marrow biopsy and aspiration with immunohistochemistry, flow cytometry, and cytogenetic and molecular markers for CML, including BCR-ABL1 by fluorescence in situ hybridization (FISH) and polymerase chain reaction (PCR) • Order peripheral blood BCR-ABL1 by FISH and PCR
Discussion	The Philadelphia chromosome (t9:22) leads to a BCR-ABL1 fusion gene. This fusion gene contains a tyrosine kinase, p210, central to the pathogenesis of CML. In acute lymphoblastic leukemia (ALL), the same translocation produces another fusion protein, p190. This subtype of ALL is known as Ph-positive ALL.[1] CML is usually diagnosed in the chronic phase, but it also has two other phases: accelerated and blast phase. The untreated chronic phase will eventually progress to a more advanced phase, usually within 3–5 years. Patients present with characteristic clinical findings secondary to large numbers of myeloid circulating progenitors, leading to splenomegaly (50%–60% of cases), leukocytosis, or even isolated thrombocytosis.

	The most common laboratory finding in chronic-phase CML is leukocytosis, with myeloid cells in all stages of maturation seen in the peripheral blood. There is frequently also an increase in basophils and eosinophils. The bone marrow is markedly hypercellular, with the myeloid-to-erythroid ratio significantly increased. The presence of additional chromosomal abnormalities (ACA), known as "major-route ACA/Ph+," such as trisomy 8, isochromosome 17q, second Ph, and trisomy 19, appearing during the course of the disease is attributable to clonal cytogenetic evolution and is associated with poor prognosis.[2]
Pearl	• Despite the significant increase in all forms of cells from all series, the percentage of blasts remains normal in chronic-phase CML
References	1. Cortes JE, Talpaz M, Kantarjian H. Chronic myelogenous leukemia: a review. Am J Med 1996;100(5):555-70. 2. Cortes JE, Talpaz M, Giles F, et al. Prognostic significance of cytogenetic clonal evolution in patients with chronic myelogenous leukemia on imatinib mesylate therapy. Blood 2003;101:3794-800.

What is accelerated-phase (AP) chronic myelogenous leukemia (CML)?

Key concept	An AP CML is a CML that is unstable due to genetic progression (clonal cytogenetic evolution) and transformation into an acute leukemia.
Action items	• In untreated patients, initiate treatment, preferably with a second-generation tyrosine kinase inhibitor • In treated patients, change therapy to a second- or third-generation tyrosine kinase inhibitor depending of the patient's circumstances • Send blood for evaluation of BCR-ABL1 tyrosine kinase mutations
Discussion	Although there is no definition of AP CML, patients are considered to be in AP if any of the following are true[1]: • The bone marrow or blood samples have >10% but <20% blasts • High blood basophil count (basophils making up ≥20% of white blood cells) • High white blood cell counts that do not decrease with treatment • Very high or very low platelet counts that are not caused by treatment • New chromosome changes in the leukemia cells Most patients evolve in sequence from the accelerated phase to the blast phase. However, up to 20% of patients can progress straight from the chronic phase to the blast phase without signs or symptoms. Blast phase is considered an acute leukemia, with >20% blasts in the peripheral blood or bone marrow or the presence of extramedullary disease (chloroma or granulocytic sarcoma).

	Half of blast-phase cases carry a myeloid phenotype, whereas the other half is split evenly between lymphoid and undifferentiated. Median survival in blast-phase CML remains poor; combination treatment with tyrosine kinase inhibitor chemotherapy followed by allogeneic stem-cell transplantation is recommended.[2] Dasatinib, nilotinib, bosutinib, and ponatinib have demonstrated activity in acute-phase and blast-phase CML. In either situation, always test for BCR-ABL1 tyrosine kinase mutations.
Pearl	• It has been established that first-generation BCR-ABL1 tyrosine kinase inhibitors such as imatinib are not as effective in controlling an accelerated-phase CML as second- and third-generation agents are
References	1. Kantarjian HM, Dixon D, Keating MJ, et al. Characteristics of accelerated disease in chronic myelogenous leukemia. Cancer 1988;61(7):1441-6. 2. Cortes JE, Talpaz M, Kantarjian H. Chronic myelogenous leukemia: a review. Am J Med 1996;100(5):555-70.

How is chronic myelogenous leukemia (CML) treated?

Key concept	Avoiding transformation is the main objective of CML treatment. Thus, achieving a complete cytogenetic response (CCyR), particularly during the first 3–6 months of therapy, is the most important prognostic factor for long-term survival. Currently there are four BCR-ABL1 tyrosine kinase inhibitors (TKIs) used for the treatment of CML: the first-generation agent imatinib and second-generation agents dasatinib, nilotinib, and bosutinib.[1] Ponatinib is considered a third-generation TKI and is not approved for frontline therapy. It is approved for salvage therapy and for patients with a TKI T315I mutation.
Clinical scenario	A 33-year-old woman is referred with a right torsed ovary. Her white blood cell count was 331,000 with a differential that includes immature forms and 7% blasts. A bone marrow aspiration and biopsy confirm the diagnosis of CML with a positive Philadelphia chromosome. She is initiated on dasatinib perioperatively and tolerates her therapy without complications for 4 years.

Action items	• Stratify the patients into one of three risk groups—low, intermediate, or high—prior to selecting treatment
	• There are two scoring systems: Sokal and Hasford (Euro) scoring systems
	  • The Sokal score uses age, spleen size, platelet count, and blast percentage in peripheral blood
	  • The Euro score includes eosinophils and basophils in the peripheral blood

Discussion	Imatinib (400 mg daily) and second-generation TKIs dasatinib (50–100 mg daily)], nilotinib (300 mg twice daily), and bosutinib (400 mg daily) are indicated in patients with a low risk score. For patients with an intermediate- or high-risk score, second-generation TKIs (dasatininb, nilotinib, and bosutinib) are indicated. In selecting a TKI, the patient's clinical situation and comorbidities may play an important role in choosing the most suitable TKI. • Imatinib has the development of peripheral edema as one of its major side effects

	• Dasatinib carries the risk of pleural effusions and platelet dysfunction[2]; patients on concomitant anticoagulants may be at an increased risk for hemorrhagic complications
	• Nilotinib can cause hyperglycemia and QT interval prolongation (monitoring of the QT interval is essential)
	  • Potassium and magnesium should be optimally replete and taken on an empty stomach twice daily
	  • Nilotinib has also been associated with peripheral artery disease, cerebrovascular accidents, cardiovascular syndromes, and pancreatitis (avoid in patients with a prior history of pancreatic inflammation)
	• Bosutinib is associated with diarrhea (70%), nausea (35%), and increased liver function
	  • Adherence to treatment is important, as interruptions lead to adverse outcomes
	• Ponatinib is suitable only for patients with the T315I mutation (in all phases of CML) and for whom no other TKI is indicated
	  • Ponatinib can cause liver dysfunction and vascular venous and arterial occlusive disease (27% of patients)
	  • Cytopenias (anemia, neutropenia, and thrombocytopenia) are managed with treatment interruptions and dose modifications
	  • GCS-F can be used, but the use of erythropoiesis-stimulating agents is not currently supported in myeloid malignancies
	• For patients with the T315I mutation and who are resistant to >2 TKIs, omacetaxine (a non-TKI CML therapy) has demonstrated safety and efficacy

Pearl	• Escalating imatinib to 800 mg in patients with low risk to achieve a better response is not indicated, given the superior benefit of using a second-generation TKI
References	1. Jabbour E, Kantarjian H. Chronic myeloid leukemia: 2014 update on diagnosis, monitoring, and management. Am J Hematol 2014;89(5):547-56. 2. O'Brien SG, Guilhot F, Larson RA, et al. Imatinib compared with interferon and low-dose cytarabine for newly diagnosed chronic-phase chronic myeloid leukemia. N Engl J Med 2003;348(11):994-1004.

How are responses to therapy evaluated and treatment monitored in patients with chronic myelogenous leukemia (CML)?

Key concept	The goal of therapy is to achieve disappearance of the Ph+ clone within at least 1 year and with a minimum of adverse events. Responses are classified into hematological (complete hematological response [CHR]), cytogenetic (complete [CCyR], partial, and minor), and molecular (major molecular response [MMR] and complete molecular response [CMR]).
Clinical scenario	A 72-year-old man presents to the emergency room. He has a white blood cell (WBC) count of 400,000 and hemoglobin of 7.7. Bone marrow biopsy confirms the presence of a Philadelphia chromosome. He is started on imatinib (Gleevec, a BCR-ABL1 tyrosine kinase inhibitor). At 1 month of treatment, he still has a very high WBC count and a BCR-ABL1 PCR of 50% (IS, international scale). It is found that he is not been compliant with treatment. After counseling, he becomes compliant and he achieves a complete hematological response within the next month. He is advised to continue treatment and to return for periodic monitoring of his response.
Action items	Evaluate patient's response using the following criteria (2013 European Leukemia Net Guidelines)[1]: • **Optimal response at 3 months:** BCR/ABL1IS $\leq$10% and/or Ph+ $\leq$35% (PCyR) • **Failure at 3 months:** No CHR and/or Ph+ >95% • **Optimal response at 6 months:** BCR/ABL1IS $\leq$1% and/or Ph+ 0% (CCyR) • **Failure at 6 months:** BCR/ABL1IS >10% and/or Ph >35% • **Optimal response at 12 months:** BCR/ABL1IS $\leq$0.1% (MMR) • **Failure at 12 months:** BCR/ABL1IS >1% and/or Ph >0% • **OPTIMAL RESPONSE AT ANY TIME:** MMR or better • **FAILURE AT ANYTIME:** Loss of CHR, loss of CCyR, or loss of MMR confirmed in two consecutive tests, one of which is >1% or mutations (clonal chromosomal abnormalities) in Ph+ cells.

Discussion	The first objective of treatment is the normalization by the third month of WBC counts to $<10 \times 10^9$/L with a normal differential, platelet count $<450 \times 10^9$/L, and disappearance of splenomegaly and other symptoms of CML (CHR). Blood counts should be performed every week until CHR is achieved, then every 3 months or as clinically indicated. At this point, the type of cytogenetic response is evaluated. Cytogenetic responses are divided into complete (0% Ph+ cells), partial (1%–35% Ph+ cells), and minor (35%–95% Ph+ cells). Cytogenetic analysis is the only test that gives reliable information regarding the presence of additional chromosomal aberrations. A follow-up bone marrow biopsy is done at 3, 6, and 12 months after starting therapy. Alternatively, if fluorescence in situ hybridization (FISH) on peripheral blood smear is negative at 6 or 12 months, further marrow exams can be omitted. Any significant change would require a marrow examination before a considering change of therapy.[2] Molecular responses are evaluated with quantitative polymerase chain reaction (PCR; usually reverse transcriptase–PCR) in the peripheral blood or bone marrow. An MMR is characterized by an BCR-ABL1/ABL1 ratio $\leq$0.1%. A CMR is characterized by undetectable transcripts of BCR-ABL1 in an assay with a sensitivity of at least 4.5 logs. BCR-ABL1 transcript levels of $\leq$1% are equivalent to a CCyR; levels of $\leq$10% are equivalent to a partial cytogenetic response. Molecular positivity above an MMR is not an indication of therapy failure. A single elevation in transcript levels should be confirmed 1–3 months later. Compliance with therapy should always be revisited first. A 5- to 10-fold increase in the BCR-ABL1 transcript indicates true relapse or emergence of mutations. Failure to achieve CHR at 3 months, partial cytogenetic response at 6 months, and CCyR at 12 months are indications for ABL kinase mutation screening.
Pearls	• An increased BCR-ABL1 PCR is not an indication to change therapy • The only true indication for a change of therapy is the recurrence of a Ph+ chromosome by FISH or cytogenetic analysis
References	1. Baccarani M, Deininger MW, Rosti G, et al. European LeukemiaNet recommendations for the management of chronic myeloid leukemia: 2013. Blood 2013;122(6):872-84. 2. Kantarjian H, Cortes J. Considerations in the management of patients with Philadelphia chromosome-positive chronic myeloid leukemia receiving tyrosine kinase inhibitor therapy. J Clin Oncol 2011;29(12):1512-6.

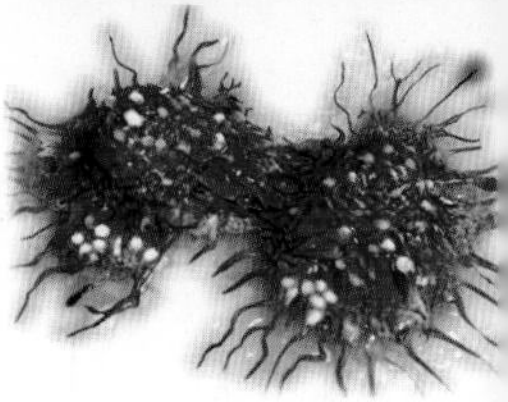

CHAPTER 14

Lymphoma

What are the differences between aggressive lymphomas and indolent lymphomas?

Key concept	One method to segregate hematological malignancies, including lymphomas, is the evolution time that the disease takes to clinically progress. Indolent lymphomas are those which evolve over years, whereas aggressive lymphomas do so over months. Indolent lymphomas are also known as low grade and aggressive lymphomas as high grade.[1]
Clinical scenario	A 65-year-old man develops enlarged cervical lymph nodes. He is completely asymptomatic. One year and a half later, he becomes anemic and develops additional enlarged lymph nodes in the axilla. An excisional biopsy is made, and he is diagnosed with follicular lymphoma, an indolent type of lymphoma.
Action item	• When facing a diagnosis of lymphoma, always obtain the grade of the tumor as estimated by the pathologist based on the Ki-67 immunohistochemistry of the disease
Discussion	The proportion of proliferating cells correlates with the immunostaining biopsy sections to determine the percentage of Ki-67 antibody–positive cells. In general, it can be said that indolent lymphomas have a Ki-67 of $\leq$30%, aggressive lymphomas between 30% and 75%, and highly aggressive lymphomas >75% Ki-67.[2] Ki-67 is a monoclonal antibody that reacts selectively with a nuclear antigen that is present only in proliferating cells in the G_1, S, and G_2 phase but is absent in the G_0 phase (resting cells).
Pearl	• Ki-67 and MIB-1 monoclonal antibodies bind different epitopes of the same proliferation-related antigen. Ki-67 and MIB-1 can be used on fixed sections.[3] MIB-1 can be used on formalin-fixed paraffin-embedded sections, after heat-mediated antigen retrieval. For this reason, it has essentially replaced Ki-67 in clinical use

References

1. Gascoyne RD, Thieblemont C, Freedman AS. Hematopathology approaches to diagnosis and prognosis of indolent B-cell lymphomas. Hematology Am Soc Hematol Educ Program 2005:299-306.
2. Ali AE, Morgen EK, Geddie WR, et al. Classifying B-cell non-Hodgkin lymphoma by using MIB-1 proliferative index in fine needle aspirates. Cancer Cytopathol 2010;118:166-72.
3. Banklfalvi A, Simon R, Brandt B, et al. Comparative methodological analysis of erbB-2/Her-2 gene dosage, chromosomal copy number and protein overexpression in breast carcinoma tissues for diagnostic use. Histopathology 2000;37:411-19.

How do I know which patients benefit from rituximab?

Key concept	B cell lymphomas represent 85% of all NHL diagnoses. B cells express a surface protein, CD20, that participates in the regulation of intracellular calcium, the cell cycle, and apoptosis. Because this protein is not shed, modulated, or internalized, it represents an ideal target for the use of monoclonal targeted therapy.[1]
Clinical scenario	A 72-year-old man was essentially asymptomatic when admitted to a hospital with severe abdominal pain. A CT of the abdomen was performed followed by a mesenteric biopsy that confirmed the diagnosis of diffuse large B cell lymphoma, germinal center subtype. His Ki-67 level was 40%. After completion of the initial staging process, the patient underwent placement of an indwelling venous catheter and initiation of systemic chemotherapy as an inpatient, given the bulkiness of his disease. He experienced a tumor lysis syndrome as a complication of his course of treatment, developing renal failure, which required temporary renal hemodialysis. After 6 courses of systemic chemotherapy combined with rituximab, he achieved complete remission.
Action items	• Always ask the pathologist to confirm expression of CD20 by immunohistochemistry in all cases of B cell lymphoma • If there is no expression of surface CD20 in the membrane of the tumor cells, there is no indication to use rituximab
Discussion	Methods of treatment of lymphoma have been until recently effective but non-specific. With the recognition that B cell lymphomas expressed cell surface proteins such as CD19, CD20, and CD22, has come the opportunity to develop monoclonal targeted antibodies against such protein that can complement the effect of more non-specific therapies. In fact, one of the most important additions to the traditional therapy of B cell lymphomas has been the incorporation of monoclonal antibody

	using rituximab. Rituximab has significantly enhanced response to therapy and overall outcomes in both indolent and aggressive lymphomas, either as initial therapy, alone when indicated or in salvage therapy.[2] Rituximab is currently approved for treatment of relapsed and refractory indolent lymphomas as single-agent therapy and as initial therapy in combination with standard chemotherapy regimens. All age groups have benefited and tolerance has been good even in the elderly patient. Given its benefits, it has opened the door for the development of other targeted therapies.
Pearl	• Administer a dose of 12.5 mg of meperidine as premedication 20 minutes prior to rituximab administration and prevent >95% of rituximab infusion reactions
References	1. Tedder TF, Engel P. CD20: a regulator of cell-cycle progression of B lymphocytes. Immunol Today 1994;15(9):450-4. 2. Hiddemann W, Kneba M, Dreyling M, et al. Frontline therapy with rituximab added to the combination of cyclophosphamide, doxorubicin, vincristine, and prednisone (CHOP) significantly improves the outcome for patients with advanced-stage follicular lymphoma compared with therapy with CHOP alone: results of a prospective randomized study of the German Low-Grade Lymphoma Study Group. Blood 2005;106(12):3725-32.

Why is it necessary to check a hepatitis panel in patients before they receive rituximab?

Key concept	Administration of rituximab to patients with active hepatitis B carries the risk of hepatitis B reactivation.
Clinical scenario	A 24-year-old patient who is HIV- and hepatitis B surface Ag–positive is going to be treated with CHOP-R for HIV-associated diffuse large B cell lymphoma. The decision is made to hold rituximab during the first course until a consultation with a hepatologist is made.
Action item	• Always check an acute hepatitis panel and consult a hepatologist if a patient is hepatitis B surface Ag positive prior to initiation of therapy with rituximab
Discussion	When patients with active hepatitis B infection are treated with rituximab, there is a clear risk of inducing hepatitis B reactivation with fulminant hepatitis, hepatic failure, and death.[1] Consultation with a hepatologist and administration of antiviral therapy should be considered if hepatitis B antigen is detectable. It is not clear why this happens, as the plasma cells which produce hepatitis B antibodies do not express CD20. For patients with hepatitis C infection, the risk has not been well defined.
Pearl	• The phenomenon of hepatitis B reactivation is not unique to rituximab: it is also observed with other types of CD20 antibodies, such as obinutuzumab and ofatumumab

References

1. Dotan E, Aggarwal C, Smith MR. Impact of rituximab (Rituxan) on the treatment of B-cell non Hodgkin lymphoma. PT 2010;35:148-57.

How many types of lymphomas are there?

Key concept	There are two types of lymphomas: B and T cell lymphomas. Hodgkin disease is a modified B cell lymphoma that does not express a B cell receptor as part of the malignant process; it thus has a definite clinical pattern and is accepted as a different category, although it strictly is a B cell lymphoma.[1]
Action item	• Always request the full profile of CDs of the tumor cells, as this may identify potential therapeutic targets
Discussion	In the hematopoietic system, there are two type of cells of lymphoid lineage origin: B cells and T cells, characterized by their specific receptor. Lymphomas are tumors of the lymphoid lineage cells. Their B or T cell origin is determined by using flow cytometry and immunohistochemistry, which allows the determination of specific surface proteins (clusters of differentiation), and therefore proper identification of the lineage.
Pearl	• In addition to identification of the type of lymphoma, the cell surface membrane protein profile can identify therapeutic targets, of which CD20 Is a prime example

References	
	1. National Comprehensive Cancer Network guidelines for lymphoma. Version 7.2017. Available at: www.nccn.org.

What are B-symptoms?

Key concept	More clinically advanced and aggressive lymphomas tend to have systemic manifestations of the disease. These manifestations include fever, night sweats, and weight loss (>10% of basal weight) and are known as "B-symptoms." Their absence is denoted by the letter A. The presence or absence of B-symptoms has prognostic significance and is reflected in the staging of these lymphomas.
Clinical scenario	A 21-year-old man is being worked up for a diagnosis of Hodgkin disease. He states that he has lost 10% of his basal body weight and that he has intermittent night sweats. The doctor tells him that he has B-symptoms.
Action item	• Always inquire for the presence of fevers, night sweats, or >10% loss of basal body weight
Discussion	The presence of B-symptoms correlates with advanced systemic disease rather than local involvement. B-symptoms are a negative prognostic factor in Hodgkin lymphoma.[1] In non-Hodgkin lymphoma, B-symptoms correlate with more widespread disease or a higher histologic grade.[2] It has been suggested that, in Hodgkin lymphoma, fever and weight loss are much more prognostically significant than night sweats. B-symptoms include: • Fever >38°C (Pel-Ebstein fever, the classic intermittent fever associated with Hodgkin disease, occurs at variable intervals of days to weeks and lasts for 1–2 weeks before resolving. However, fever associated with lymphoma can follow virtually any pattern.) • Drenching sweats, especially at night • Unintentional weight loss of >10% of normal body weight over a period of ≤6 months

	B-symptoms are so called because Ann Arbor staging of lymphomas includes both a number (I–IV) and a letter (A or B).[1] "A" indicates the absence of systemic symptoms, whereas "B" indicates their presence. The significance of A-status in non-Hodgkin lymphoma is less clear, although B-symptoms tend to correlate with disease that is either more widespread or of a higher histologic grade.[3] It has been suggested that in Hodgkin lymphoma, fever and weight loss are much more prognostically significant than night sweats. In one series of patients with early stage Hodgkin disease, the presence or absence of night sweats had no impact on cure rates and outcome. However, fever and weight loss had a pronounced negative impact on cure and survival rates, regardless of treatment modality.
References	1. Gobbi PG, Cavalli C, Gendarini A, et al. Reevaluation of prognostic significance of symptoms in Hodgkin disease. Cancer 1985; 56:2874-80. 2. Anderson T, Chabner BA, Young RC, et al. Malignant lymphoma: the histology and staging of 473 patients at the National Cancer Institute. Cancer 1982;50(12):2699-707. 3. Carbone PP, Kaplan HS, Musshoff K, et al. Report of the Committee on Hodgkin's Disease Staging Classification. Cancer Res 1971;31(11):1860-1.

Does the Ann Arbor staging system apply to both Hodgkin and non-Hodgkin lymphoma?

Key concept	In both non-Hodgkin and Hodgkin disease, the extent of disease at diagnosis is the most important single guide to prognosis and treatment.
Clinical scenario	A 22-year-old man develops palpable bilateral cervical lymph nodes. A biopsy reveals classical Hodgkin disease. He has had evening fevers for ~3 weeks. He asks what other tests are necessary before starting treatment.
Action items	Criteria for TNM clinical staging: • Physical examination and history • Urinalysis • Chest X-ray • Blood chemistries • Bone marrow biopsy • PET-CT scan Criteria for TNM pathologic staging: • All of the clinical studies above, plus • Biopsy of accessible extranodal primary site(s) Staging laparotomy (including splenectomy, wedge liver biopsy, and multiple lymph node biopsies) is not required but may be used for additional staging information if indicated. Otherwise, liver biopsy or other biopsies may be performed to determine distant metastases.

Discussion	In July 1971, the traditional staging for Hodgkin lymphoma was initially presented at the Ann Arbor Symposium on Staging of Hodgkin Lymphoma. Under the Ann Arbor System, clinical staging includes all the non-invasive procedures. Pathologic staging is based on findings made as a result of laparotomy or mediastinotomy.[1] Staging accomplishes two important objectives in the management of lymphomas: prognosis and therapeutic guidance, and it facilitates communication among treating physicians. In 1988, revisions to the Ann Arbor staging system were made.[2] The main changes include: • Allowed use of CT scanning to assess disease involvement below the diaphragm • For stage II disease, the number of anatomic nodal sites is indicated by a subscript (eg, stage II_3) • For stage III disease, upper and lower abdominal involvement are subdivided as stage III_1 and III_2, respectively • Bulky disease is denoted by X, defined as >one-third widening of the mediastinum at the T5–6 level or >10 cm maximum dimension of the nodal mass • Unconfirmed/uncertain complete remission (CRu) denotes the presence of residual imaging abnormality but the absence of pathologically confirmed residual disease
Pearls	• If a PET CT scan at the end of treatment is positive in a patient with Hodgkin disease and there are no other symptoms, this usually indicates the presence of residual disease • If there are symptoms, this usually indicates something other than residual Hodgkin disease • The definition of empirically "bulky" disease has been reduced from 7-cm maximum dimension of the nodal mass to 5 cm
References	1. Carbone PP, Kaplan HS, Mushoff K, et al. Report of the Committee on Hodgkin's Disease staging classification. Cancer Res 1971; 31:1860-1. 2. Lister TA, Crowther D, Sutcliffe SB, et al. Report of a committee convened to discuss the evaluation and staging of patients with Hodgkin's disease: Cotswolds Meeting. J Clin Oncol 1989;7:1630-6.

I have a patient with HIV/AIDS and a new lymphoma diagnosis: what type could it be?

Key concept	Just as in primary immunodeficiency, where there is an increased incidence of malignancies associated with a lack of surveillance of the immune system, in HIV the same happens as a direct effect of the pathogenesis of HIV infection.[1]
Clinical scenario	A 34-year-old man with a diagnosis of multiple substance abuse and untreated HIV disease presents with a 4 × 5 cm (major diameter) mass in the superior gingival region above the right canine tooth. A PET/CT scan is highly positive only in that area. A biopsy confirms the diagnosis of a plasmablastic diffuse large B cell lymphoma involving the superior right maxillary gingiva. After proper staging of his lymphoma and HIV disease, the patient starts on highly active anti-retroviral therapy (HAART), prophylaxis for opportunistic infections, and systemic chemotherapy with rituximab-DA-EPOCH.
Action items	• Always make sure patient is treated with the appropriate HAART regimen • Always make sure to screen for viral hepatitis and take appropriate measures based on results • Always make sure the appropriate prophylactic regimen to prevent opportunistic infections is started • Always make sure that STDs and other potential comorbid conditions are treated
Discussion	HIV infection is characterized by a rapid destruction of memory cells of the gut-associated lymphoid tissue (GALT). Once HIV is integrated into the genome of susceptible cells, there is a gradual destruction of the immune system. This early senescence of the immune system is implicated in changes at a molecular level resulting in loss of control of oncogenic viruses and associated with the malignant transformations observed in AIDS. The development of non-Hodgkin lymphomas (NHLs) in HIV patients is similar to that of malignancies associated with other congenital or post-transplant immunodeficiency disorders.[2] Under such conditions, most of these malignancies consist of NHL and Kaposi sarcoma (KS). In the case of HIV, immunodeficiency and cofactors including oncogenic

	viruses, chronic antigenic stimulation, and cytokine overproduction are responsible for the development of AIDS-related NHL malignancies. In contrast to AIDS-associated KS, no one has yet found HIV sequences in tumor cells of AIDS-related NHLs, although PCR analysis has revealed the presence of HIV in infiltrating T cells. For patients with severe HIV immunodeficiency, the oncogenic nature of both Epstein–Barr virus (EBV) and human herpesvirus–8 (HHV-8) is responsible for the development of the immunoblastic subtype of diffuse large B cell lymphoma, primary central nervous system (PCNS) lymphoma, plasmablastic lymphoma of the oral cavity, and primary effusion lymphoma. The last of these often results from coinfection with HHV-8 and EBV. These lymphomas are the result of active oncogenic viruses released from control by an effective immune surveillance.
Pearls	• If a brain biopsy cannot be performed in an HIV patient suspected of having a PCNS lymphoma, a negative toxoplasmosis serology, the presence of EBV DNA by PCR in the cerebral spinal fluid and a positive single-photon emission CT–thallium scan of the brain have high specificity for diagnosis of PCNS lymphoma • In HIV patients receiving prophylaxis, the best prevention for *Pneumocystis jirovecii* is either daily dapsone or atovaquone, as they do not further suppress the bone marrow
References	1. Rios A, Hagemeister FB. Acquired immunodeficiency syndrome–related cancer. In: *MDACC Manual of Oncology*. 3rd ed. Columbus, OH: McGraw-Hill Education; 2016;933. 2. Vajdic CM, van Leeuwen MT. What types of cancers are associated with immune suppression in HIV? Lessons from solid organ transplant recipients. Curr Opin HIV/AIDS 2009;1:35-41.

Is a bone marrow evaluation required for all lymphoma patients?

Key concept	A bone marrow biopsy with aspirate is essential in all lymphoma patients who are to receive treatment.
Clinical scenario	A 52-year-old woman was found to have an elevated white blood cell count during her routine health examination. A flow cytometry was done and confirmed the diagnosis of small lymphocytic lymphoma (SLL)/chronic lymphocytic leukemia (CLL). She is started on treatment. No bone marrow aspiration and biopsy is done, as all the clinical and laboratory information required for initiation of treatment is available.
Action item	• Unless the patient has SLL/CLL, always order a bone marrow aspiration and biopsy for immunohistochemistry, flow cytometry, cytogenetic analysis, and a molecular lymphoma panel
Discussion	The bone marrow evaluation has two objectives in the management and treatment of patients with lymphoma: • as part of the staging of the disease • to aid in planning the patient's therapy, including the need for vigorous central nervous system prophylaxis, particularly in intermediate or high-grade lymphomas with bone marrow involvement In general, bone marrow involvement occurs in 39% of low-grade, 36% of intermediate-grade, and 18% of high-grade lymphomas. The only exceptions to this rule are patients with SLL/CLL, whose disease can be diagnosed by flow cytometry alone, and patients with indolent lymphomas, in whom the decision for observation is made on a clinical basis, as it would not change therapy.[1,2]
Pearl	• Bilateral core marrows are indicated in the cases where radioimmunotherapy is considered

References

1. Lister TA, Crowther D, Sutcliffe SB, et al. Report of a committee convened to discuss the evaluation and staging of patients with Hodgkin's disease: Cotswolds Meeting. J Clin Oncol 1989;7:1630-6.
2. Conlan MG, Bast M, Armitage JO, et al. Bone marrow involvement by non-Hodgkin's lymphoma: the clinical significance of morphologic discordance between the lymph node and bone marrow. Nebraska Lymphoma Study Group. J Clin Oncol 1990;8(7):1163-72.

If my patient has central nervous system (CNS) lymphoma, will intravenous R-CHOP treat it?

Key concept	CNS lymphoma may refer to primary CNS lymphoma or secondary CNS lymphoma metastasis from a systemic lymphoma. In either case, the blood-brain barrier is a formidable obstacle to must drugs, and the levels achieved by using systemic therapy of lymphoma are not sufficient to become therapeutically efficacious.[1]
Clinical scenario	A 48-year-old right-handed woman experiences gradual onset of weakness in her right upper and lower extremities. Her husband noted that at breakfast the patient felt well but by the end of the meal, she was unable to move her right upper and lower extremities. He also noted that her speech was slightly slow and slurred. The patient's family called the neurosurgery clinic and was brought immediately to the emergency room. The patient denied changes in vision, nausea, vomiting, headache, or sensory changes. A stereotactic biopsy confirmed the diagnosis of diffuse large B cell (DLBC) lymphoma PCNS. She was started on high-dose methotrexate with rituximab and dexamethasone and had a dramatic improvement in her condition.
Action items	• Order an acute hepatitis panel (patient will receive a higher than average dose of rituximab) • Order HIV test • In view of the new observations with checkpoint immune inhibitors, order gene sequencing
Discussion	PCNS lymphomas represent 1%–2% of all brain tumors. Approximately 95% of PCNL tumors are CD20+ and DLBCL, with T cell tumors being less common. They occur in immunocompetent and immunodeficient patients, especially following organ transplantation, and in advanced HIV disease, usually when the patient reaches <100 CD4+ cells/dL.[1] Clinically, these patients present with raised intracranial pressure, stroke, or encephalopathy. Given the fact that rituximab has significant therapeutic impact in patients with DLBC lymphoma, and considering that there is an associated disruption of the blood-brain barrier in newly diagnosed PCNSL, rituximab has been incorporated

	into the therapeutic platform of high-dose methotrexate and radiotherapy.[2] In immunocompetent patients, the dose of high-dose methotrexate can be as high as 8 g/m^2 and in immunocompromised patients, between 3 and 4 g/m^2. In both situations, the rituximab is given at a dose of 500 mg/m^2; patients usually receive four courses of treatment before considering the use of brain radiotherapy in the most appropriate modality for the patient's specific condition. More recently, it has been found that PCNS lymphoma has unique differences from systemic DLBCL, including a high frequency of 9p24 copy gain and increased PD1 ligand expression, as well as a chromosomal translocation resulting in PD-L1/PD-L2 deregulation. Based on these findings, five patients with PCNS lymphoma have been treated with checkpoint immune inhibitors with spectacular outcomes.[3] It is possible that this therapeutic modality will be the backbone of the future standard of care for this disease.
Pearls	• The standard for imaging diagnosis of cerebral masses is MRI with and without contrast • In immunocompromised patients, the most frequent cause of cerebral masses is cerebral toxoplasmosis
References	1. Rubenstein JL, Gupta NK, Mannis GN, et al. How I treat CNS lymphomas. Blood 2013;122:2318-30. 2. Chamberlain MC, Johnston SK. High-dose methotrexate and rituximab with deferred radiotherapy for newly diagnosed primary B-cell CNS lymphoma. Neuro-Oncol 2010; 12:736-44. 3. Beth C. Checkpoint inhibition in CNS lymphoma. Inside Blood Commentary 2017;129:3046.

If a lymphoma is causing cord compression, do I refer for surgery, radiation, or chemotherapy?

Key concept	Malignant spinal cord compression is secondary to metastasis of the malignant tumor to the spine with erosion of the epidural space and compression of the spinal cord. Regardless of its cause, it must be treated immediately.[1]
Clinical scenario	A 63-year-old man was about to start treatment for the relapse of a high-grade non-Hodgkin lymphoma. He experienced an acute worsening of his pain over the prior 48–72 hours. A MRI of the spine showed a paravertebral right lesion. He was treated with chemoradiation, with excellent recovery of neurological function after a short program of physical therapy.
Action items	• Start dexamethasone as soon as there is a clinical suspicion of cord compression • Order a whole-spine MRI with contrast if kidneys function allows it • Always consult a neurosurgeon, although the main treatment usually is chemotherapy and radiotherapy either concurrently or sequentially administered
Discussion	In addition to the erosion of the epidural space, in 15% of the cases a paravertebral lesion enters the spinal canal through a intervertebral foramen (neuroblastomas or lymphomas). In less-frequent cases, there is actual destruction of bone, with vertebral body collapse and fragments of bone compressing the cord. The two consequences are demyelination and vascular damage. Of these two, vascular damage is the most deleterious. The most common presentation is back pain (>90%) in the setting of an established diagnosis of a lymphoma. In 10%–15% of cases, the cord compression will be the initial presentation of the disease. The pain can have different patterns associated with the lesion's anatomic location. MRI of the whole spine is the standard for diagnosis, followed by CT myelography, as there are often multiple lesions.[1] Plain films are not helpful at all. Anti-inflammatory

	steroids should be started immediately and, in the case of lymphomas, these do have a therapeutic benefit. There is no evidence that high-dose steroids are of any increased therapeutic benefit. A typical dose schedule is 10–16 mg of dexamethasone IV bolus followed by 4–6 mg every 4 hours with taper once specific treatment is initiated. In the case of lymphomas, due to their sensitivity to chemotherapy and radiotherapy, these two modalities concurrently and or sequentially are preferred. Surgery can be used in unusual cases where the diagnosis is uncertain or there is spine instability.[2]
Pearl	• Patients who only have back pain and a normal neurological examination can have imaging completed in 48–72 hours
References	1. Behl D, Hendrickson WA, Moynihan TJ. Oncologic emergencies. Crit Care Clin 2010;26:181-205. 2. Grimm S, Chamberlain M. Hodgkin's lymphoma: a review of neurological complications. Adv Hematol 2011;2011:624578.

What type of biopsy is needed to diagnose a nodal lymphoma?

Key concept	In managing and treating lymphomas, the most important step is an accurate pathologic diagnosis.[1]
Clinical scenario	A 45-year-old man presents with large retroperitoneal mass and bilateral axillary nodes. He tells his physician that if a biopsy needs to be done, he prefers to undergo excision of one of the axillary lymph nodes. His physician agrees.
Action item	• Always review the physical findings and imaging studies before deciding how to approach the histological diagnosis
Discussion	The correct pathological of a lymphoma is a complex histological and molecular biology evaluation which by necessity requires sufficient tissue for it to be properly performed. For this reason, core biopsies and fine-needle aspiration are not ideal, even though they are popular due to availability of the techniques. Whenever possible, an incisional or excisional biopsy is recommended to firmly establish the diagnosis of a lymphoma.[1] Immunophenotypic analysis is required for a complete diagnosis; although in most institutions this is done by immunohistochemistry, ideally it can be done at the time of biopsy at institutions were flow cytometry is readily available.
Pearl	• When reviewing the flow cytometry of a sample, B cell CDs (clusters of differentiation) have two digits (eg, CD19, CD22, and CD20), and T cell CDs have one (eg, CD3, CD4, CD5, CD7, and CD8).

References

1. Dunphy CH. Applications of flow cytometry and immunohistochemistry to diagnostic hematopathology. Arch Pathol Lab Med 2004;128:1004-22.

Lymphomas associated with infection: mucosa-associated lymphoid tissue (MALT) lymphomas

Key concept	Chronic stimulation of lymphocytes can cause certain types of lymphomas. Specifically, chronic stimulation by infectious pathogens or inflammation is part of the etiology of marginal zone lymphomas (MZLs). MZLs originate from lymphocytes of the marginal zone of lymphoid follicles from the spleen, lymph nodes, and mucosal lymphoid tissues (MALT lymphomas).[1]
Clinical scenario	An 83-year-old woman was diagnosed with a stage II Lugano classification MALT lymphoma of the stomach (involvement of the mucosa and eroding into the lamina propria). The tumor was *Helicobacter pylori* negative and had a t(11;18) translocation. After a complete staging, she received involved-field radiation therapy (IFRT), which in Lugano stages I/II disease is associated with an overall response rate of >90% and a complete remission (CR) rate of 99% with a failure-free survival rate of 100%. She remains in complete remission 3 years after treatment.
Action items	• In stomach MALT, always test for *H. pylori* and test molecular markers in search of t(11;18). translocation • In splenic MZL, always test for hepatitis C • Stage the patient based on the Lugano classification
Discussion	Marginal zone lymphocytes are specialized in antigen recognition; hence their strategic position in the follicles of the spleen, mucosal tissue, and lymph nodes. There are three subtypes of MZL: MALT lymphomas (gastric and non-gastric), nodal MZL, and splenic MZL. In 50% of cases, MALT lymphomas are in the GI tract, and 80% of the GI tract MALT lymphomas are located in the stomach. In order of frequency, non-gastric MALT lymphomas occur in the lung, the eyes (conjunctiva and surrounding

	mucosa), and skin. Nodal MZL behaves like other nodal lymphomas. It is commonly associated with autoimmune disorders such as Sjögren syndrome. Splenic MZL is characterized by splenomegaly and pancytopenia. Splenic hilar lymph nodes are often involved, with sparing of peripheral lymph nodes.[2] Chronic infection with *H. pylori* has been associated with gastric MALT lymphoma, *Chlamydia psittaci* with ocular MZL, and hepatitis C with splenic MALT lymphoma in 30% of cases and ~35% of non-gastric MALT lymphomas. When associated with t(11;18) and t(1;14) translocation, MALT lymphomas are usually less likely to respond to *H. pylori* eradication with antibiotic therapy.[3] For these types of lymphoma, IFRT can induce >90% CRs. For splenic MZL, treatment of hepatitis C for those with the infection is indicated, and rituximab or splenectomy for those not infected with hepatitis C. Finally, nodal MZLs are treated with the same strategy used to treat follicular lymphomas.
Pearl	• The MYD88 L265P somatic mutation widely prevalent in patients with Waldenstrom macroglobulinemia (lymphoplasmacytic lymphoma) can be used to differentiate it from MZL
References	1. Kahl B, Yang D. Marginal zone lymphomas: management of nodal, splenic, and MALT NHL. Hematology Am Soc Hematol Educ Program 2008;2008:359-64. 2. Isaacson PG, Chott A, Nakamura S, et al. Extranodal marginal zone lymphoma of mucosa associated lymphoid tissue (MALT lymphoma). In: Swerdlow SH, Campo E, Harris NL, et al., eds. *WHO Classification of Tumours of Haematopoietic and Lymphoid Tissues.* 4th ed. Lyon: IARC; 2008:185-7. 3. Auer IA, Gascoyne RD, Connors JM, et al. t(11;18)(q21:q21) is the most common translocation in MALT lymphomas. Ann Oncol 1997; 8:979-85.

A patient with an indolent lymphoma now has B-symptoms and increased lactate dehydrogenase (LDH): do I need to re-biopsy?

Key concept	Histological transformation (HT) is a frequent event in patients with indolent lymphomas.
Clinical scenario	A 67-year-old man with a history of indolent follicular lymphoma was under observation for 2 years when a surveillance PET CT scan showed a new focal FDG uptake in the right oropharynx and the retroperitoneal area. A right tonsillectomy confirmed a diagnosis of HT to diffuse large B cell lymphoma (DLBCL). After completion of a staging work-up, he received therapy with CHOP-R, completing 6 courses of treatment. He is 6 months post completion of therapy and in complete remission.
Action items	• In patients in whom an HT is suspected, a complete restaging should be immediately initiated • The best areas for re-biopsy are those of increased metabolic uptake with discordant growth
Discussion	The incidence of histological transformation varies among different series. In general, the most frequent type of indolent lymphoma is follicular lymphoma. It has also been described in small lymphocytic/chronic lymphocytic leukemia (SLL/CLL), lymphoplasmacytic lymphoma (LPL), and marginal zone lymphoma (MZL), among others. Usually the transformation is to an aggressive, higher grade DLBC. The criteria for consideration of a case of HT are: rapid discordant lymphadenopathy growth, unusual sites of extra-nodal involvement, a sudden increase in LDH, hypercalcemia, or the presence of new B-symptoms.[2] In general, patients who are naïve to chemotherapy have good outcomes with R-CHOP. Patients who present with HT after receiving ≥1 lines of chemotherapy should receive standard salvage chemotherapy followed by stem cell transplantation.[3]
Pearl	• Always administer intrathecal therapy in patients with HT, regardless of the stage and size of the HT at presentation

References

1. Bernstein SH, Burack WR. The incidence, natural history, biology, and treatment of transformed lymphomas. Hematology Am Soc Hematol Educ Program 2009:532-41.
2. Al-Tourah AJ, Gill KK, Chhanabhai M, et al. Population-based analysis of incidence and outcome of transformed non-Hodgkin's lymphoma. J Clin Oncol 2008:26(32):5165-9.
3. Montoto S. Treatment of patients with transformed lymphoma. Hematology Am Soc Hematol Educ Program 2015: 625-30.

Why are checkpoint immune inhibitors used mainly for Hodgkin lymphoma and not non-Hodgkin lymphomas?

Key concept	Tumors that have a genetic dependency on the PD1 pathway for survival are more susceptible to the therapeutic targeting of this pathway. The Reed-Sternberg (RS) cells found in Hodgkin lymphoma have a genetically determined overexpression of PD1 ligands on their surface, making them a suitable target for checkpoint immune inhibitors.
Clinical scenario	A 24-year-old man has a history of recurrent fevers up to 101°F associated with severe night sweats, fatigue, and a dry cough. A PET-CT scan shows extensive lymphadenopathy in the mediastinum, supraclavicular, and cervical regions. He had previous exposure to substandard doses of ABVD (11 weekly doses in addition to other natural remedies in an alternative therapy clinic). His disease continued to progress with compression of the brachial plexus. A supraclavicular lymph node biopsy shows the presence of nodular sclerosis–type classical Hodgkin lymphoma. After a restaging of his disease, he is started on a combination of nivolumab-brentuximab, achieving a complete remission in 2 months, followed by a successful autologous hematopoietic stem cell transplant at 6 months after initiating this new combination treatment.
Action item	• Obtain baseline thyroid function, adrenal function as measured by free serum cortisol, and a good clinical neurological evaluation prior to initiation of therapy with checkpoint inhibitors
Discussion	It is known that RS cells have an amplification of 9p24.1, which leads to induction of PD1 ligand transcription. This copy-number–dependent mechanism causes the overexpression of PD1 ligands on the surface of RS cells. In addition, infection of RS cells by Epstein–Barr virus is a co-factor that contributes to additional overexpression of PD-L1. As a result of these two mechanisms, there is increased RS surface expression of PD-L1. In initial translational studies, the targeting of this pathway led to overall responses of 87% that were durable. In contrast, responses observed in non-Hodgkin

	lymphoma were only ≤10%. More recently, in the salvage setting it has been shown that there is synergy between brentuximab and checkpoint immune inhibitors, making this combination extremely attractive to use in relapsed Hodgkin lymphoma.
Pearl	• It is not necessary to confirm PD-L1 overexpression to initiate salvage therapy with checkpoint inhibitors in Hodgkin lymphoma
References	1. Armand P. Immune checkpoint blockade in hematological malignancies. Blood 2015;125(22):3393-400. 2. Herrera AF, Moskowitz AJ, Bartlett NL, et al. Interim results of brentuximab vedotin in combination with nivolumab in patients with relapsed or refractory Hodgkin lymphoma. Blood 2018;131(11):1183-94.

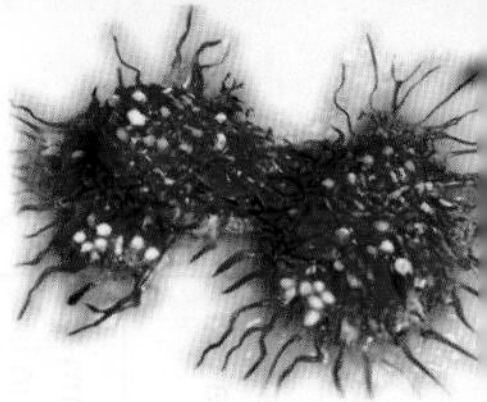

CHAPTER 15

Plasma Cell Disorders

What tests do I order if I have a patient with high total protein levels in serum and normal or low albumin levels?

Key concept	The cardinal feature of plasma cell disorders is the abnormal increased production of monoclonal antibodies. Thus, abnormal elevation of serum proteins should always raise suspicion of a plasma cell neoplasia.
Clinical scenario	A 65-year-old woman presents with a history of anemia of recent onset. A complete physical examination is unrevealing. Complete blood chemistry shows an elevated total protein. Serum albumin is normal. Serum electrophoresis is ordered.
Action item	• Order a serum electrophoresis, a serum immune-electrophoresis, and a urine spot for Bence-Jones protein
Discussion	Multiple myeloma (MM) is a malignant neoplasm of plasma cells that accounts for 1.8% of all cancers and ~17% of all hematological malignancies in the United States. It is most frequently diagnosed among people aged 65–74 years, with the median age being 69 years. The American Cancer Society has estimated close to 30,000 cases of myeloma newly diagnosed in 2017. The approximate death rate is 12,000 deaths per year.[1] For a patient to be diagnosed with MM, they must have not only a plasma cell disorder but also end-organ damage attributable to the plasma cell disorder. This includes at least one of the CRAB criteria (hyper-**C**alcemia, **R**enal disease, **A**nemia, and **B**one disease) classically used to define symptomatic MM. Anemia occurs in 73% of patients. Bone pain is common (60% of patients), and 50% of patients have an elevated serum creatinine. Renal disease results from light precipitated complexes obstructing the distal convoluted tubules. Other causes of renal disease include nephrocalcinosis, amyloidosis, heavy-chain disease, and light-chain disease. Hypercalcemia >11 mg/dL is present in 10% of patients. This requires hydration with isotonic saline and bisphosphonate therapy with zoledronic acid or pamidronate in moderate or severe cases. Calcitonin can also be used to rapidly reduce serum calcium levels. Other symptoms include fatigue (32%) and

	weight loss (20%). Because of immune dysfunction, patients are at risk for infections. About 7%–18% of patients may present with extramedullary plasmacytomas. Less common symptoms include fever, splenomegaly, hepatomegaly, and lymphadenopathy.
Pearl	• If there is elevated serum protein, the critical differentiation to be made is whether the elevation is associated with a monoclonal gammopathy or is a nonspecific elevation of the gamma region associated with a chronic inflammatory process
References	1. Kyle Ra, Gertz MA, Witzig TE, et al. Review of 1027 patients with newly diagnosed multiple myeloma. Mayo Clin Proc 2003;78:21-33.

What is the difference between monoclonal gammopathy of undetermined significance (MGUS) and multiple myeloma (MM)?

Key concept	MM is always preceded by a gammopathy of either undetermined significance or a state of evident progression and transformation to a myelomatous state without end organ damage, or what is known as "smoldering MM." Only when there is end organ damage (anemia, kidney damage, hypercalcemia, or bone lesions) attributable to the proliferating plasma cells with its correspondent monoclonal gammopathy can this clinical condition be definitively diagnosed as a case of MM.
Clinical scenario	A 62-year-old man has been followed up for MGUS for 5 years. During previous evaluations, there has been no evidence of end organ damage and <10% monoclonal plasma cells in the bone marrow aspiration and biopsy. This time, the plasma cells are 20%, and a complete work-up including a bone MRI of the skeleton reveals no evidence of end organ damage. His doctor informs him that he will continue to be monitored and that he has now the diagnosis of smoldering MM.
Action items	• Evaluation work-up in a patient with a monoclonal gammopathy to determine absence of end organ damage includes (in addition to specific tests related to the monoclonal gammopathy itself): • Complete blood count (anemia) • Comprehensive metabolic panel with serum creatinine and blood urea nitrogen (kidney damage) • Serum calcium (hypercalcemia) • Bone marrow survey by MRI (radiographic evidence of bone lesions)[1]
Discussion	Plasma cell neoplasias start as a monoclonal process that progress from MGUS to smoldering MM to MM. This clonal evolution, which occurs over the course of years, depends on interactions of the tumor cells with the bone marrow microenvironment. When it causes end organ damage, the disease ceases to be MGUS and/or smoldering MM and becomes multiple myeloma.[2]

Pearl	• The best imaging technique for early detection of bone lesions is MRI, which does not require contrast media
References	1. Rajkumar SV, Dimopoulos MA, Palumbo A, et al. International Myeloma Working Group updated criteria for the diagnosis of multiple myeloma. Lancet Oncol 2014;15(12):e538-48. 2. Ghobrial IM, Landgren O. How I treat smoldering multiple myeloma. Blood 2014;124 (23):3380-8.

Can multiple myeloma present as a solid mass?

Key concept	A mass can be part of multiple plasma cell lesions and thus not multiple myeloma. However, when clonal proliferation of plasma cells occurs as a single solitary mass, it is not called multiple myeloma but plasmacytoma.[1]
Clinical scenario	A 57-year-old woman develops neurological symptoms compatible with cord compression. An MRI of the spine shows a solitary mass at the level of T-7. She undergoes successful surgical decompression. The histopathologic diagnosis of the mass is plasmacytoma. Her surgery is followed by local radiotherapy and placement on a surveillance program for a plasma cell disorder.
Action items	The following tests are to be done prior to the definitive treatment of a solitary plasmacytoma if the mass is not causing an acute emergency at presentation: • Serum complete blood count • Electrophoresis for β_2 microglobulin • Serum creatinine • Serum lactate dehydrogenase • Complete metabolic profile • Serum free light chains • Serum immunoelectrophoresis • Pro-BNP 24-hour protein excretion with urine electro- and immunoelectrophoresis • Bone marrow aspiration and biopsy • Complete MRI bone survey

Discussion	Malignant proliferation of plasma cells can present as a solitary mass known as a plasmacytoma. The mass can be located in bone, in which case it is called an osseous plasmacytoma. If situated at a site other than bone, solitary plasmacytomas are classified as extraosseous. Once a clinical diagnosis of plasmacytoma is made, the patient should undergo the same complete work-up as a patient with suspected multiple myeloma, to ensure that it is a solitary lesion. Both osseous and extraosseous solitary plasmacytomas are treated the same. Options include radiotherapy, chemotherapy, surgery, and combinations thereof. In general, patients who receive localized radiotherapy have a lower rate of local relapse.[2]
Pearls	• In plasmacytomas where the paraprotein associated to it disappears with treatment, the prognosis is good • If paraprotein persists, it can do so for years, and patients must be closely followed as if they have monoclonal gammopathy of undetermined significance
References	1. Soutar R, Lucraft H, Jackson G, et al. Guidelines on the diagnosis and management of solitary plasmacytoma of bone and solitary extramedullary plasmacytoma. United Kingdom Myeloma Forum. Br J Hematol 2004;124:717-26. 2. Knowling MA, Harwood AR, Bergsagel DE. Comparison of extramedullary plasmacytoma with solitary and multiple plasma tumors of bone. J Clin Oncol 1983;1:255-62.

How do I monitor a patient receiving treatment for multiple myeloma (MM)?

Key concept	The therapeutic objective in MM is the complete disappearance of the malignant plasma cells of the bone marrow and of the systemic effects of monoclonal gammopathy, optimally with restoration of the end-organ damaged functions to the closest to baseline prior to diagnosis.[1]
Clinical scenario	A 70-year-old man developed an M spike and elevated κ light-chain by serum protein electrophoresis. He presented with weakness, weight loss of >10% of basal weight, and constipation with hypercalcemia. A bone scan showed an acute osteoblastic lesion in right 5th and 8th ribs representing healing fractures. There were acute osteoblastic changes in L3 and L4. A staging work-up bone marrow aspiration showed plasma cell dyscrasia (with immature morphology) of 66%, κ light chain restricted, consistent with plasma cell myeloma, and CD138-positive plasma cells approaching 80% of cells with κ light chain restriction. He received local radiotherapy to the spine and was started on bortezomib, dexamethasone, and lenalidomide. After 4 courses of treatment and serological staging during courses 2 and 3, a complete re-staging of bone marrow showed no morphologic or immunophenotypic evidence of residual myeloma. Immunophenotyping of bone marrow aspirate by flow cytometry showed that plasma cells accounted for ~1% of the cells analyzed, with no evidence of cytoplasmic light chain restriction. These results indicate no evidence of monoclonal plasma cells by flow cytometry. There was still serum evidence of monoclonal gammopathy. He was considered to have a very good partial remission.

Discussion	The International Myeloma Working Group has guidelines to standardize response criteria in MM and to define disease progression. This facilitates comparisons of outcomes between treatment centers and results reporting in clinical trials. The new guidelines include determination of minimal residual disease by the use of next-generation sequencing and flow cytometry in the bone marrow. Assessment of response with M-protein measurements using serum protein electrophoresis, urine protein electrophoresis, and serum free light-chain assay is recommended prior to each cycle of therapy. Bone marrow biopsy is necessary to monitor disease in the absence of measurable M-protein in the serum or urine or to document a complete or stringent complete response. Serial imaging assessments may be required if soft tissue plasmacytomas are present at baseline. After 4–6 courses of therapy, candidates for stem cell transplant should be evaluated and the transplants done if indicated. Alternatively, primary therapy can be continued until the best response is achieved. Maintenance therapy or observation can be considered beyond maximal response.[2]
Pearl	• Patients who have 2 or 3 monoclonal peaks are treated the same as patients who have 1 peak of monoclonal protein
References	1. Moreau P. How I treat myeloma with new agents. Blood 2017;130(13):1507-13. 2. Durie BG, Harousseau JL, Miguel JS, et al. International uniform response criteria for multiple myeloma. Leukemia 2006;20:1467-73.

What tests do I order if a patient has high total protein levels in the serum and normal or low albumin levels?

Key concept	The immunoglobulin light chain is the small polypeptide subunit of an immunoglobulin (Ig). A typical antibody is composed of two I) heavy chains and two Ig light chains: • A kappa (κ) chain, encoded by the immunoglobulin kappa locus (IGK@) on chromosome 2 • A lambda (λ) chain, encoded by the immunoglobulin lambda locus (IGL@) on chromosome 22
Clinical scenario	A 70-year-old man with advanced multiple myeloma is treated with 4 courses of bortezomib, dexamethasone, and lenalidomide. His re-staging bone marrow shows no morphologic or immunophenotypic evidence of residual myeloma. Flow cytometry shows that plasma cells account for ~1% of the cells analyzed, with no evidence of cytoplasmic light chain restriction. His kappa:lambda free light chain ratio decreases from 4442 to 1.65. He is declared to have a stringent complete response.
Discussion	Antibodies are produced by B lymphocytes, each expressing only one class of light chain. Once set, light chain class remains fixed for the life of the B lymphocyte. In a healthy individual, the total kappa:lambda ratio is roughly 2:1 in serum (measuring intact whole antibodies) or 1:1.5 if measuring free light chains. A highly divergent ratio is indicative of a neoplasm. The exact normal ratio of kappa to lambda, according to a novel polyclonal free light chain assay, ranges from 0.26 to 1.65. This is a very sensitive test for screening and follow-up of plasma cell disorders. It has prognostic value in all plasma cell disorders. According to International Myeloma Working Group Uniform Response Criteria, a normal free light chain ratio is required to document a stringent complete response.[1,2]
Pearls	• Both the kappa and lambda chains can increase proportionately, maintaining a normal ratio; this is usually indicative of something other than a blood cell dyscrasia, such as kidney disease • Determination of the free light chain ratio cannot replace 24-hour urine protein electrophoresis for monitoring patients with urinary M-protein

References

1. Dispenzieri A, Kyle R, Merlini G, et al. International Myeloma Working Group guidelines for serum-free light chain analysis in multiple myeloma and related disorders. Leukemia 2009;23:215-24.
2. Merlini G, Palladini G. Differential diagnosis of monoclonal gammopathy of undetermined significance. Hematology Am Soc Hematol Educ Program 2012;595-603.

What are immunomodulatory drugs (iMDs)?

Key concept	iMDs are a group of compounds consisting of two portions: phthalimide and glutarimide, in which only the glutarimide portion is modified. Currently there are three iMDs: thalidomide, lenalidomide, and pomalidomide. They possess immunomodulatory activities that include anti-inflammatory, anti-angiogenic, and anti-proliferative properties. They are widely used in the treatment of multiple myeloma (MM).[1]
Clinical scenario	A 56-year-old woman presents with symptoms of fatigue and tiredness. A serum electrophoresis showed an IgG kappa of 5.8 g/dL, and a bone survey shows lytic lesions in the pelvic area. After completion of a staging work-up she is started on treatment. After 5 courses of therapy with a proteasome inhibitor, dexamethasone, and lenalidomide, she undergoes an autologous stem cell transplant, with neuropathy and zoster as complications of her treatment. Four years later, her disease recurs, and a second autologous transplant is done, achieving a complete remission. She is placed on maintenance lenalidomide and a surveillance program for relapse and potential secondary malignancies.
Discussion	Thalidomide and its analogs, lenalidomide (CC-5013, Revlimid, Celgene, NJ, USA) and pomalidomide (CC4047, Actimid, Celgene, NJ, USA), belong to the family of iMDs. Both lenalidomide and pomalidomide are potent inhibitors of tumor necrosis factor–α and are better tolerated than thalidomide. iMDs are used in the treatment of all stages of MM (newly diagnosed, transplant-eligible and -ineligible patients, relapsed myeloma, and post-transplant maintenance).[2] The primary adverse events associated with lenalidomide are myelosuppression and thromboembolic complications. These are managed with dose modifications, administration of granulocyte colony-stimulating factor, and thromboprophylaxis. There is debate regarding the increased risk of developing second primary malignancies (SPMs) with the use of lenalidomide. SPMs observed in patients receiving lenalidomide include acute myeloid leukemia and myelodysplastic syndrome.

Pearl	In general, any anti-thrombotic therapy (low-molecular-weight heparin, direct anticoagulants, anti-platelet aggregation agents, or aspirin) is effective in preventing thrombosis in patients receiving lenalidomide. Which one to use depends on patient condition and availability.
References	1. Chang X, Zhu Y, Shi C, et al. Mechanism of immunomodulatory drugs' action in the treatment of multiple myeloma. Acta Biochim Biophys Sin (Shanghai) 2014;46(3):240-53. 2. Kumar SK, Rajkumar SV, Dispenzieri A, et al. Improved survival in multiple myeloma and the impact of novel therapies. Blood 2008;111(5):2516-20.

What type of stem cell therapy/transplant (SCT) is offered to selected patients with multiple myeloma (MM)?

Key concept	The treatment plan of patients newly diagnosed with MM should always include high-dose therapy with stem cell support (stem cell transplant or SCT), when feasible.[1]
Clinical scenario	A 56-year-old woman presents with symptoms of fatigue and tiredness. A serum electrophoresis showed an IgG kappa of 5.8 g/dL, and a bone survey shows lytic lesions in the pelvic area. After completion of a staging work-up she is started on treatment. After 5 courses of therapy with a proteasome inhibitor, dexamethasone, and lenalidomide, she undergoes an autologous stem cell transplant, with neuropathy and zoster as complications of her treatment. Four years later, her disease recurs, and a second autologous transplant is done, achieving a complete remission. She is placed on maintenance lenalidomide and a surveillance program for relapse and potential secondary malignancies.
Action items	• The initiation of treatment for a new patient with MM should always include the early evaluation and discussion with the transplant program of the plan for high-dose therapy with SCT
Discussion	The three types of SCT offered to patients with MM are: • Single autologous SCT • Tandem SCT, which involves a second course of high-dose therapy and SCT within 6 months of the first course • Allogeneic SCT Allogeneic SCT can be done after prior myeloablative therapy or after non-myeloablative therapy. Although all types of SCT are appropriate in different clinical settings, all candidates for high-dose chemotherapy must have adequate liver, renal, pulmonary, and cardiac function. In the past, radiotherapy was an important tool in the performance of SCT. It has now been abandoned, as chemotherapy regimens have equivalent efficacy and less toxicity.[2]

Pearls	• Non-ablative allogeneic transplant is not adequate therapy by itself, and it should be done after maximal tumor control or after an autologous SCT • Patients started on bortezomib need prophylaxis for *Pneumocystis jiroveci* and herpetic infections as well as pneumococcal immunization due to the inhibition of NF-κB pathway by bortezomib
References	1. Fermand JP, Katsahian S, Divine M, et al. High-dose therapy and autologous blood stem-cell transplantation compared with conventional treatment in myeloma patients aged 55 to 65 years: long-term results of a randomized control trial from the Group Myelome-Autogreffe. J Clin Oncol 2005;23(36):9227-33. 2. Kumar SK, Dispenzieri A, Lacy MQ, et al. Continued improvement in survival in multiple myeloma: changes in early mortality and outcomes in older patients. Leukemia 2014;28(5):1122-8.

What are the priorities in choosing an anti-myeloma regimen?

Key concept	The priority in choosing treatment for a patient newly diagnosed with multiple myeloma (MM) is not only to treat the MM but also to be able to perform stem cell transplant (SCT).
Clinical scenario	A 70-year-old man with advanced MM is treated with 4 courses of bortezomib, dexamethasone, and lenalidomide. His re-staging bone marrow shows no morphologic or immunophenotypic evidence of residual myeloma. Flow cytometry shows that plasma cells account for ~1% of the cells analyzed, with no evidence of cytoplasmic light chain restriction. His kappa:lambda free light chain ratio has decreased from 4442 to 1.65. He is declared to have a stringent complete response. The patient is in excellent physical condition and is referred for consideration of SCT.
Action items	• Determine liver, renal, pulmonary, and cardiac function at the time of diagnosis • Engage the assistance of an SCT transplant specialist in evaluating the potential candidacy of the patient for SCT if indicated
Discussion	MM is an incurable disease in which the longest-term outcomes are best seen in patients who are able to undergo SCT. However, age, comorbidities, and the effects of the disease stage and presentation significantly influence the appropriateness of patients for SCT. Additionally, certain classes of therapeutic agents, such as nitrosoureas and alkylating agents, may compromise the stem cell reserve and should be avoided in potential candidates for SCT. Thus, matching the patient with a therapeutic regimen that does not compromise the potential for SCT is a top priority in choosing treatment. Other factors can influence the therapeutic decision: for example, proteasome inhibitors containing regimens are of great value in patients with renal compromise (35%).[1]
Pearl	• Advanced age and renal dysfunction are not absolute contraindications for a SCT; thus, unless absolutely evident, all MM patients should be considered for SCT evaluation

References

1. Harousseau JL, Attal M, Avet-Loiseau H, et al. Bortezomib plus dexamethasone is superior to vincristine plus doxorubicin plus dexamethasone as induction treatment prior to autologous stem-cell transplantation in newly diagnosed multiple myeloma: results of the IFM 2005-01 phase III trial. J Clin Oncol 2010;28(30):4621-9.

How is multiple myeloma (MM) staged?

Key concept	Staging is an important tool assisting in the risk stratification of patients and is one of the prognostic tools used to assess therapy and its outcome.
Clinical scenario	A 70-year-old man is diagnosed with MM. His serum albumin is 4.0 g/dL, and his β_2 microglobulin is 2.0 mg/L. He has standard risk-chromosomal abnormalities. His physician tells him that his disease is Revised-ISS (R-ISS) stage I.
Discussion	Because MM is a heterogeneous disease, staging, as with other malignant disorders, can provide insights into the biology of the disease and expected course. In addition, staging can help stratify patients in clinical trials and may help guide therapy [eg, bortezomib in patients with t(4;14) and del 13q mutations]. In 2005 the International Myeloma Working Group established the International Staging System (ISS). This staging system was based on the analysis and review of >10,000 patients across 17 different centers. The two strongest correlates of median survival were β_2 microglobulin and albumin. The patients were categorized into three stages based on serum levels at diagnosis. The ISS is the current preferred staging method and has supplanted the previously used Durie-Salmon staging system. This latter system included observer-dependent variables that added subjectivity, such as degree of lytic bone lesions. Risk as measured by chromosomal abnormalities and lactate dehydrogenase (LDH) values was added later to the three stages of ISS, creating the Revised-ISS (R-ISS). In this regime, standard risk is defined as having no high-risk chromosomal abnormalities such as the presence of del 17(17p) and/or translocation t(4:14) and or translocation t(14:16). The ISS should not be extrapolated to patients with monoclonal gammopathy of undetermined significance or smoldering MM. The three stages are: R-ISS I, serum β_2 microglobulin <3.5 mg/L, serum albumin >3.5 g/dL, serum LDH <upper limit of normal, and standard-risk chromosomal abnormalities; R-ISS stage II, not R-ISS stage I or III; and R-ISS stage III, serum β_2 microglobulin >5.5 mg/L, high-risk chromosomal abnormalities by FISH, or serum LDH >upper limit of normal.

Pearl	• β_2 microglobulin is renally excreted; thus, high levels may be found in the presence of renal failure
References	1. Palumbo A, Avet-Loiseau H, Oliva S, et al. Revised International Staging System for multiple myeloma: a report from the International Myeloma Working Group. J Clin Oncol 2015;33:2863-9.

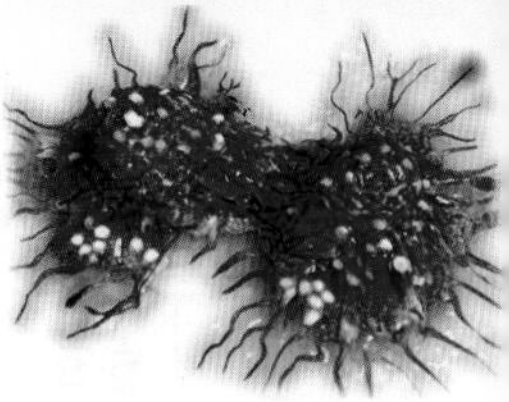

CHAPTER 16

Myeloproliferative Neoplasms

What are myeloproliferative neoplasms (MPNs)?

Key concept	MPNs include myelofibrosis (MF), polycythemia vera (PV), and essential thrombocythemia (ET). They are characterized by being Philadelphia chromosome–negative.
Clinical scenario	A 56-year-old woman is admitted to the emergency room with a severe case of pharyngitis. In addition to her symptom of pharyngitis, a peripheral blood count reveals 1×10^6 platelets/dL. She is told she has ET. Blood is drawn for determination of JAK2 mutations.
Action items	• Schedule bone marrow aspiration and biopsy • Obtain blood for determination of JAK2 mutations • Start patient on acetylsalicylic acid (low-dose aspirin)
Discussion	MPNs are a group of heterogeneous disorders that are characterized by a risk of transformation to acute myeloid leukemia and are collectively Philadelphia chromosome–negative. The profile varies for each type, but indications often include constitutional symptoms, fatigue, pruritus, weight loss, splenomegaly, and laboratory abnormalities such as erythrocytosis, thrombocytosis, and leukocytosis. Patients with MF have worse survival than patients with PV and ET. MPNs are diagnosed by identifying driver mutations such as JAK2, CALR, and MPL mutations.[1]
Pearl	• MPNs are not associated with chromosomal abnormalities

References

1. Mesa R, Miller CB, Thyne M, et al. Myeloproliferative neoplasms (MPNs) have a significant impact on patients' overall health and productivity: the MPN Landmark survey. BMC Cancer 2016;16:167.

What are the molecular abnormalities that occur in myeloproliferative neoplasms (MPNs)?

Key concept	The mutations associated with MPNs are: JAK2 mutations, the thrombopoietin receptor (MPL), and the calreticulin gene (CALR).[1]
Discussion	JAK2 V617F (exon 14) accounts for >90% of patients with PV and 60% of patients with ET or MF. Exon 12 JAK2 mutations account for 2%–3% of patients with PV. MPL mutations are reported in 5%–8% of MF patients and 1%–4% of ET patients. The CALR gene has two types of mutations in the exon 9: type 1 and type 2. Type 1 is frequent in MF patients and type 2 in ET patients. CALR gene mutations account for 60%–80% of ALL JAK2/MPL-negative ET and MF patients. Other mutations such as EZH2 and TP53 have also been reported in MPN patients.[2]
Pearls	• Patients with CARL mutations have better prognosis than those with JAK2/MPL mutations, and those with CARL mutations type 1 have better survival than those with type 2 • Patients with CARL mutations have better prognosis than those with triple-negative MPNs • CALR type 1 mutations are 52 base pair deletions, and CALR type 2 are 5 base pair insertions

References

1. Kralovics R, Passamonti F, Buser AS, et al. A gain-of-function mutation of JAK2 in myeloproliferative disorders. N Engl J Med 2005;352(17):1779-90.
2. Beer PA, Campbell PJ, Scott LM, et al. MPL mutations in myeloproliferative disorders: analysis of the PT-1 cohort. Blood 2008;112(1):141-9.

How is polycythemia vera (PV) diagnosed?

Key concept	The 2016 World Health Organization (WHO) criteria for diagnosis of PV requires 3 major criteria or the first 2 major criteria and the minor criterion.
Clinical scenario	A 56-year-old woman is admitted to the emergency room with a severe case of pharyngitis. In addition to her symptom of pharyngitis, a peripheral blood count reveals a hemoglobin (Hgb) level of 18 g/dL. Bone marrow biopsy reveals panmyelosis. Peripheral blood and bone marrow is positive for a JAK2 exon 12 mutation. She is diagnosed with PV.

Action items	When diagnosing PV, confirm the presence of all 3 major criteria or the first 2 and the minor criterion[1]:
	• MAJOR CRITERIA
	  • Hgb >16.5 g/dL (hematocrit [Hct] >49%) in men and >16 g/dL (Hct >48%) in women
	  • Bone marrow biopsy with panmyelosis with pleomorphic mature megakaryocytes
	  • Presence of JAK2 mutations
	• MINOR CRITERION
	  • Subnormal erythropoietin level

Discussion	The recent changes in the criteria for PV diagnosis were made because patients with so-called masked PV have a worse prognosis than patients with classical cases. For this reason, criteria levels of Hgb and Hct have been reduced. Bone marrow biopsy is a requirement except in obvious cases that meet the higher, previous levels for Hgb and Hct WHO criteria from 2008 (Hgb >18.5 g/dL/Hct 55% men and Hgb >16 g/dL/Hct 49% in women). It is required to differentiate PV from essential thrombocythemia with polycythemia in the context of decreased levels of Hgb and Hct for diagnosis.[2]

Pearls	• Measurement of red cell mass is not a requirement, as it is not available in most centers • While leg ulcers can occur at any time during hydroxyurea treatment, they are most commonly seen with chronic use
References	1. Alvarez-Larrán A, Angona A, Ancochea A, et al. Masked polycythaemia vera: presenting features, response to treatment and clinical outcomes. Eur J Haematol 2016;96(1):83-9. 2. Barosi G, Mesa RA, Thiele J, et al. Proposed criteria for the diagnosis of post-polycythemia vera and post-essential thrombocythemia myelofibrosis: a consensus statement from the International Working Group for Myelofibrosis Research and Treatment. Leukemia 2008;22(2):437-8.

How is polycythemia vera (PV) treated?

Key concept	Cytoreduction is important in PV to avoid cardiovascular complications. Hematocrit (Hct) ideally should be <45%.
Clinical scenario	A 56-year-old woman is admitted to the emergency room with a severe case of pharyngitis. In addition to her symptom of pharyngitis, a peripheral blood count reveals a hemoglobin level (Hgb) of 18 g/dL. Bone marrow biopsy reveals panmyelosis. JAK2 exon 12 mutation is positive in peripheral blood and bone marrow. She is diagnosed with PV. She is started on hydroxyurea 1.5 g/day. After 2 months, her Hgb is 14.5g/dL (Hct 45%). She is advised to continue treatment.
Discussion	Hydroxyurea is the most common drug used in first-line therapy of PV.[1] Ruxolitinib is used as a second-line therapy on the basis of the results of two large randomized clinical trials.[2] Interferons, which are known for their capacity to induce molecular remissions, may also be used as initial therapy. Interferons are becoming preferred in younger patients due to their lack of leukemogenicity. A complete response requires a Hct <45% and no phlebotomy, platelets $<400 \times 10^9$/L, leukocytes $<10 \times 10^9$/L, and no disease-related symptoms. The need for phlebotomy, uncontrollable myeloproliferation, and failure to reduce splenomegaly to <10 cm below the left costal margin, or myelosuppression with the doses needed for complete or partial response, indicates resistance or intolerance to hydroxyurea.
Pearl	• Intolerance to hydroxyurea can be manifested by leg ulcers, mucocutaneous manifestations, gastrointestinal symptoms, pneumonitis, or fever at any dose of hydroxyurea

References	1. Vannuchi AM. How I treat polycythemia vera. Blood 2014;124:3212-20. 2. Verstovsek S, Vannuchi AM, Griesshammer M, et al. Ruxolitinib versus best available therapy in patients with polycythemia vera: 80-week follow-up from the RESPONSE trial. Hematologica 2016;101:821-9.

How is essential thrombocythemia (ET) diagnosed and treated?

Key concept	ET is diagnosed when there is persistent thrombocytosis with a predisposition to thrombosis and bleeding. ET remains a diagnosis of exclusion. Median age of diagnosis is 55–60 years, and the female:male ratio is 2:1.
Clinical scenario	A 56-year-old woman is admitted to the emergency room with a severe case of pharyngitis. In addition to her symptom of pharyngitis, a peripheral blood count reveals 1×10^6 platelets/dL. She is told that she has ET. Blood is drawn for determination of JAK2 mutations. She is scheduled for a bone marrow aspiration and biopsy.
Action items	To make the diagnosis of ET, patients must meet the 2008 WHO criteria: • Sustained platelet count $\geq 450 \times 10^9$/L • Bone marrow biopsy specimen showing proliferation mainly of the megakaryocytic lineage with increased numbers of enlarged, mature megakaryocytes • No significant increase or left shift of neutrophil granulopoiesis or erythropoiesis • Does not meet WHO criteria for polycythemia vera, primary myelofibrosis, chronic myeloid leukemia, myelodysplastic syndrome, or other myeloid neoplasm • Demonstration of JAK2V617F or other clonal marker or, in the absence of a clonal marker, no evidence for reactive thrombocytosis Diagnosis of ET requires meeting all four criteria.[1]
Discussion	Therapy for ET is intended to prevent morbidity and mortality caused by thromboembolic events. All patients should be advised about smoking cessation. The two major classes of drugs used in ET are antiplatelet therapy (aspirin [ASA], 75–100 mg/day) and cytoreductive therapy (hydroxyurea 2 g/day for body weight <80 kg).

	There are four categories of risk, for each of which there is a general approach for treatment
	• Very low risk:
	  • Younger patients, with no history of thrombosis and wild-type JAK2 genes
	  • Observation is appropriate
	• Low risk:
	  • $<$60 years old, with no history of thrombosis but with JAK2 mutations
	  • Low-dose ASA is indicated
	• Intermediate risk:
	  • Patients $<$60 years old, no history of thrombosis with cardiovascular factors (smoking included) and platelet counts $>1000 \times 10^9$/L
	  • Low-dose ASA is indicated
	• High risk:
	  • Patients $\geq$60 years old or history of thrombosis
	  • Cytoreductive therapy and low-dose ASA are used[2]

Pearl	• If intermediate and high-risk patients have $>1.5 \times 10^9$/L platelets when using ASA, always test to rule out von Willebrand disease
References	1. Tefferi A, Thiele J, Orazi A, et al. Proposals and rationale for revision of the World Health Organization diagnostic criteria for polycythemia vera, essential thrombocythemia, and primary myelofibrosis: recommendations from an ad hoc international expert panel. Blood 2007;110(4):1092-7. 2. van Genderen PJ, Mulder PG, Waleboer M, et al. Prevention and treatment of thrombotic complications in essential thrombocythaemia: efficacy and safety of aspirin. Br J Haematol 1997; 97(1):179-84.

What is primary myelofibrosis (PMF), and how is it diagnosed?

Key concept	PMF is a clonal disorder characterized by myeloid cell proliferation, megakaryocytic atypia, bone marrow (BM) fibrosis, a leukoerythroblastic peripheral blood picture, extramedullary hematopoiesis (EMH), and splenomegaly. It can occur either de novo or as a late complication of polycythemia vera (PV) or essential thrombocythemia (ET) with an intense marrow stromal reaction, including collagen fibrosis, osteosclerosis, and angiogenesis.
Clinical scenario	A 78-year-old patient chronically treated with hydroxyurea for several years develops anemia and severe splenomegaly. He becomes severely fatigued and has fevers and weight loss. A bone marrow biopsy reveals 15% blasts and evidence of megakaryocyte proliferation and atypia, accompanied by reticulin and collagen fibrosis. A diagnosis of PV myelofibrosis is made.

Action items	Make sure the patient meets 2008 WHO criteria for diagnosis of PMF.[1]
	• MAJOR CRITERIA
	  • Presence of megakaryocyte proliferation and atypia, usually accompanied by either reticulin and/or collagen fibrosis or, in the absence of significant reticulin fibrosis, the megakaryocyte changes must be accompanied by an increased bone marrow cellularity characterized by granulocytic proliferation and often decreased erythropoiesis (ie, prefibrotic cellular-phase disease)
	  • Not meeting WHO criteria for PV, chronic myeloid leukemia, myelodysplastic syndrome, or another myeloid neoplasm
	  • Demonstration of JAK2617VF or another clonal marker (eg, MPL515WL/K) or, in the absence of a clonal marker, no evidence of bone marrow fibrosis due to underlying inflammatory or other neoplastic diseases
	• MINOR CRITERIA
	  • Leukoerythroblastosis
	  • Increased serum lactate dehydrogenase

	• Anemia • Palpable splenomegaly Diagnosis requires meeting all three major criteria and at least two minor criteria.
Discussion	The release of growth-promoting factors such as vascular endothelial growth factor, platelet-derived growth factor, basic fibroblast growth factor, and transforming growth factor β from proliferating atypical megakaryocytes promotes fibrogenesis and angiogenesis. Some 50%–60% of PMF patients have a JAK2 mutation. Thrombopoietin receptor (encoded by MPL, the myeloproliferative leukemia virus oncogene) mutations are found in 5%–10% of patients, and CALR mutations in 25%. Median age at diagnosis is 64 years. Clinical presentation includes leukocytosis or splenomegaly (80% of patients, often extending into the pelvis). There is severe fatigue with constitutional symptoms (weight loss, pruritus, low-grade fever, and night sweats). Myeloproliferation leads to extra-medullary erythropoiesis with hepatosplenomegaly, with pain, early satiety, portal hypertension, anemia, and thrombocytopenia. Peripheral blood smear shows teardrop red cells and leukoerythroblastosis. Leukopenia and thrombocytopenia are seen during the later stages of the disease. Transformation to acute myeloid leukemia occurs in 10%–20% of patients within the first 10 years from diagnosis. Median survival after transformation is 5 months. There are thrombotic and cardiovascular complications, infections, bleeding, and portal hypertension.[2]
Pearl	• PMF is distinguished clinically from PV and ET by the development of anemia in nearly all patients, a higher incidence of splenomegaly, greater symptom burden, and greater risk of leukemic transformation
References	1. Tefferi A, Thiele J, Orazi A, et al. Proposals and rationale for revision of the World Health Organization diagnostic criteria for polycythemia vera, essential thrombocythemia, and primary myelofibrosis: recommendations from an ad hoc international expert panel. Blood 2007;110:1092-7. 2. Rumi E, Pietra D, Pascutto C, et al. Clinical effect of driver mutations of JAK2, CALR, or MPL in primary myelofibrosis. Blood 2014;124(7):1062-9.

How is myelofibrosis (MF) treated?

Key concept	The FDA approved the JAK1/2 inhibitor ruxolitinib in 2011. Before this, treatment of MF was unsatisfactory and was mostly based on cytoreductive and symptomatic therapy. The decision how to treat MF, regardless of primary disease or post-ET or -PV, is based on the result of two prognostic scoring systems, the IPSS and the D-PISS.[1]
Action items	The International Prognostic Scoring System (IPSS) is designed to be used at diagnosis, and the Dynamic IPSS (D-IPSS), at any point in the disease course. Both are based on clinical and laboratory characteristics: • age (>65 years) • constitutional symptoms (yes/no) • hemoglobin (<10 g/dL) • leukocyte count (>25 × 10^9/L) • circulating blasts (≥1%) In the IPSS system, all factors are given a score of 1, whereas in the D-IPSS, hemoglobin <10 g/dL is given 2 points. There are four risk groups: • low risk (0 points) • intermediate-1 risk (1 point IPSS; 1–2 points D-IPSS) • intermediate-2 risk (2 points IPSS; 3–4 points D-IPSS) • high risk (≥3 points IPSS; 5–6 points D-IPSS)

	The median survival time for each IPSS risk group is 63, 46, 15, and 5 months, respectively. Cytogenetic abnormalities are found in approximately half of the patients with primary MF. Common abnormalities include del(13q), del(20q), trisomy 8 or 9, and abnormalities of chromosome 1 (partial trisomy). Unfavorable cytogenetics include abnormalities of chromosomes 5 or 7 or complex (≥3) cytogenetics, and very unfavorable cytogenetics include any abnormality of chromosome 17. Asymptomatic patients with low or intermediate-1 risk should be observed. Intermediate-2 or high-risk patients can be treated with ruxolitinib and other measures as described below.[2]
Discussion	Prior to ruxolitinib, hydroxyurea and cladribine were used to control hyperproliferation, with only transient effects. Oral alkylating agents induce myelosuppression and are associated with transformation to acute myeloid leukemia. Corticosteroids, erythroid-stimulating agents, and androgens are helpful in treatment of anemia. Patients with low serum erythropoietin (Epo; <125 U/L) can be given subcutaneous injections of Epo (40,000 U/week). Corticosteroids (prednisone 0.5–1.0 mg/kg/day) or androgens (testosterone) can also be helpful.
Pearls	• Although splenectomy or splenic radiation may help with symptom control or improve blood cell count, they carry significant adverse effects • Ruxolitinib is contraindicated in patients with active or latent tuberculosis
References	1. Cervantes F, Dupriez B, Pereira A, et al. New prognostic scoring system for primary myelofibrosis based on a study of the International Working Group for Myelofibrosis Research and Treatment. Blood 2009;113(13):2895-901. 2. Verstovsek S, Mesa RA, Gotlib J, et al. A double-blind, placebo-controlled trial of ruxolitinib for myelofibrosis. N Engl J Med 2012;366(9):799-807.

CHAPTER 17

Myelodysplastic Syndromes

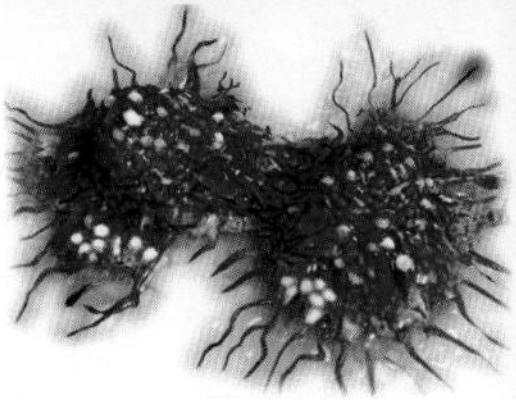

What are myelodysplastic syndromes (MDSs)?

Key concept	MDSs are a group of heterogeneous myeloid hematopoietic disorders characterized by ineffective hematopoiesis and increased risk of transformation to acute myelogenous leukemia (AML). Most patients with MDS die of causes related to the disease. The median age of patients with MDS is 70–75 years.[1]
Clinical scenario	A 71-year-old man is admitted to a hospital with generalized weakness and dyspnea on exertion. On physical examination, the abdominal reveals no organomegaly. His hemoglobin level is 6 g/dL, and the rest of his blood work is normal. There is no obvious evidence of blood loss. A bone marrow examination shows normocellular marrow with dysplastic changes in the megakaryocytes and erythroid series. Increased promyelocytes with granules (14.6%), eosinophils (5.6%), and basophils (7%) are observed. Karyotype is normal (46,XX). Diagnosis is MDS with eosinophilia and basophilia (refractory cytopenia with multilineage dysplasia).

Action items	Review whether a patient diagnosed with MDS meets minimal diagnostic criteria[2]:
	• Stable cytopenia (6 months, or 2 months if there is a specific MDS karyotype or bilineage dysplasia)
	• Exclusion of other disorders as cause of cytopenia and/or dysplasia or both
	• At least 1 of the 3 MDS-related (decisive) criteria:
	  • Dysplasia (>10% in ≥1 of 3 major bone marrow lineages)
	  • A blast count of 5%–19%
	  • Specific karyotype, such as del(5q), del(20)q, +8, or −7del (7q)
	• Co-criteria help to confirm diagnosis:
	  • Abnormal bone marrow immune histology, immunohistochemistry
	  • Abnormal flow cytometry
	  • Abnormal CD34 expression

	• Fibrosis • Myeloid clonality • Dysplastic megakaryocytes
Discussion	MDS is usually suspected when there is cytopenia in a routine peripheral blood count. A bone marrow aspiration and biopsy follows, with a manual count of blasts, which is essential for risk assessment. Cytogenetic analysis assists in predicting risk and selecting therapy. Risk is calculated using the International Prognostic Scoring System (IPSS). Patients with low and intermediate-1 (INT-1) scores are treated to improve transfusion needs. Patients with higher scores, intermediate-2 (INT-2) or higher, are treated with interventions patterned after AML therapy. The revised IPSS score (IPSS-R) includes a new cytogenetic risk classification that divides patients into 5 categories. It is used more for prognosis than for deciding therapy, since all the approved treatments for MDS have been approved in clinical trials using the IPSS.
Pearl	• IPSS criteria are used to decide therapy and IPSS-R criteria to evaluate prognosis
References	1. Montalban-Bravo G, Garcia-Manero G. Myelodysplastic syndromes: 2018 update on diagnosis, risk-stratification and management. Am J Hematol 2018;93:129-47. 2. Valent P, Horny HP, Bennett JM, et al. Definitions and standards in the diagnosis and treatment of the myelodysplastic syndromes: consensus statements and report from a working conference. Leuk Res 2007;31(6):727-36.

What is included in the evaluation of a patient with a myelodysplastic syndrome (MDS)?

Key concept	A clear picture of the MDS patient's clinical status is essential for diagnosis, prognosis, and to establish treatment.[1]
Clinical scenario	A 50-year-old woman is seen in the clinic with pancytopenia. On physical examination, the only relevant findings are pallor of mucosal surfaces and fatigue. The peripheral blood count reveals pancytopenia. There is a remote history of treatment with systemic chemotherapy for breast cancer. Tests are ordered to evaluate her for MDS.
Discussion	The diagnosis of MDS starts with an abnormal complete blood count. It is followed by a bone marrow aspiration and biopsy. The aspiration allows study of the cellular morphology and percentage of blasts in the marrow. The biopsy permits study of the marrow cellularity and architecture. The presence of dysplasia establishes the diagnosis. An additional and essential evaluation is bone marrow cytogenetics. Other useful laboratory testing includes serum erythropoietin, vitamin B12 level, red blood cell (RBC) folate level, serum ferritin, iron, and total iron binding capacity.[2] Additional genetic screening should be considered for patients with familial cytopenias. Screening for paroxysmal nocturnal hemoglobinuria, HLA-DR15 positivity, and STAT3 mutant cytotoxic T cell clones is useful to select patients for immunosuppressive therapy. Finally, it should be noted that flow cytometry data from the bone marrow cannot replace the experienced hematopathologist's morphologic determination of the blast percentage.
Pearl	• RBC folate levels reflect folate stores, and serum folate levels reflect recent nutrition

References

1. Tefferi A, Vardiman JW. Myelodysplatic syndromes. N Engl J Med 2009;361:1872-85.
2. Dunn DE, Tanawattanacharoen P, Boccuni P, et al. Paroxysmal nocturnal hemoglobinuria cells in patients with bone marrow failure syndromes. Ann Intern Med 1999;131:401-8.

What is the prognostic stratification of patients with myelodysplastic syndromes (MDSs)?

Key concept	The development of clinical systems allows an accurate prognostication of individual patients into low- and high-risk categories. This is essential to guide management and treatment decisions. It also allows the study of investigational drug protocols.
Clinical scenario	A 71-year-old man is admitted to the hospital with generalized weakness and dyspnea on exertion. The abdominal examination reveals no organomegaly. His hemoglobin level is 6 g/dL, and all other blood work is normal. There is no obvious evidence of blood loss. A bone marrow examination shows normocellular marrow with dysplastic changes in the megakaryocytes and erythroid series. Increased promyelocytes with granules (14.6%), eosinophils (5.6%), and basophils (7%) are observed. Karyotype is normal (46,XX). The diagnosis is MDS with eosinophilia and basophilia (refractory cytopenia with multilineage dysplasia). The patient is told his International Prognostic Scoring System (IPSS) score is 1 and that he has a low-risk MDS.
Discussion	The prognosis of MDS patients is heterogeneous. The IPSS is a system developed in 1997 for staging MDS.[1] It rates 3 factors: • The percentage of blasts in the bone marrow (scored on a scale from 0 to 2) • Chromosome abnormalities (scored from 0 to 1) • The patient's blood counts (scored as 0 or 0.5) Each factor is given a score, with the lowest scores having the best outlook. Then the scores for the factors are added together to make the IPSS score. The IPSS puts people with MDS into 4 groups: • Low risk: 0 • Intermediate-1 risk (Int-1): 0.5–1

	• Intermediate-2 risk (Int-2): 1.5–2 • High risk: ≥2.5 The risk associated with cytogenetic abnormalities is good if there is a normal diploid karyotype, isolated del(5q), isolated del(20q), or isolated-Y. Poor risk abnormalities are defined as abnormalities involving chromosome 7 or complex karyotypes with the presence of ≥3 karyotypic abnormalities. All other cytogenetic abnormalities are considered intermediate risk. Patients classified as IPSS low and Int-1 risks are generally considered to have low-risk MDS, and patients classified as having IPSS Int-2 and high to have high-risk MDS. In 2012, an international consortium developed a new MDS classification known as IPSS-R (Revised). It includes different cutoff points for cytopenias and incorporates the cytogenetic MDS score. The IPSS-R divides patients into five risk categories (very low, low, intermediate, high, and very high). It has good predictive value but is not useful to determine therapy.
Pearl	• The IPSS has been used for defining outcomes in response to therapies, whereas the IPPSS-R is used for prognosis, since it has not been used to validate any therapeutic intervention, unlike the IPSS[2]
References	1. Greenberg P, Cox C, LeBeau MM, et al. International scoring system for evaluating prognosis in myelodysplastic syndromes. Blood 1997;89(6):2079-88. 2. Greenberg PL, Tuechler H, Schanz J, et al. Revised International Prognostic Scoring System for myelodysplastic syndromes. Blood 2012;120(12):2454-65.

How are myelodysplastic syndromes (MDSs) treated?

Key concept	Low-risk MDSs are typically treated more conservatively than higher risk MDSs. Thus, the major therapeutic aim for patients in the lower-risk group is hematological improvement. For those in the higher-risk group, alteration of the disease natural history is the main objective.
Clinical scenario	A 50-year-old woman is seen in the clinic with pancytopenia. On physical examination, the only relevant findings are pallor of mucosal surfaces and fatigue. The peripheral blood count reveals pancytopenia. There is a remote history of treatment with systemic chemotherapy for breast cancer. Tests are ordered to evaluate her for MDS. She is found to have low-risk MDS with isolated del(5q). She is started on lenalidomide treatment.
Discussion	Once the diagnosis of MDS is confirmed and the patient stratified according to the IPSS into low- and high-risk MDS, the choices of therapy can be made. The goals of therapy in MDS vary in different patient populations. The treatment should consider the patient's age, comorbidities, and disease risk. For patients with lower-risk disease, the use of growth factors, lenalidomide if they have deletion (5q), and azanucleosides should be considered, particularly if they fail replacement and/or supportive therapy. Treatment of anemia with transfusions and prevention of iron overload with chelation (deferoxamine, deferasirox, and, more recently, deferiprone) should be aggressively used. The use of erythropoietin-stimulating agents such as recombinant human Epo or the longer-acting darbapoietin, with or without granulocyte colony-stimulating factor, has been found to provide clinical benefit to patients in the lower-risk group with symptomatic anemia. For thrombocytopenia, platelet transfusion is the first choice. Active investigation is ongoing into the use of trombopoietin receptor agonists (eg, romiplostin and eltrombopag). However, neither of these agents is approved for use in MDS, and there is concern about stimulation of leukemic blasts (this concern is expected to be resolved through the outcome of ongoing clinical trials). High-risk MDS has a poor prognosis and forms a continuum with acute myeloid leukemia. For these patients choices include allogenic

	stem cell transplant, acute myelogenous leukemia–like therapy, and azanucleosides. Finally, there is a group of patients with low-risk MDS in whom the use of immunosuppressive therapy (anti-thymocyte globulin, cyclosporine, and lenalidomide) appears to have noticeable benefit. Lower-risk MDS patients who are best candidates for this type of therapy have HLA-DR15 histocompatibility type, marrow hypoplasia, normal cytogenetics, low-risk disease, evidence of paroxysmal nocturnal hemoglobinuria, or with STAT3 mutant cytotoxic T cell clones.
Pearl	• Red blood cell folate levels reflect folate stores, and serum folate levels reflect recent nutrition
References	1. Montalban-Bravo G, Garcia-Manero G. Myelodysplastic syndromes: 2018 update on diagnosis, risk-stratification and management. Am J Hematol 2018; 93:129-47. 2. Cheson BD, Greenberg PL, Bennett JM, et al. Clinical application and proposal for modification of the International Working Group (IWG) response criteria in myelodysplasia. Blood 2006;108(2):419-25.

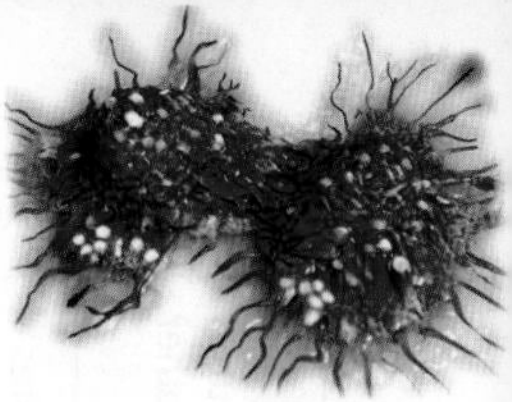

CHAPTER 18

Guidelines for Supportive Care

What are different measures of performance status?

Key concept

Performance status is a measure of functional capacity that is used as a clinical parameter to estimate survival in cancer patients.[1] There are two metrics—Eastern Cooperative Oncology Group (ECOG) performance status and Karnofsky Performance Status (KPS)—used by oncologists and other medical professionals and for entry into clinical trials.[1,2]

Clinical scenario

A 58-year-old woman with metastatic pancreatic cancer is unable to perform self-care and requires aid with daily activities of living, including bathing herself. She presents for follow-up with her oncologist. What is her performance status?

Action items

KARNOFSKY STATUS	KARNOFSKY GRADE	ECOG GRADE	ECOG STATUS
Normal, no complaints	100	0	Fully active, able to carry on all pre-disease performance without restriction
Able to carry on normal activities; minor signs or symptoms of disease	90	1	Restricted in physically strenuous activity but ambulatory and able to carry out work of a light or sedentary nature (eg, light house work or office work)
Normal activity with effort, some signs or symptoms of disease	80	1	

	Able to care for self; unable to carry out normal activity or do active work	70	2	Ambulatory and capable of all self-care but unable to carry out any work activities; up and about >50% of waking hours
	Requires occasional assistance, but able to care for most needs	60	2	
	Requires considerable assistance and frequent medical care	50	3	Capable of only limited self-care, confined to bed or chair >50% of waking hours
	Disabled; requires special care and assistance	50	3	
	Severely disabled; hospitalization indicated, although death not imminent	30	4	Completely disabled; cannot carry out any self-care; totally confined to bed or chair
	Very sick; hospitalization necessary; active supportive treatment necessary	20	4	
	Moribund; fatal processes progressing rapidly	10	4	
	Dead	0	5	Dead
References	1. Zubrod CG, Schneiderman M, Frei E, et al. Appraisal of methods for the study of chemotherapy of cancer in man: comparative therapeutic trial of nitrogen mustard and triethylene thiophosphoramide. J Chron Dis 1960;11(1):7-33. 2. Oken MM, Creech RH, Tormey DC, et al. Toxicity and response criteria of the Eastern Cooperative Oncology Group. Am J Clin Oncol 1982;5:649-55.			

How do I address fertility in young patients who plan to receive chemotherapy?

Key concept	The treatment of cancer in patients of reproductive age can be associated with the risk of infertility.
Clinical scenario	A 34-year-old woman was started on rituximab-DA EPOCH treatment for a primary B cell lymphoma of the mediastinum after diagnosis and completion of a staging work-up. She completed 6 courses of chemotherapy. Six months later, she became pregnant and delivered a healthy baby.
Action item	• Men and women of reproductive age who are going to be treated with systemic chemotherapy/ radiotherapy should undergo counseling sessions with a reproductive specialist or genetic counselor[1]
Discussion	Infertility in patients treated for cancer can be caused by injury to the organs of the reproductive tract and to the hypothalamic pituitary-gonadal axis. The use of cytotoxic agents, radiotherapy, and surgery, as well as the disease process itself, can all be associated with infertility. Factors that influence the overall fertility outcome in patients with cancer include the patient's age, the type and stage of cancer, the cumulative doses and types of chemotherapy and hormonal agents used, and the extent of surgery and radiotherapy. It is always advisable to provide patients with fertility counseling; there are circumstances when the priority to treat overrides this consideration. This situation has led to significant experience in patients of reproductive age who undergo even the most dose-intensive regimens showing a moderate effect on fertility, and most patients are able to conceive after a recovery period, usually of ~6 months. Still, it is important that every patient with reproductive capacity undergo counseling with a fertility expert or genetic counselor.[2]
Pearls	• Chemotherapy-induced amenorrhea does not predict the inability of a woman to get pregnant • For this reason, woman of reproductive potential receiving chemotherapy should practice a recognized and established method of contraception

References

1. Armuand GM, Rodriguez-Wallberg KA, Wettergren L, et al. Sex differences in fertility-related information received by young adult cancer survivors. J Clin Oncol 2012;30:2147-53.
2. Niemasik EE, Letourneau J, Dohan D, et al. Patient perceptions of reproductive health counseling at the time of cancer diagnosis: a qualitative study of female California cancer survivors. J Cancer Surviv 2012; 6:324-32.

How is chemotherapy-induced nausea/vomiting (CINV) best managed?

Key concept	Principles of antiemetic support include preventive measures prior to chemotherapy administration and management of acute, delayed, anticipatory, and breakthrough CINV.[1,2] The mechanisms of nausea include triggering the vomiting center in the medulla and chemoreceptor trigger zone, vagal stimulation within the pharyngeal and gastrointestinal tract, and cerebral cortex.[1,2] Effective antiemetics block different pathways of nausea and are active against serotonin and dopamine receptors.[1,2]
Clinical scenario	A 45-year-old woman with a history of stage III breast cancer is receiving adriamycin and cyclophosphamide. She has a history of morning sickness with prior pregnancies and does not drink alcohol. She is concerned about nausea and vomiting associated with her chemotherapy regimen. What medications can be administered prior to chemo?
Action items	• Acute onset of CINV usually occurs within a few minutes to several hours after drug administration and peaks by around 5–6 hours after administration[1,2] • Delayed onset of CINV usually occurs >24 hours after drug administration and can vary from 48 hours up to 6–7 days later, depending on the drug[1,2] • Anticipatory CINV is associated with prior episodes of nausea/vomiting[1,2] • Breakthrough CINV is associated with nausea/vomiting that occurs despite prophylactic medications[1,2]

TYPE OF AGENT	DRUG EXAMPLES	SIDE EFFECTS	PEARLS
Serotonin (5-HT3) receptor antagonists	Palonosetron, granisetron, ondansetron	Mild headaches, mild transaminase elevation, and constipation	• Should be used in conjunction with dexamethasone for regimens that are moderate-emetogenic potential • Depending on the dose and route of administration, there can be QT prolongation that should be monitored while on therapy
Neurokinin (NK)-1 antagonists	Aprepitant, fosaprepitant, netupitant	Mild headaches, anorexia, fatigue, diarrhea, hiccups, and mild transaminase elevation	Should be used in conjunction with a 5-HT3 antagonist ± dexamethasone

(continued on following page)

(continued from previous page)

Dopamine receptor antagonists**	Phenothiazines (promethazine, prochlorperazine)	Sedation and dry mouth	Caution if used in conjunction with metoclopramide and/or haloperidol due to concern for extrapyramidal symptoms
	Metoclopramide	Drowsiness, fatigue, and tardive dyskinesia	Metoclopramide reserved for patients intolerant of or refractory to 5-HT3-receptor antagonists, dexamethasone, and aprepitant
	Haloperidol	Monitor for QT prolongation	Should administer at lower doses in order to produce antiemetic effect versus antipsychotic effect
Steroids	Dexamethasone	Dyspepsia, hyperglycemia, and insomnia	Use of steroids is not recommended in immunotherapies or cellular therapies
Atypical antipsychotics**	Olanzapine	• Fatigue, drowsiness, sedation, and dystonia • Monitor for QT prolongation	Caution if used in conjunction with metoclopramide and/or haloperidol due to concern for extra-pyramidal symptoms

Benzodiazepines**	Lorazepam	Sedation, dizziness	Used to treat anxiety and reduce the risk of anticipatory CINV
Other	Scopolamine**	Dry mouth, dizziness, fatigue, drowsiness, and headaches	Can be used in patients in whom nausea/vomiting associated with positional changes or movement or excessive secretions
	Cannabinoids**	Sedation, euphoria, dizziness, dysphoria, and hallucinations	Recommended for patients intolerant of or refractory to 5-HT3-RA or steroids and aprepitant

***Caution should be exercised with use of these agents in elderly patients who are at high risk for falls or are frail due to associated CNS depression.*

(continued on following page)

(continued from previous page)

DEGREE OF EMETOGENIC POTENTIAL[2]	TYPE OF AGENT
High (>90%)	IV: cisplatin, mechlorethamine, streptozotocin, cyclophosphamide, carmustine, dacarbazine PO: hexamethylmelamine, procarbazine
Moderate (30%–90%)	IV: oxaliplatin, cytarabine, carboplatin, ifosfamide, cyclophosphamide, doxorubicin, daunorubicin, epirubicin, idarubicin, irinotecan, azacytidine, bendamustine, clofarabine, alemtuzumab PO: cyclophosphamide, temozolomide, vinorelbine, imatinib
Low (10%–30%)	IV: paclitaxel, docetaxel, mitoxantrone, liposomal doxorubicin, ixabepilone, topotecan, etoposide, pemetrexed, methotrexate, mitomycin, gemcitabine, cytarabine <1000 mg/m^2, 5-fluorouracil, temsirolimus, bortezomib, cetuximab, trastuzumab, panitumumab PO: capecitabine, tegafur-uracil, fludarabine, etoposide, sunitinib, everolimus, lapatinib, lenalidomide, thalidomide
Minimal (<10%)	IV: bleomycin, busulfan, 2-chlorodeoxyadenosine, fludarabine, vinblastine, vincristine, vinorelbine, bevacizumab PO: chlorambucil, hydroxyurea, L-phenylalanine mustard, 6-thioguanine, methotrexate, gefitinib, erlotinib, sorafenib

References	
	1. National Comprehensive Cancer Network guidelines for antiemesis. Version 2.2017. Available at: www.nccn.org. 2. Feyer P, Jordan K. Update and new trends in antiemetic therapy: the continuing need for novel therapies. Ann Oncol 2010;22(1):30-8.

How is chemotherapy-related diarrhea managed?

Key concept	Diarrhea is a common side effect of chemotherapy, including traditional cytotoxic agents such as 5-fluorouracil and irinotecan, targeted agents such as tyrosine kinase inhibitors (including sorafenib and sunitinib), and immunotherapy agents such as nivolumab and ipilumumab.[1] Thorough evaluation of the etiology of the diarrhea, including history and physical examination, must be pursued in order for the correct treatment to be initiated. Factors including diet, conditions such as Crohn disease or diverticulitis, and medications can contribute to diarrhea. Laboratory evaluation to rule out malabsorption or infectious causes with stool cultures of *Clostridium difficile* or other bacterial, viral, or parasitic organisms is also important.[2] Mechanisms of chemotherapy-related diarrhea (CRD) occur through three different pathophysiologic mechanisms[2]: • Diarrhea due to altered gastrointestinal motility: increased GI motility results in decreased absorptive capacity and increased stool volume • Exudative diarrhea: there is disruption of epithelium caused by surgery or chemotherapy drugs, which leads to water and electrolyte leakage • Osmotic diarrhea: there is an increase of intraluminal osmotic substances leading to water absorption • Secretory diarrhea: there is an increase secretion of electrolytes caused by luminal secretagogues or reduced absorptive capacity Management of CRD includes decrease or discontinuation of the chemotherapy agent, increased oral hydration (up to ≥3 L of electrolyte-containing fluids a day), the BRAT (bananas, rice, applesauce, and toast) or a bland diet, and anticholinergic medications, including loperamide and diphenoxylate-atropine. If the patient is unable to tolerate oral intake, IV fluids and possible hospitalization should be considered. Somatostatin analogs such as octreotide can also be given to control/decrease diarrhea.[1,2] Diarrhea associated with certain tumors such as neuroendocrine tumors or pheochromocytoma can be treated using similar agents. In addition, diarrhea associated with carcinoid syndrome can also be treated with telotristat ethyl.[1,3]

Clinical scenario	A 63-year-old man with a history of a mesenteric mass underwent evaluation with biopsy showing a low-grade neuroendocrine tumor. He reports a 30-lb weight loss and diarrhea. He states up to 4–5 bowel movements a day. What is the next step of management?
Action items	• The most common anti-diarrheal agents include loperamide and diphenoxylate-atropine, which are anticholinergic agents that decrease GI motility and secretion[1,2] • Octreotide is a somatostatin analog that inhibits serotonin release and secretion of gastrin, vasoactive intestinal polypeptide, glucagon, secretin, motilin, and pancreatic polypeptide and increases intestinal absorption[1,2] • Telotristat ethyl is an oral medication that blocks tryptophan hydroxylase, which converts tryptophan to 5-hydroxytryptophan, which is then converted to serotonin; an international, multicenter, randomized, double-blind, placebo-controlled phase 3 trial (TELESTAR)[1] demonstrated that telotristat decreased bowel movements in patients with carcinoid syndrome with diarrhea not controlled by somatostatin analogs[3] • Early recognition of immune-mediated diarrhea is important in order to initiate corticosteroids[1,4]
Pearls	• In general, secretory diarrhea characteristically continues despite fasting, is associated with stool volumes >1 L/day, and occurs day and night, in contrast to osmotic diarrhea • If there is a concern for infectious diarrhea, anti-diarrheal agents must be used with caution due to possible development of ileus, which can be life-threatening[2]
References	1. National Comprehensive Cancer Network guidelines for palliative care. Version 2.2017. Available at: www.nccn.org. 2. Richardson G, Dobish R. Chemotherapy induced diarrhea. J Oncol Pharm Pract 2007;13(4):181-98. 3. Kulke MH, Hörsch D, Caplin ME, et al. Telotristat ethyl, a tryptophan hydroxylase inhibitor for the treatment of carcinoid syndrome. J Clin Oncol 2016;35(1):14-23. 4. Weber JS, Dummer R, de Pril V, et al. Patterns of onset and resolution of immune-related adverse events of special interest with ipilimumab. Cancer 2013;119(9):1675-82.

How is chemotherapy-related constipation managed?

Key concept	Constipation is a common symptom experienced by cancer patients. Opiate-induced constipation is the leading cause. Constipation can also be a side effect of chemotherapy (ie, vincristine) and other adjunctive medications, including antiemetics, antacids, and anticholinergic medications (ie, antidepressants).[1] Thorough evaluation of constipation must be pursued, including ruling out mechanical obstruction from malignancy versus fecal impaction versus an underlying medical disorder (ie, hypothyroidism) in order for the correct treatment to be initiated.[1] A prophylactic stool regimen including either laxatives or stool softeners should be initiated in patients who are prescribed narcotics for management of cancer-related pain.[1] A peripherally acting mu-opioid receptor antagonist (ie, methylnaltrexone or naloxegol) can be used to treat opiate-related constipation but should be AVOIDED in patients with postoperative ileus or mechanical bowel obstruction.[1]
Clinical scenario	A 58-year-old woman with metastatic pancreatic cancer is currently on palliative chemotherapy with gemcitabine and nab-paclitaxel. She has severe mid-epigastric pain that radiates to her back and takes extended-release morphine sulfate 60 mg twice daily and requires breakthrough medications with 30 mg of morphine sulfate immediate release every 4 hours. She has been compliant with bisacodyl daily but has developed abdominal distention and pellet-like stools. What is the next step of management?
Action items	• Different agents can be used to help with constipation, including stimulant laxatives (ie, senna and bisacodyl) that act to evoke gut muscle contraction and reduce gut water absorption versus osmotic laxatives (ie, magnesium sulfate, lactulose, and polyethylene glycol) that cause gut distention, promoting peristalsis, versus rectal suppositories[2] • Fluid balance with an oral intake of at least 2 liters of fluid per day is an important component of preventing and treating constipation[3]

	• For patients on chronic opioids and who are not responsive to laxatives, methylnaltrexone or naloxegol can be used to help with constipation while preserving the analgesic effect[1]
References	1. National Comprehensive Cancer Network guidelines for palliative care. Version 2.2017. Available at: www.nccn.org. 2. Mancini I, Bruera E. Constipation in advanced cancer patients. Support Care Cancer 1998;6(4):356-64. 3. Sykes NP. The pathogenesis of constipation. J Support Oncol 2006;4(5):213-8.

How do I manage a patient with cancer cachexia?

Key concept	Cancer cachexia is a multisystem syndrome characterized by weight loss, anorexia, loss of muscle mass, systemic inflammation, insulin resistance, and functional decline. Cancer cachexia is a marker of poor outcome with no current standard of care.
Clinical scenario	A 72-year-old man presents with increasing jaundice, abdominal pain, early satiety, and 50-lb weight loss. He is noted to have temporal wasting and low serum albumin. CT scan demonstrates a large mass on the pancreatic head with metastasis to the liver. Biopsy confirms adenocarcinoma of pancreas. The patient reports a significant decline in functional status and poor appetite.
Action items	• Monitor weight loss in newly diagnosed cancer patients and those on active treatment • Measure C-reactive protein, serum albumin, and interleukin-6 levels • Counsel patients and family about cancer cachexia and its clinical implications
Discussion	Clinically, cachexia is defined through a consensus definition of weight loss of ≥5% of body weight in the past 6 months, or ≥2% in those with body mass index (BMI) of <20 kg/m^2.[1] Patients with certain types of cancers—such as lung, pancreas, esophagus, and head & neck—are more likely to experience weight loss/cachexia than are patients with breast cancer or sarcomas. Patients with cachexia experience loss of muscle mass and systemic inflammation. Cancer cachexia management remains an unmet need in oncology. Progestins such as megestrol acetate and short-course corticosteroids have been shown to improve weight gain in cancer patients.[2] Currently, there are no FDA-approved drugs available for the management of cancer cachexia. Anamorelin, a ghrelin agonist, has been shown to increase lean body mass in patients with cancer cachexia but provides no functional improvement or survival advantage.[3]

Pearl	• Heat-shock proteins 70 and 90 have recently been shown to be the main drivers of cancer cachexia[4]
References	1. Fearon K, Strasser F, Anker SD, et al. Definition and classification of cancer cachexia: an international consensus. Lancet Oncol 2011;12:489-95. 2. Yavuzsen T, Davis MP, Walsh D, et al. Systematic review of the treatment of cancer-associated anorexia and weight loss. J Clin Oncol 2005;23:8500-11. 3. Temel JS, Abernethy AP, Currow DC, et al. Anamorelin in patients with non-small-cell lung cancer and cachexia (ROMANA 1 and ROMANA 2): results from two randomised, double-blind, phase 3 trials. Lancet Oncol 2016;17:519-31. 4. Zhang G, Liu Z, Ding H, et al. Tumor induces muscle wasting in mice through releasing extracellular Hsp70 and Hsp90. Nat Commun 2017;8(1):589.

What is palliative care, and how is it incorporated into oncology management? What is involved in the goals of care discussion?

Key concept	Palliative care involves group of health-care professionals who aim to improve symptoms related to cancer, such as pain, and provide psychological support for patients diagnosed with advanced cancer.[1] Traditionally, palliative care has been introduced in patients with advanced, metastatic cancer during the latter stages of the clinical course, which appeared to be ineffective in improving quality of life or delivery of care for patients. A phase 3 randomized control study of metastatic non–small-cell lung cancer conducted by Temel et al[2] demonstrated that early initiation of palliative care improved quality of life and longer median survival (compared to standard of care[#]).[2]
Clinical scenario	During a discussion between a 59-year-old man with metastatic pancreatic cancer and his oncologist, the patient requests to know about his prognosis and states, "I'm tired of being sick all the time." This patient has had 2 lines of treatment with mFOLFIRINOX (5-fluorouracil, irinotecan, oxaliplatin, and leucovorin) and gemcitabine/nab-paclitaxel over the span of 8 months. He has had chronic back pain due to the pancreatic head mass and has had celiac plexus nerve block to palliate his pain. His recent scans show progressive disease. What should the oncologist discuss with the patient?
Action items	• The goals of care discussion involves an interdisciplinary team of physicians including palliative care specialists, oncologists, social work, nurses, and chaplains, who review with the patient (and patient's family or caregivers) the current status and prognosis of malignancy, current physical and psychological symptoms, and the patient's social, cultural, and spiritual beliefs and values[3] • The goals include optimizing the quality of life (defined by physical, psychological, social, and spiritual domains, Figure 18-1), reducing suffering, maintaining function (as much as possible), and providing support for families and loved ones[3,4]

- When initiating the goals of care discussion, a thorough and empathetic understanding of what the patient and family knows and understanding their expectations and hopes is important and can facilitate realistic goals[4]

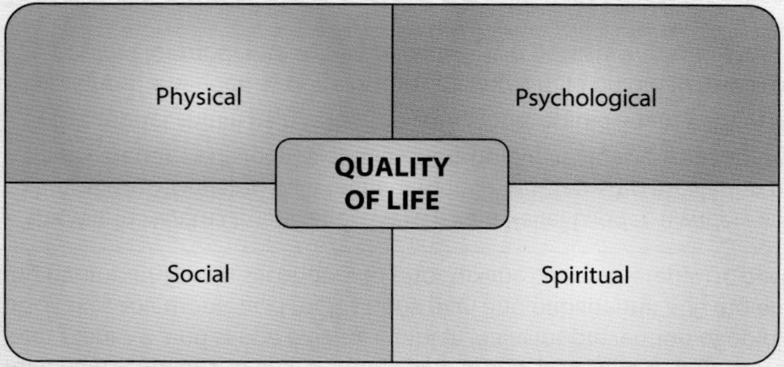

Figure 18-1. Facets of quality-of-life measures.

Pearl

- Predictions for estimated survival have been found to be only 20% accurate; >60% of physicians tend to be overly optimistic vs <20% overly pessismistic[4]

References

1. Ahmedzai SH, Costa A, Blengini C, et al. A new international framework for palliative care. Eur J Cancer 2004;40(15):2192-200.
2. Temel JS, Greer JA, Muzikansky A, et al. Early palliative care for patients with metastatic non–small-cell lung cancer. N Engl J Med 2010;363(8):733-42.
3. *Clinical Practice Guidelines for Quality Palliative Care*. 3rd ed.; 2013. Available at: https://www.hpna.org/multimedia/NCP_Clinical_Practice_Guidelines_3rd_Edition.pdf.
4. Stone MJ. Goals of care at the end of life. Proc Baylor Univ Med Center 2001;14(2):134-7.

[#]Standard of care was considered when the patient, family, or oncologist requested palliative care services.

How do I manage cancer-related pain in patients with advanced malignancies?

Key concept	Pain is a commonly encountered symptom of advanced malignancies and should be managed in an effective and comprehensive manner. General knowledge in the different components of pain and identifying the nature, severity, type, and location of our patients' pain can help us deliver adequate palliative care and alleviate their symptoms.
Clinical scenario	A 42-year-old man with chronic pain secondary to his metastatic castrate-resistant prostate cancer and metastasis to the axial skeleton and pelvic lymph nodes is seen in the clinic. His pain regimen, effectively controlling his symptoms, consists of extended-release morphine sulfate 60 mg orally every 12 hours, immediate-release morphine sulfate 15 mg, 1 tablet orally every 6 hours as needed for a pain score of 1–6 on a numeric pain rating scale, and 2 tablets every 6 hours as needed for a pain score >6, and senna 8.6 mg, 2 tablets daily for prevention of opioid-induced constipation. He also takes zoledronic acid for his bony pain and gabapentin 300 mg orally 3 times daily for preexisting neuropathic pain secondary to prior taxane chemotherapy. He declines palliative chemotherapy.
Action items	• The World Health Organization (WHO) Pain Relief Ladder, a widely adopted tool in approaching clinical cancer-related pain management, is a three-step escalation process of treating pain using three categories of agents: opioids, non-opioid analgesics, and adjuvant agents • In this model, initial pain is treated with a non-opioid agent with or without an adjuvant agent • Escalation, if needed, is done by introducing a mild opioid for mild to moderate pain and a stronger opioid for moderate to severe pain if pain persists or progresses
Discussion	The following are general principles in using different agents for cancer-related pain management. <u>Non-opioid analgesic agents (WHO Pain Relief Ladder Step 1)</u> • Used for mild to moderate pain

- Acetaminophen or non-steroidal anti-inflammatory drugs
- May add an adjuvant agent
- Escalate to an opioid if persistent or increasing pain

Opioid analgesic agents

- Morphine and oxycodone are common starting points for short-acting opioids
- When combining short and long-acting opioids, the short-acting opioid is dosed at 10%–20% of the daily long-acting dose and is used for breakthrough "rescue" pain[1]
- When converting from frequent short-acting opioids to long-acting opioids, start with 50%–100% of the total daily dose of the short-acting opioid
- If pain is controlled and adverse toxicities of opioids occur, a 10%–20% dose reduction should be attempted[2]
- If a significant adverse toxicity occurs (eg, marked sedation), a 50%–75% dose reduction may be warranted[2]
- Transdermal fentanyl is an option when oral intake is not possible; it should not be used in opioid-naive patients or when frequent titrations are needed
- When converting from one opioid to another, use morphine equianalgesic charts to calculate dosage
- Use morphine, hydromorphone, and hydrocodone with caution in patients with fluctuating renal function
- Conversion to methadone should only be done by a specialist, given its variable pharmacokinetics and toxicities
- The management of pain crisis may warrant intravenous (IV) opioids via frequent boluses of patient-controlled analgesic pumps

(continued on following page)

	(continued from previous page)
	Adjuvant agents[1]
	• Oral corticosteroids: acute nerve compression, visceral distention, increased intracranial pressure, soft tissue infiltration
	  • Example: dexamethasone 4–8 mg orally twice or thrice daily
	• IV corticosteroids: acute spinal cord compression, severe increased intracranial pressure
	  • Example: dexamethasone 10–20 mg IV every 6 hours
	• Anticonvulsants: neuropathic pain
	  • Examples: gabapentin, carbamazepine, clonazepam
	• Tricyclic antidepressants: neuropathic pain
	  • Examples: nortriptyline, desipramine
	• Bisphosphonates: bone pain from metastases
	  • Examples: zoledronic acid, pamidronate
	• Scopolamine or octreotide is used for pain syndromes as a result of bowel spasms from obstruction

Pearls	• Most cancer-related pain in patients with advanced cancers is chronic • In one study evaluating opioid dependence rates among cancer patients, 0 of 100 patients developed opioid dependence[3] • When using the transdermal route, drug delivery is increased by fever or direct heat application to the skin; by contrast, impaired absorption is observed in cachectic patients with limited subcutaneous tissue[4] • Initiating methadone may warrant hospitalization for titration and cardiac monitoring • The Faces Pain Rating Scale can be used to evaluate pain intensity in non-verbal patients

References

1. Kamal A, Abernethy A. Palliative and end-of-life care. In: *American Society of Clinical Oncology Self-Evaluation Program.* 4th ed.; 2015:530-5.
2. National Comprehensive Cancer Network guidelines for adult cancer pain. Version 1.2018. Available at: www.nccn.org.
3. Passik SD, Kirsh KL, Donaghy KB, et al. Pain and aberrant drug-related behaviors in medically ill patients with and without histories of substance abuse. Clin J Pain 2006;22(2):173-81.
4. Heiskanen T, Mätzke S, Haakana S, et al. Transdermal fentanyl in cachectic cancer patients. Pain 2009;144(1-2):218-22.

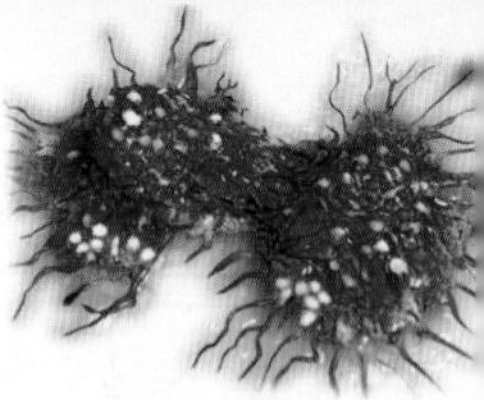

CHAPTER 19

Oncologic Emergencies

What is the clinical scope and management for brain metastases?

Key concept	Brain metastases are common sequelae of solid tumors (lung, breast, melanoma, renal, and colorectal). Lung cancer has the highest number of brain metastases; however, melanoma has the highest propensity to metastasize to brain. Although their exact incidence is unknown, about 8%–10% of patients with cancer will manifest brain metastasis, with an expected growing incidence as a function of increased life expectancy.[1,2] Management is primarily local, owing to limited penetration of most systemic agents through the blood-brain barrier. The historical standard of care (whole-brain radiation therapy [WBRT]) is being rapidly replaced by focal techniques such as stereotactic radiosurgery (SRS) and surgical resection, alone or in combination.[1,3]
Clinical scenario	A 48-year-old woman with a history of stage 2 triple-negative (ER– PR– Her-2-Neu–) breast cancer treated 3 years prior presents with headache and seizure. Imaging demonstrates a solitary 2-cm lesion in the left motor cortex.

Action items	• Assess prognosis; although the historical expected survival duration for patients with brain metastases is <1 year, at present multiple factors are used to assess prognosis, including
	  • the extent of intracranial disease (number and volume of metastases)
	  • the extent of extracranial disease (primary site control and/or presence of extracranial metastases)
	  • histology and radiosensitivity
	  • performance status[1,3]
	• A customized treatment plan should be tailored for each patient based on the above factors and should be discussed in a multidisciplinary team including medical oncology, radiation oncology, and neurosurgery[1,3]

Discussion	SRS offers a convenient method for the treatment of brain metastases that differs from traditional fractionated WBRT in both scope and adverse-effect profile. Published studies describe local control rates ranging from 70% to 90% for brain tumors smaller than 2 cm, dependent on histology. The control rates are lower for larger lesions, and sometimes a decision is made to combine surgery with SRS for such tumors.[1,3] SRS is preferred to WBRT due to comparable long-term overall survival,[3] as well to decreased neurocognitive decline. Studies, including the most recent North Central Cancer Treatment Group N0574 trial, have demonstrated a decline in cognitive function in patients who received WBRT and SRS versus SRS alone.[4] A recently published meta-analysis denoted decreased overall survival for patients receiving WBRT versus SRS alone, presumably due to neurocognitive dysfunction.[5] Trials are being performed to determine the maximum number of lesions that can safely be treated with SRS. At present, the number is typically 4, but recent series have described a favorable safety profile in treating up to 10 brain metastases.[6]
Pearls	• SRS is an emerging option for the treatment of brain metastases • Palliative WBRT remains the standard of care for widely disseminated central nervous system disease, leptomeningeal disease, or poor performance status[1,3]
References	1. National Comprehensive Cancer Network (NCCN) guidelines for central nervous system cancers. Version 1.2017. Available at: https://www.nccn.org. 2. Barnholtz-Sloan JS, Sloan AE, Davis FG, et al. Incidence proportions of brain metastases in patients diagnosed (1973 to 2001) in the Metropolitan Detroit Cancer Surveillance System. J Clin Oncol 2004;22(14):2865-72. 3. Lin X, DeAnglis LM. Treatment of brain metastases. J Clin Oncol 2015;33(30):3475-84. 4. Badiyan SN, Regine WF, Mehta M. Stereotactic radiosurgery for treatment of brain metastases. J Oncol Pract 2016;12(8):703-12. 5. Sahgal R, Aoyama H, Kocher M, et al. Phase 3 trials of stereotactic radiosurgery with or without whole-brain radiation therapy for 1 to 4 brain metastases: individual patient data meta-analysis. Int J Radiat Oncol Biol Phys 2015;91(4):710-7. 6. Li J, Brown PD. The diminishing role of whole-brain radiation therapy in the treatment of brain metastases. JAMA Oncol 2017;3(8):1023-4.

How should I manage a patient with febrile neutropenia?

Key concept	Cancer patients undergoing cytotoxic chemotherapy are at a risk of developing febrile neutropenia, which can be fatal if not treated quickly. Often, an offending infectious agent is not identified, but empiric treatment with antibiotics is justified to avoid clinical deterioration to sepsis and even death. Fever is defined as a documented oral temperature of ≥38.3°C (≥100.4°F). A patient is considered neutropenic when absolute neutrophil count (ANC) is <500/mm³ or <1000/mm³ but expected to be <500/mm³ within 48 hours.[1,2] The patient may not have focal signs of infection, but it is important to do a thorough physical examination to find the source of infection.[1,2]
Clinical scenario	A 65-year-old woman with stage 3B HER2+ ER+ PR+ breast cancer undergoing neoadjuvant chemotherapy with trastuzumab, pertuzumab, and docetaxel presents with fever up to 101°F (38°C) and chills. CBC shows WBC of 1.0 and absolute neutrophil count of 200. What is the next step in management?
Action items	• Draw at least 2 sets of blood culture • If an intravascular device (eg, an intravenous catheter) is present, a blood culture should be drawn from it as well • Other infectious evaluation includes urinalysis, urine cultures, and chest X-ray • Site-specific cultures should be obtained if needed (ie, stool culture if experiencing diarrhea) • Patients should be admitted if they are considered high risk (eg, anticipated neutropenia >7 days, clinically unstable, medical comorbidities, hepatic or renal impairment, and significant mucositis)

	• Initial intravenous antibiotics should be broad spectrum (eg, cefepime, piperacillin/tazobactam, or carbapenem) • Vancomycin can be used if gram-positive infection is suspected, especially in the presence of an intravascular device • Vancomycin can be discontinued if culture remains negative for gram-positive infection • If fever persists for 4–7 days, antifungal coverage should be considered
Discussion	Risk factors for febrile neutropenia include the rapidity of ANC decrease, decreased renal function, cardiovascular comorbidities, and elevated alkaline phosphatase, bilirubin, or aspartate aminotransferase levels. Empiric antibiotics can be given in the inpatient or outpatient setting based on initial risk factor assessment (Figure 19-1).[2] Low-risk patients can be managed as outpatients with oral antibiotics (eg, ciprofloxacin + amoxicillin/clavulanate). If fever persists or the patient clinically deteriorates, they should be admitted to the hospital.[2] Use of colony-stimulating factors is discussed in Chapter 1, Cancer Pharmacology.

(continued on following page)

(continued from previous page)

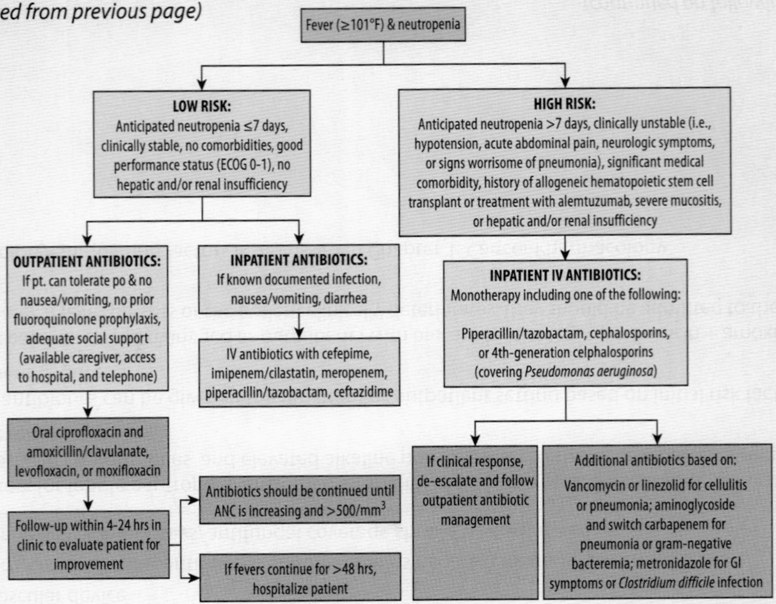

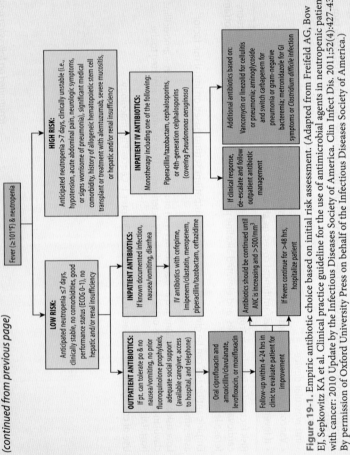

Figure 19-1. Empiric antibiotic choice based on initial risk assessment. (Adapted from Freifeld AG, Bow EJ, Sepkowitz KA et al. Clinical practice guideline for the use of antimicrobial agents in neutropenic patients with cancer: 2010 Update by the Infectious Diseases Society of America. Clin Infect Dis. 2011;52(4):427-431. By permission of Oxford University Press on behalf of the Infectious Diseases Society of America.)

Pearls	• Empiric antibiotics for initial management of febrile neutropenia have reduced the risk of chemotherapy-related mortality[1,2] • Intravenous catheter should be removed if blood cultures become positive for *Staphylococcus aureus, Pseudomonas aeruginosa,* fungi, or mycobacteria[1] • The nadir in ANC occurs 5–10 days after the last dose (for most outpatient chemotherapy regimens)[1] • Gram-positive cocci are the most common cause of culture-positive cases of febrile neutropenia, such as *S. aureus*, *Staphylococcus epidermidis* (especially in patients with indwelling devices), *Streptococcus pneumoniae*, *Streptococcus pyogenes*, *Streptococcus viridans*, and *Enterococcus faecalis* and *faecium*[1] • Digital rectal exam should be AVOIDED owing to possible bacterial translocation upon manipulation[1,2]
References	1. Lewis MA, Hendrickson AW, Moynihan TJ. Oncological emergencies: pathophysiology, presentation, diagnosis and treatment. CA Cancer J Clin 2011;61:287-314. 2. National Comprehensive Cancer Network guidelines for prevention and treatment of cancer-related infections. Version 1.2018. Available at: www.nccn.org.

How should I manage a patient with malignant spinal cord compression (MSCC)?

Key concept	MSCC is observed with many tumors, but is especially seen in patients with breast, prostate, lung, and renal cell cancers and in those with non-Hodgkin lymphoma. It is a medical emergency that requires urgent attention. Early detection is important, because pretreatment neurological status determines the likelihood of the patient regaining function after treatment. Most patients with MSCC have a known history of cancer, but 5%–25% of cases present for the first time. The most common site of MSCC is the thoracic spine, followed by the lumbosacral and cervical spine. Common symptoms include back pain, tenderness on percussion over the affected area, motor weakness, sensory impairment, urinary retention, and overflow incontinence. Patients may also demonstrate hyper-reflexia, spasticity, or loss of sensation.[1]
Clinical scenario	A 68-year-old man with metastatic castrate-resistant prostate cancer with diffuse bony metastasis presenting with worsening back pain and MRI demonstrates a T11 compression fracture resulting in cord compression. What are the next steps in management?
Action items	• MRI is the standard for detecting MSCC and should cover the entire length of the spine[1] • Corticosteroids should be initiated to reduce swelling around the spinal cord[1] • Surgical decompression followed by radiation leads to a significantly higher chance of ambulation and improved overall survival than with radiation alone[1,2] • Those unable to undergo surgery are treated with palliative radiation alone[1] • Bisphosphonates or antibodies targeting the receptor activator of nuclear factor κB ligand are also given[1]

Discussion	MSCC results from extrinsic compression due to following mechanisms: • Posterior extension through the spinous or transverse processes or into vertebral body • Anterior extension of a mass arising from the dorsal elements • Growth of a mass invading the vertebral foramen The common route of spread is hematogenous.
Pearls	• Patients with back pain and neurological findings should undergo a spine MRI immediately • Those with back pain only and suspected MSCC should undergo spine MRI within 48–72 hours • There is no benefit of using high-dose dexamethasone (96 mg) compared with a 10- to 16-mg intravenous bolus
References	1. Lewis MA, Hendrickson AW, Moynihan TJ. Oncological emergencies: pathophysiology, presentation, diagnosis and treatment. CA Cancer J Clin 2011;61:287-314. 2. Patchell RA, Tibbs PA, Regine WF, et al. Direct decompressive surgical resection in the treatment of spinal cord compression caused by metastatic cancer: a randomised trial. Lancet 2005;366:643-8.

How should I manage superior vena cava (SVC) syndrome?

Key concept	Early recognition of signs and symptoms of SVC syndrome can lead to timely management to reduce the morbidity and mortality from these situations. SVC syndrome occurs most often in patients with lung cancer, breast cancer, lymphomas (ie, primary mediastinal lymphoma), thymomas, and germ cell tumors.[1,2]
Clinical scenario	A 73-year-old male smoker presents with a 1-week history of worsening facial swelling and right arm swelling. He is seen in the emergency room after experiencing a near-syncopal episode. On physical exam, he has facial swelling and venous distention in the neck veins. CT of the chest w/ contrast shows a large right 7-cm hilar lung mass causing compression on the SVC (Figure 19-2). What are the potential treatment options? 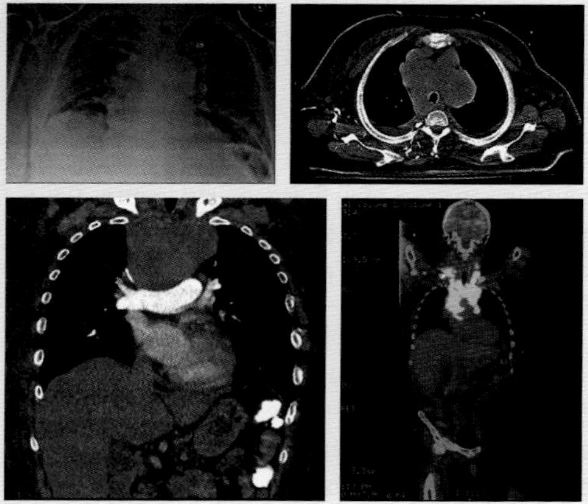 **Figure 19-2.** Clockwise: Top left, Chest X-ray showing a superior mediastinal mass and bilateral paratracheal lymphadenopathy and prominent aortic arch and mass effect on trachea. Top right, CT chest (axial view) showing mediastinal lymphadenopathy resulting in obstruction of the SVC and extensive right chest wall collateral veins. Bottom left, CT chest (coronal view) showing widened mediastinum from the lymphadenopathy. Bottom right, PET scan showing numerous FDG-avid mediastinal lymphadenopathy and prevascular and subcarinal lymph nodes.

Action items	• Initial recognition of SVC syndrome may be made on physical findings and chest X-ray[1,3] • Prompt recognition of symptoms and imaging with CT or MRI can confirm diagnosis • Immediate treatment in a patient presenting with airway compromise requires endotracheal intubation • Palliation of compression can include endovascular stenting, chemotherapy (if presenting in a non-emergency setting), and radiation
Discussion	Extrinsic compression on the SVC can result in obstructed blood flow to adjacent venous systems, including the azygos and internal mammary gland, causing facial plethora, chemosis, dilated chest wall veins, and edema of the arms. The severity of the symptoms depends on how quickly the obstruction occurs.
Pearls	• The management of SVC syndrome depends on the severity of symptoms, the response to intervention (ie, radiation or stent placement), and treatment of the underlying malignancy[1-3] (Figure 19-3) • Steroids and diuretics are of uncertain benefit for the management of SVC syndrome[1-3]

(continued on following page)

(continued from previous page)

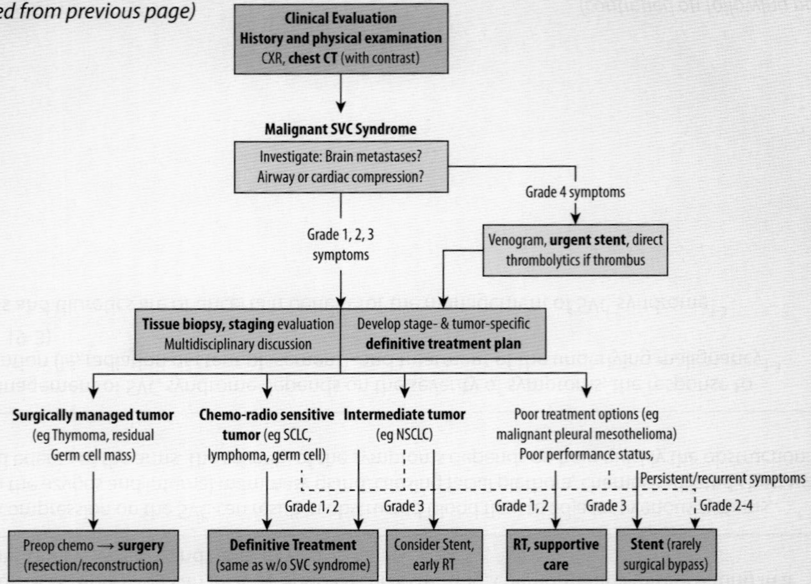

Figure 19-3. Proposed management of SVC syndrome based on grading system. (Reproduced with permission from Yu JB, Wilson LD, Detterbeck FC. Superior vena cava syndrome – a proposed classification system and algorithm for management. J Thorac Oncol 2008;3(8):811-814. Copyright © Elsevier.)

References

1. Lewis MA, Hendrickson AW, Moynihan TJ. Oncologic emergencies: pathophysiology, presentation, diagnosis, and treatment. CA Cancer J Clin 2011;61(5):287-314.
2. National Comprehensive Cancer Network guidelines for prevention and treatment of cancer-related infections. Version 1.2018. Available at: www.nccn.org.
3. Yu JB, Wilson LD, Detterbeck FC. Superior vena cava syndrome—a proposed classification system and algorithm for management. J Thoracic Oncol 2008;3(8):811-4.

How should I manage malignancy-associated hypercalcemia?

Key concept	Up to one-third of cancer patients can experience hypercalcemia related to their underlying malignancy. It is more likely to be seen in patients with cancers of lung, breast, and kidney, as well as those with multiple myeloma and adult T cell leukemia/lymphoma. Cancer patients admitted with hypercalcemia have a 30-day mortality approaching 50%.[1]
Clinical scenario	A 62-year-old man with IgG multiple myeloma presents with bony pain and worsening fatigue and lethargy. His blood work reveals a calcium of 12 and albumin of 2.5. What is the next step in management?
Action items	Patients with advanced malignancy may have elevated calcium discovered on routine labs. Often they present with nonspecific symptoms and signs of fatigue, confusion, generalized weakness, and bone pain. Serum calcium should be adjusted for hypoalbuminemia to estimate the correct calcium value.[1] • Patients with symptomatic hypercalcemia should be admitted to the hospital • Aggressive intravenous hydration is the mainstay of therapy • After adequate hydration, loop diuretics such as furosemide are given • Bisphosphonates such as pamidronate and zoledronic acid are given • Calcitonin can also quickly lower serum calcium levels • Glucocorticoids can also be used, especially in patients with lymphoma • The receptor activator of nuclear factor κB ligand antibody denosumab is also used to lower serum calcium levels[1] • See "Management guide for malignancy-associated hypercalcemia" below for further treatment options

Discussion	Hypercalcemia is caused by the following mechanisms[1]: • Parathyroid hormone–related peptide (PTHrP) is released by the tumor into the systemic circulation, causing bone resorption and renal retention of calcium (most common mechanism) • Bony metastases stimulate osteoclasts via local paracrine stimulation of osteoclasts, leading to bone resorption • Tumor secretion of vitamin D analogs
Pearls	• Thiazide diuretics such as hydrochlorothiazide should be avoided, as they can cause patients to retain calcium[1] • Ionized calcium is the most reliable laboratory test with which to detect hypercalcemia; other lab tests can be obtained, including PTH and PTHrP levels • In the setting of hypoalbuminemia, calcium should be corrected using the following formula[1]: • Calcium in mg/dL = measured total calcium in mg/dL + 0.8 (4 – measured albumin in g/dL)
References	1. Lewis MA, Hendrickson AW, Moynihan TJ. Oncological emergencies: pathophysiology, presentation, diagnosis and treatment. CA Cancer J Clin 2011;61:287-314.

Management guide for malignancy-associated hypercalcemia[1]

MEDICATION	DOSE	IMMEDIATE EFFECT OF HYPERCALCEMIA	PEARLS
Normal saline	Infuse at a rate of 300–500 mL/hr until euvolemic	Rapid hydration and restoration to euvolemia will result in increased urine output (therefore increased calciuresis)	Use caution in patients with congestive heart failure
Furosemide	20–40 mg IV every 12–24 hr	Within 5–15 min and duration is ~2 hr	Should AVOID other diuretics, especially thiazides, as this can increase calcium uptake
Pamidronate	60–90 mg IV	Within 48–96 hr on infusion and nadirs at 1 week	• Needs to be adjusted based on renal function • If glomerular filtration rate <30 m/L/min or serum creatinine >3.0 mg/dL, bisphosphonates should be AVOIDED due to risk of acute tubular necrosis
Zoledronic acid	4 mg IV		

Calcitonin	4–8 IU/kg SC or IM every 12 hr	Within 12–24 hr	• Repeat used can result in tachyphylaxis • Intranasal calcitonin has no efficacy in treatment of malignancy-associated hypercalcemia
Steroids	Hydrocortisone 100 mg IV every 6 hr or prednisone 60 mg PO daily	Within 3–5 days	• Can be considered in patients with lymphoma presenting with hypercalcemia • Mechanism of action is direct lympholytic effect and inhibition of calcitriol production by macrophages

IM, intramuscular; IV, intravenous; PO, oral; SC, subcutaneous.

[1]Lewis MA, Hendrickson AW, Moynihan TJ. Oncological emergencies: pathophysiology, presentation, diagnosis and treatment. CA Cancer J Clin 2011;61:287-314.

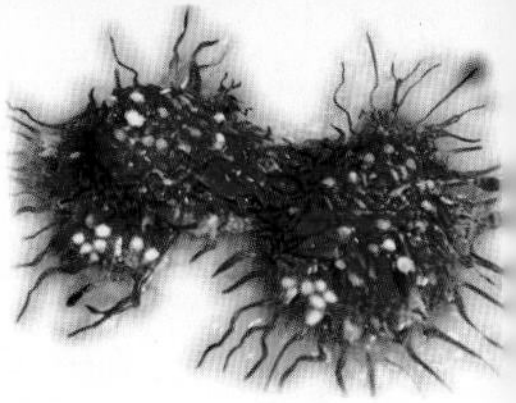

CHAPTER 20

Genetic and Familial Assessment for Hereditary Cancer Syndromes

What is hereditary breast and ovarian cancer (HBOC) syndrome, and how is it managed?

Key concept	Around 5%–10% of cancers are hereditary. Genetic testing is helpful to identify high-risk patients and families who may benefit from increased screening, chemoprevention, and risk-reducing surgeries. HBOC is an autosomal dominant condition caused by a mutation in *BRCA1* or *BRCA2*. Families with HBOC have combinations of breast, ovarian, prostate, and pancreatic cancers and possibly melanoma, sometimes at younger ages. These families are commonly Ashkenazi Jewish (carrier frequency of 1/40), but this is a differential diagnosis regardless of ancestry (1/400–1/800 in Europeans).
Clinical scenario	A 60-year-old woman with stage IV pancreatic cancer and a prior history of stage I invasive ductal carcinoma of the right breast at age 39, post-mastectomy, with a family history of ovarian cancer in paternal aunt at age 79 and a paternal male cousin with prostate cancer at age 65 through unaffected uncle. She has two daughters and wants to know whether her children need to get genetic testing.
Action items	• Educated genetic counseling process: discussion between genetic counselor, patient, and physician about possible cancer risks and management prior to pursuing genetic testing for educated testing decision, including post-test counseling to discuss the management plan • Genetic testing to be offered to adults only (age 25 years, as screening begins at this age, although if family planning is earlier, may start as young as age 18 years) • Offer **comprehensive** testing to the patient first (prior to family): individuals affected with cancer are more informative testing candidates • This will likely include a panel to address breast, ovarian, and pancreatic gene overlap • Risk assessment: if the patient meets criteria for genetic testing, per NCCN guidelines, offer testing[1] • Management if results are positive[1-7]

GENE	LIFETIME CANCER RISK	SPECIALIST	MANAGEMENT
BRCA1/2	Female breast: 50%–87%	Breast surgeon, breast medical oncologist	OPTIONS: ↑ Surveillance: mammogram alternating with breast MRI every 6 mo Risk reduction: chemoprevention, bilateral mastectomy
	Second breast primary: 65%		
	Male breast: 6%–8%	PCP	Self breast and clinical breast exams every 12 mo at age 35, mammograms begin at age 40
BRCA1	Ovarian: 44%	High-risk gynecologic oncologist	↑ Surveillance: Consider baseline CA125, TVUS at age 30 RECOMMENDATION: Bilateral salpingo-oophorectomy at age 35–40 (if post-bilateral mastectomy, complete at age 40–45)
BRCA2	Ovarian: 27%		
BRCA1	Prostate: 16%	PCP	Annual prostate-specific antigen and digital rectal exam at age 40
BRCA2	Prostate: 20%–30%		
BRCA1	Pancreas: 4%	High-risk GI medical oncologist	Consider pancreatic screening if meet CAPS3 and ACG criteria (based on family history of pancreatic cancer)
BRCA2	Pancreas: 5%–10%		
BRCA1/2	Melanoma: 1%–6%	Dermatologist	Annual skin exam

(continued on following page)

(continued from previous page)

Discussion	Patients with suspected hereditary conditions should meet with a genetic counselor and/or physician to pursue genetic counseling and testing (a blood test) to clarify their cancer risk management recommendations. There are several tests to choose from, and test selection should take into consideration the cancer primaries in each patient's personal and family medical history to allow for a comprehensive testing approach. There are at least 17 hereditary breast cancer risk genes, 24 hereditary ovarian cancer risk genes, 13 hereditary pancreatic cancer risk genes, 9 hereditary prostate cancer risk genes, and 12 hereditary melanoma risk genes. Of these, *TP53* and *BRCA1/2* overlap with all of them, and there is overlap among each of these genes into other organ risks but many that do not (ie, many pancreatic cancer risk genes that do not increase breast cancer risk and vice versa). The most likely scenario when evaluating any patient is that cancers are not related, given the rarity of hereditary conditions; however, the identification of a mutation in *BRCA1/2* or in a comparatively lower risk gene requires significant cancer risk management changes for prevention to ideally stop the family cancer pattern.
Pearls	• Identification of germline mutation(s) can lead to risk-reducing medication, breast/prostate/ovarian/pancreatic/dermatological screening, and risk-reducing surgeries (breast/ovaries) • Patients with *BRCA1/2* germline mutations may benefit from a PARP inhibitor treatment regimen for HBOC-associated cancer(s) • Utilizing a genetic counselor for pre-test and post-test counseling is highly beneficial for assessment and interpretation of risk and management • Long-term follow-up in a high-risk clinic may be beneficial

References

1. National Comprehensive Cancer Network guidelines for genetic/familial high-risk assessment: breast and ovarian. Version 1.2018. Available at: www.nccn.org.
2. Canto MI, Harinck F, Hruban RH, et al. International Cancer of the Pancreas Screening (CAPS) Consortium summit on the management of patients with increased risk for familial pancreatic cancer. Gut 2013;62(3):339-47.
3. Syngal S, Brand RE, Church JM, et al. ACG clinical guideline: genetic testing and management of hereditary gastrointestinal cancer syndromes. Am J Gastroenterol 2015;110(2):223-62.
4. Ford D, Easton DF, Stratton M, et al. Genetic heterogeneity and penetrance analysis of the BRCA1 and BRCA2 genes in breast cancer families. The Breast Cancer Linkage Consortium. Am J Hum Genet 1998;62(3):676-89.
5. Tai YC, Domchek S, Parmigiani G, Chen S. Breast cancer risk among male BRCA1 and BRCA2 mutation carriers. J Natl Cancer Inst 2007;99(23):1811-4.
6. Struewing JP, Hartge P, Wacholder S, et al. The risk of cancer associated with specific mutations of BRCA1 and BRCA2 among Ashkenazi Jews. N Engl J Med 1997;336(20):1401-8.
7. van Asperen CJ, Brohert RM, Meijers-Heijboer EJ, et al. Cancer risks in BRCA2 families: estimates for sites other than breast and ovary. J Med Genet 2005;42(9):711-9.

What are common hereditary breast and ovarian syndromes and genetic etiologies?

Key concept	Around 5%–10% of breast cancers and 10%–20% of ovarian cancers are hereditary. Genetic testing is helpful to identify high-risk patients and families who may benefit from increased screening, chemoprevention, and risk-reducing surgeries. There are at least 24 genes associated with increased ovarian cancer risk and at least 17 genes associated with increased breast cancer risk.
Clinical scenario	A 41-year-old woman is seen due to a recent diagnosis of invasive ductal carcinoma of the left breast. She has a family history of ovarian cancer in her paternal grandmother at age 78 and breast cancer in two paternal aunts at ages 57 and 48. What genetic testing should be discussed?
Action items	• Educated genetic counseling process: discussion between genetic counselor, patient, and physician about possible cancer risks and management prior to pursuing genetic testing for educated testing decision, including post-test counseling to discuss the management plan • Genetic testing to be offered to adults only (age 25 years, as screening begins at this age, although if family planning is earlier, may start as young as 18 years) • Offer **comprehensive** testing to the patient first (prior to family): individuals affected with cancer are more informative testing candidates • This will likely include a panel to address breast and ovarian gene overlap: *ATM, BARD1, BRCA1/2, BRIP1, CDH1, CHEK2, EPCAM, MLH1, MRE11A, MSH2, MSH6, NBN, PALB2, PMS2, PTEN, RAD50, RAD51C, RAD51D, SMARCA4, STK11*, and *TP53* (*NF1* and *MutYH* are also on these breast panels, although currently no change in management is recommended for these patients based solely on this finding)[1-3] • Risk assessment: if the patient meets criteria for genetic testing, per NCCN guidelines, offer testing[1] • Management if results are positive

Discussion	

Discussion

Genes on current testing panels can be separated into high-risk, moderate/high-risk genes:

- ***HIGH-RISK GENES*** such as *BRCA1/2* with respect to the breast cancer risk management will have options of increased surveillance as well as risk-reduction options
  - *BRCA1/2* are known to confer increased risks of pancreatic, prostate, male breast cancer, and melanoma as well[1]
  - Ovarian cancer risk recommendations are clearer for *BRCA1/2* for recommendation of bilateral salpingo-oophorectomy after childbearing is complete, close to 35–40 years of age or 40–45 years if bilateral mastectomy is completed[1]
- ***MODERATE/HIGH-RISK GENES*** *(ATM* and *PALB2)* confer an 18%–52% and 35%–58% risk of breast cancer, respectively
  - Patients can minimally be offered increased surveillance or risk reduction, based on additional factors such as family history
  - *ATM*: breast and pancreas; *PALB2*: breast, pancreas, possibly ovarian, male breast, and prostate[4,5]
- ***MODERATE-RISK GENES*** *(BARD1, BRIP1, CDH1, CHEK2, MRE11A, NBN, PTEN, RAD50, RAD51C, RAD51D, STK11,* and *TP53)* confer risks closer to 20%–40% and will have more of an increased surveillance management recommendation if based solely on genetic risk[1]
  - *CHEK2*: breast, prostate, colon, and possibly male breast
- *PALB2* and ***MODERATE RISK GENES*** which include ovarian cancer risk: the ovarian cancer risk is not as well quantified for many of these genes and is left more based on the personal/family history, literature, and discussion between healthcare providers and patients until guidelines are clearer for this population[1,2]

(continued on following page)

	(continued from previous page)
	• *ATM, PALB2,* and *CHEK2* genes increase cancer risks outside of the breast/ovarian spectrum (unlike most moderate-risk genes, except *PTEN, TP53, STK11*, and *CDH1* which have well-known cancer phenotypes)
	  • *ATM*: breast and pancreas
	  • *PALB2*: breast, pancreas, possibly ovarian, male breast, and prostate
	  • *CHEK2*: breast, prostate, colon, and possibly male breast
	• Of note, the genes associated with Lynch syndrome are also to be analyzed with ovarian cancer, although there is not currently a breast cancer risk associated with Lynch syndrome[1-8]

Pearls	• Patients with a personal and/or family history of breast and/or ovarian cancer should be offered a comprehensive genetic test to assess for the at least 24 genes associated with breast/ovarian cancer • Identification of germline mutation(s) can lead to risk-reducing medication, increased screening, and risk-reducing surgeries • If patients have been tested in the past and were negative, be sure to review prior testing to see whether updated testing is available to them, as there could be a missed mutation that may lead to preventative cancer risk approaches in the family
References	1. National Comprehensive Cancer Network guidelines for genetic/familial high-risk assessment: breast and ovarian. Version 1.2018. Available at: www.nccn.org. 2. Walsh T, Casadei S, Lee MK, et al. Mutations in 12 genes for inherited ovarian, fallopian tube, and peritoneal carcinoma identified by massively parallel sequencing. Proc Natl Acad Sci USA 2011;108(44):18032-7. 3. Buys SS, Sandbach JF, Gammon A, et al. A study of over 35,000 women with breast cancer tested with a 25-gene panel of hereditary cancer genes. Cancer 2017;123(10):1721-30. 4. Ahmed M, Rahman N. ATM and breast cancer susceptibility. Oncogene 2006;25(43):5906-11. 5. Antoniou AC, Casadei S, Heikkinen T, et al. Breast-cancer risk in families with mutations in PALB2. N Engl J Med 2014;37(6):497-506.

6. Schoolmeester JK, Moyer AM, Goodenberger ML, et al. Pathologic findings in breast, fallopian tube and ovary specimens in non-BRCA hereditary breast and/or ovarian cancer syndromes: a study of 18 patients with deleterious germline mutations in RAD51C, BARD1, BRIP1, PALB2, MUTYH or CHEK2. Hum Pathol 2017;70:14-26.
7. Pritzlaff M, Summerour P, McFarland R, et al. Male breast cancer in a multi-gene panel testing cohort: insights and unexpected results. Breast Cancer Res Treat 2017;161(3):575-86.
8. Erkko H, Xia B, Nikkila J, et al. A recurrent mutation in PALB2 in Finnish cancer families. Nature 2007;446(7133):316-9.

What are common colorectal cancer (CRC) syndromes and associated cancers?

Key concept	Around 5%–10% of CRCs are hereditary. Genetic testing is helpful to identify high-risk patients and families who may benefit from increased screening, chemoprevention, and risk-reducing surgeries. There are at least 17 genes associated with CRC syndromes, many of which are also polyposis syndromes.
Clinical scenario	A 30-year-old man presents with stage IIIC colon cancer. His first colonoscopy identified an infiltrating mass in his sigmoid colon which blocked 60% of his colon, making the surgeon unable to go past the mass. Three polyps were identified as well: two 2-mm tubular adenomas and a 3-mm hyperplastic polyp. Patient is a poor historian but reports that his mother died of colon cancer and his maternal grandfather's sister died from a GI bleed.
Action items	• Educated genetic counseling process: discussion between genetic counselor, patient, and physician about possible cancer risks and potential management changes prior to pursuing genetic testing for educated testing decision, including post-test counseling to discuss the management plan • Discuss possible differentials for CRC syndromes and offer comprehensive testing: *CRC without polyposis:* Lynch syndrome—*MLH1, MSH2, MSH6, PMS2, EPCAM* *POLD1* Li-Fraumeni syndrome—*TP53* *CHEK2* Hereditary diffuse gastric cancer syndrome—*CDH1* *CRC with polyps* Familial atypical polyposis (FAP)/attenuated FAP (AFAP)—*APC* Juvenile polyposis syndrome (JPS)—*BMPR1A, SMAD4* Peutz-Jeghers syndrome (PJS)—*STK11*

	POLE *GREM1* *MutYH*-associated polyposis (MAP)—*MutYH* *PTEN*—hamartomatous polyposis syndrome—*PTEN* • Risk assessment: evaluate for mucocutaneous hyperpigmentation (inside lip/cheeks), possibility for abnormal immunohistochemical (IHC) analysis for MMR on pathology, inquire about personal/family history of frequent nosebleeds, history of polyposis, history of abnormal female breast screening in family and confidence of colon cancer vs. other type of primaries in reported relatives • Manage based on patient's genetic testing results with regard to increased screening, chemoprevention, and risk-reducing surgeries
Discussion	• Prior to 2013, tiered genetic testing was the approach for genetic evaluation. However, now we are able to assess patients through cancer genetic panels to clarify risk assessment through at least 17 genes, although most can be further assessed in clinic • Absence of mucocutaneous hyperpigmentation on the inside of the lip can significantly reduce likelihood of PJS, as it is a hallmark of the condition • Many hospitals should have universal IHC analysis for mismatch repair (MMR) proteins for colon tumor tissue per 2016 NCCN guidelines to prescreen for features suggestive of Lynch syndrome. If normal IHC, this will significantly reduce likelihood of Lynch[1] • *CHEK2* and *CDH1* are also of low suspicion based on lack of family history of higher risk–associated cancers within the gene spectrum. *CHEK2* families tend to have prostate cancer and female breast cancers in addition to colon cancer, although the last is the lowest at 7%–9%. *CDH1* families typically have diffuse gastric cancer and may have lobular breast cancer. Some have colon cancer, although this is not a hallmark cancer. Also, some *CDH1* families, as of recently, were found to have breast cancer(s) without a personal or family history of gastric cancer at time of diagnosis[1-3] *(continued on following page)*

(continued from previous page)

- *POLD1* remains a differential diagnosis for early onset colon cancers, as these families present with colon and possibly endometrial cancers[4]
- Young age and an inability to see the colon beyond the sigmoid on colonoscopy contraindicate ruling out polyposis conditions WITHOUT genetic testing. Primary suspicions: AFAP, JPS, *POLE;* low suspicion: *TP53;* unlikely suspicion: *GREM1*, MAP, *PTEN*
- Approximately 30% of patients have de novo *APC* mutations are de novo, thus increasing concern of AFAP; alternatively, his maternal family history could be part of the differential as well. *APC* could also lead to further evaluation of his GI tract as well as other surveillance including the thyroid, desmoid tumors, and assessment for congenital retinal pigment epithelial hypertrophy (CHRPE). *POLE* is also associated with colon polyposis and increased risk of colon cancer[1,4]
- JPS genes can lead to juvenile polyps, as well as other polyp pathologies, but *SMAD4* also has a phenotype overlap with hereditary hemorrhagic telangiectasia, which can have symptoms of epistaxis, telangiectasias, arteriovenous malformations, and visceral lesions (some of which can lead to GI bleeds)[1]
- Given patient's age of diagnosis, *TP53* is a differential, even though *TP53* has an ~2.3% incidence of CRC and the patient does not meet *TP53* NCCN criteria; however, given the age at diagnosis, family history, low incidence of CRC in *TP53* mutation carriers, and that 30% of *TP53* mutation carriers are de novo, there is a slight suspicion[1,5]
- Based on patient's presentation, *GREM1* is not likely, as it is associated with mixed-polyp pathology in one polyp, and is not a differential diagnosis based on current phenotype of *GREM1* mutation carriers. Based on the patient having a family history of colon cancer in multiple successive generations, MAP is also unlikely, as it is an autosomal recessive condition. Given that *PTEN* phenotype has several NCCN criteria to meet to qualify for testing and patient currently only has CRC and does not meet others, this is not a differential diagnosis[1,6]

Pearls	• Patients with a personal and/or family history of early onset colon cancer (with or without polyposis) can have several differential diagnoses; with regard to genetic testing; given that many of these genes can lead to increased cancer risk beyond the colon and even beyond the GI tract, a genetic panel should be considered for these patients • If genetic testing is negative, recommendations should be made based on familial risk for the family • If genetic testing is negative, encourage patients to consider returning for updated testing in a few years in case new genes may provide genetic etiology and change of management recommendations for the patient/family • There are hereditary GI conditions that do not have candidate genes at this time • Utilizing a genetic counselor for pre-test and post-test counseling is highly beneficial for assessment and interpretation of risk and management • Long-term follow-up may be beneficial for patients in high-risk clinics
References	1. National Comprehensive Cancer Network guidelines for genetic/familial high-risk assessment: colorectal cancer. Version 3.2017. Available at: www.nccn.org. 2. Xiang HP, Geng HP, Ge WW, et al. Meta-analysis of CHEK2 1100delC variant and colorectal cancer susceptibility. Eur J Cancer 2011;47(17):2546-51. 3. Petridis C, Shinomiya I, Kohut K, et al. Germline CDH1 mutations in bilateral lobular carcinoma in situ. Br J Cancer 2014;110(4):1053-7. 4. Bellido F, Pineda M, Aiza G, et al. POLE and POLD1 mutations in 529 kindred with familial colorectal cancer and/or polyposis: review of reported cases and recommendations for genetic testing and surveillance. Genet Med 2016;18(4):325-32. 5. Rengifo-Cam, W, Shepherd HM, Jasperson KW, et al. Colon pathology characteristics in Li-Fraumeni syndrome. Clin Gastroenterol Hepatol 2018;16(1):140-1. 6. Liberman S, Walsh T, Schechter M, et al. Features of patients with hereditary mixed polyposis syndrome caused by duplication of GREM1 and implications for screening and surveillance. Gastroenterology 2017;152(8):1876-80.

What is the hereditary evaluation for breast and pancreatic cancer?

Key concept	Around 5%–10% of cancers are hereditary. Genetic testing is helpful to identify high-risk patients and families who may benefit from increased screening, chemoprevention, and risk-reducing surgeries. At least 17 genes are associated with increased breast cancer risk, and 13 genes are associated with increased pancreatic cancer risk, 6 of which are known to overlap: *BRCA1, BRCA2, PALB2, ATM, STK11, TP53*. The use of panels for hereditary cancer risk analysis can identify high-risk families and who warrants a change in their cancer risk management.
Clinical scenario	A 72-year-old woman with stage III pancreatic cancer and a prior history of stage I invasive ductal carcinoma of the right breast at age 54 years, post-mastectomy with a family history of breast cancer in her mother, two maternal aunts, and one paternal cousin, as well as pancreatic cancer in one maternal cousin was seen in the clinic. She had previously had *BRCA1/2* genetic testing in 2004, which was negative. Does she warrant further genetic testing?
Action items	• Educated genetic counseling process: discussion between genetic counselor, patient, and physician about possible cancer risks and possible management changes prior to pursuing genetic testing for educated testing decision, including post-test counseling to discuss the management plan • Genetic testing to be offered to adults only (age 25 years, as screening begins at this age, although if family planning is earlier, may start as young as age 18 years) • Prior testing: testing for *BRCA1/2* was updated in 2008 to include rearrangement analysis; testing prior to that time should be repeated, using either an updated *BRCA1/2* panel or updated panels available starting in 2013 (depending on insurance coverage review of prior testing after 2008, testing may still not have been full coverage) • Offer **comprehensive** testing to the patient first (prior to family); individuals affected with cancer are more informative testing candidates • This will likely include a panel to address breast/pancreatic gene overlap

	• Risk assessment: • Given prior *BRCA1/2* testing, there is a lower likelihood of mutation being identified in *BRCA1/2* through rearrangement (deletion/duplication analysis), as only 15% of mutation carriers are detected through this methodology • *STK11* is unlikely if patient lacks mucocutaneous hyperpigmentation[1] • Personal and family medical history do not meet *TP53* testing criteria, and although the patient has two primaries, given the lack of *TP53* common cancers, this is a low suspicion[1] • *PALB2* functions similarly to *BRCA2* and remains a differential diagnosis[2–8] • *ATM* is associated with pancreatic cancer and female breast cancer risk in the heterozygous state[9] If that patient meets criteria for genetic testing per NCCN guidelines, offer testing[1]
Discussion	Patients with suspected hereditary conditions should meet with a genetic counselor and/or physician to pursue genetic counseling and testing (a blood test) to clarify their cancer risk management recommendations. Testing options include personal and family history as well as gene differentials. Insurance coverage can also play a role in test selection. *BRCA1/2* are high-risk genes associated with breast and ovarian cancer as well as other cancers, including pancreatic, prostate, and a slight risk of melanoma.[1,2] Since 2013, other genes have been discovered to be associated with these types of cancers; testing for them can be offered to patients with similar phenotypes, as *BRCA1/2* may not be the contributing factor, but rather may be at the high-risk end of the group of genes that should be assessed for comprehensive risk analysis. *(continued on following page)*

(continued from previous page)

PALB2 has been reported to be associated with at least 35%–58% female breast cancer risk and increased pancreatic cancer risk. It has also been reported in individuals with ovarian cancer, male breast cancer, and prostate cancer, thus further suggesting that it has similar functionality to *BRCA2*.[2-8] *ATM* is associated with 18%–52% lifetime risk of female breast cancer and increased risk of pancreatic cancer. *ATM* mutation carriers are also counseled to avoid radiation, given its likelihood to mutate when exposed to radiation.[9,10]

Pearls

- Genetic risk assessment should be a comprehensive approach with regard to cancer primaries
- Due to updates in germline genetics since 2013, families suspicious for *BRCA1/2* mutations should be offered a panel to address high-risk and moderate-risk genes[1,10–12]
- *PALB2* functions similarly to *BRCA2*; due to its pancreatic cancer risk, if found in individuals with close relatives with pancreatic cancer, testing for it should be offered high-risk pancreatic screening[2,7]
- *ATM* mutation carriers should avoid radiation unless absolutely necessary for their care (ie, MRI vs. CT for imaging)[1,9,10]

References

1. National Comprehensive Cancer Network guidelines for genetic/familial high-risk assessment: breast and ovarian. Version 1.2018. Available at: www.nccn.org.
2. Canto MI, Harinck F, Hruban RH, et al. International Cancer of the Pancreas Screening (CAPS) Consortium summit on the management of patients with increased risk for familial pancreatic cancer. Gut 2013;62(3):339-47.
3. Antoniou AC, Casadei S, Heikkinen T, et al. Breast-cancer risk in families with mutations in PALB2. N Engl J Med 2014;371(6):497-506.
4. Jones S, Hruban RH, Kamiyama M, et al. Exomic sequencing identifies PALB2 as a pancreatic cancer susceptibility gene. Science 2009:324:217.
5. Slater EP, Langer P, Niemczyk E, et al. PALB2 mutations in European familial pancreatic cancer families. Clin Genet 2010;78:490-4.

6. Tischkowitz MD, Sabbaghian N, Hamel N, et al. Analysis of the gene coding for the BRCA2-interacting protein PALB2 in familial and sporadic pancreatic cancer. Gastroenterology 2009;137:1183-6.
7. Schneider R, Slater EP, Sina M, et al. German national case collection for familial pancreatic cancer (FaPaCa): ten years experience. Fam Cancer 2011;10:323-30.
8. Antoniou AC, Casadei S, Heikkinen T, et al. Breast-cancer risk in families with mutations in PALB2. N Engl J Med 2014;37(6):497-506.
9. Ahmed M, Rahman N. ATM and breast cancer susceptibility. Oncogene 2006;25(43):5906-11.
10. Swift M, Morrell D, Massey RB, et al. Incidence of cancer in 161 families affected by ataxia-telangiectasia. N Engl J Med 1991;325(26):1831-6.
11. Walsh T, Casadei S, Lee MK, et al. Mutations in 12 genes for inherited ovarian, fallopian tube, and peritoneal carcinoma identified by massively parallel sequencing. Proc Natl Acad Sci USA 2011;108(44):18032-7.
12. Heikkinen K, Karppinen SM, Soini Y, et al. Mutation screening of Mre11 complex genes: indication of RAD50 involvement in breast and ovarian cancer susceptibility. J Med Genet 2003;40(12):e131.

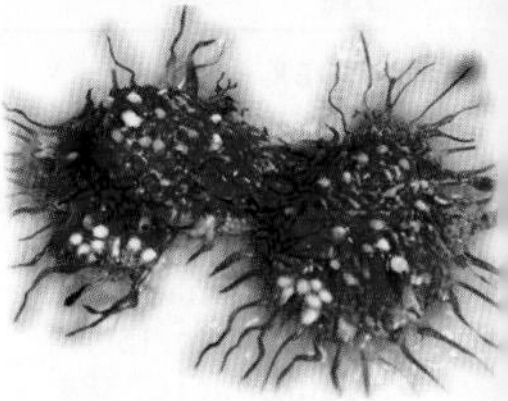

INDEX

Note: Page number followed by f indicates figure.

D

F

G

H

K

L

M

N

R

U

V